Progress
in
Drug Metabolism

Volume 12

Progress
in
Drug Metabolism

Volume 12

Edited by
G. G. Gibson
Department of Biochemistry
University of Surrey
Guildford
Surrey GU2 5XH
UK

Taylor & Francis
London · New York · Philadelphia
1990

UK   Taylor & Francis Ltd, 4 John St., London WC1N 2ET

USA   Taylor & Francis Inc., 1900 Frost Road, Suite 101, Bristol, PA 19007

© 1990 Taylor & Francis Ltd

British Library Cataloguing in Publication Data

Progress in drug metabolism. — Vol. 12 (1990)—.
   1. Man. Drugs. Metabolism
   I. Title
   615.7

   ISBN 0 85066 8069

Library of Congress Catalogue Card Number:

84-642984

Typeset by Mathematical Composition Setters,
7 Ivy Street, Salisbury, Wiltshire.
Printed in Great Britain by Burgess Science Press.
Basingstoke, Hants.

Contents

Preface

This volume opens with a discussion of the role of the kidney in xenobiotic biotransformation by Tarloff, Goldstein and Hook. As these authors correctly state, the kidney as a xenobiotic-metabolizing organ has historically been neglected with the majority of investigators in the field of xeno-biochemistry focusing their attention on the liver. This neglect has now been partially offset by this excellent contribution which details what we currently know about renal xenobiotic-metabolizing enzymes. In addition to considering the 'classical' Phase I and II xenobiotic-metabolizing enzymes, the authors have highlighted recent developments in renal glutathione conjugation and the subsequent processing of these adducts, the latter sometimes being referred to as Phase III biotransformation. The authors have also considered the prostaglandin H synthetase-dependent cooxidation of xenobiotics, a topic that has attracted much attention in recent years. It would appear that organs, which exhibit a relatively low (in absolute terms) complement of the major oxidative enzymes (like the kidney), have developed auxiliary systems, including prostaglandin H synthetase, to combat the influx of potentially harmful drugs and chemicals. Conversely, this enzyme system can also activate xenobiotics. The contributors to this chapter have not confined themselves to describing the enzymology of the kidney, but have also considered the pharmacological and toxicological responses to renally-produced metabolites. Quite clearly, the clinical manifestations and importance of these latter responses cannot be over-emphasized and the authors themselves have made substantial contributions to this area. In particular, if xenobiotic-dependent nephrotoxicity is identified either in morphological or urinary analysis terms, then how do medicinal chemists proceed in designing new drugs devoid of nephrotoxic potential? One way to approach this problem is to gain a full understanding of the comparative biological activities of the parent compound and the corresponding metabolites, further emphasizing the important contribution made by xenobiochemists in rationalizing the molecular mechanisms of drug-induced, site-specific nephrotoxicity.

The second chapter by Regårdh and his colleagues reflects the recent interest in drug modulation of calcium flux across biological membranes. In particular, these authors have detailed the pharmacokinetics and biotransformation of 1,4-dihydropyridine calcium antagonists, both in man and experimental animal species. This class of compounds is an excellent example of drugs that are extensively metabolized and exhibit first pass phenomenon resulting in a generally low systematic bioavailability, an important factor to be taken into consideration in their clinical pharmacology. Not only is metabolism of these compounds extensive, but several biotransformation pathways exist including dehydrogenation of the 1,4-dihydropyridine ring to the corresponding pyridine, ester hydrolysis, side-chain hydroxylation, nitro reduction, decarboxylation and subsequent conjugation reactions. The oxidation to the corresponding pyridine is particularly important as this metabolite exhibits very little pharmacological activity as compared to the active parent compound. The majority of these drugs exist as optical enantiomers because of the chiral nature of one of dihydropyridine ring carbon atoms. The presence of such optical enantiomers has proved important in clinical use as it has been demonstrated that enantiomer selectivity exists in both pharmacological activity and biotransformation/clearance parameters. Although much information has already been gained on the importance of drug isomerism in activity and disposition, it is clear that this will continue to be an important emphasis in the years to come. The current contribution by these Swedish authors also reviews the importance of disease states, genetic variability, age and drug interactions for these calcium channel blockers, and as such, forms a very comprehensive overview of this important class of compounds.

The topic of drug absorption across the nasal mucosa and the mechanisms involved is the subject of the timely contribution by Fisher. The nasal application of drugs clearly is advantageous when one considers that many drugs, although pharmacologically active *per se*, exhibit low activity when administered by the oral route, primarily because of instability in the acidic environment of the stomach or extensive first pass metabolism in the gut wall and/or liver. Accordingly, many classes of drugs have been formulated for nasal administration, notably peptide-based pharmaceuticals. The oxidative biotransformation potential of the nose is quite large and when expressed as cytochrome P450 content per gram tissue, is second only to that of the liver. Knowledge of the protein biochemistry and substrate specificity of the nasal cytochrome(s) P450 is not as well developed as for the liver, primarily because its existence in the nasal elipethelia has only been recently demonstrated in the earlier part of this decade. However, because of the importance of the nose as a first portal of entry for airborne, environmental contaminants and nasal drug delivery, it is clear that this tissue will receive much more attention from pharmacologists and xenobiochemists in the future. Fisher's erudite contribution covers the topics of gross anatomy, enzymology and mechanisms of nasal drug absorption, thus pulling together much valuable information of interest to those concerned with drug metabolism.

It has often been stated that advancement of knowledge in the field of drug metabolism is rate-limited by development of sensitive and specific analytical techniques for drugs and particularly their metabolites. This is certainly true in the case of nuclear magnetic resonance (NMR) spectroscopy, as elegantly described in the contribution by Preece and Timbrell. These authors cover the remarkable progress made in this field in recent years and they have provided a coherent analysis of both the advantages and disadvantages of this potentially powerful analytical technique. As the authors point out themselves, the judicious use of labelled compounds not only provides direct structural assignment of drugs and their metabolites in body fluids, but can also be used in the whole body situation. An added advantage of this NMR approach is that when drugs are analysed in body fluids, such as urine, it is also possible to identify simultaneously normal urinary constituents, thereby indirectly assessing the influence of the drug on the excretion of endogenous compounds which may have pharmacological or toxicological significance. Clearly, NMR spectroscopy is a relatively specialist technique involving high cost equipment and it is encouraging to know that exponents of this technique are applying their expert skills to xenobiochemistry in substantial numbers, a situation which we all hope will continue to develop. Preece and Timbrell have considered most multinuclear NMR approaches in use today and provided many examples of drug and metabolite analysis by this spectroscopic technique; in addition they have avoided the pitfall of placing too technical a slant to their contribution.

The ultimate goal of medicinal chemists and toxicologists is to understand in molecular, physical or chemical terms, the contribution made by particular functional groups or even atoms to the biological activity or toxicity of drugs and chemicals. The contribution by Lewis brings these topics together in his discussion of molecular orbital-generated, quantitative structure activity relationships (MO-QSAR). This topic developed from the pioneering work of Corwin Hansch approximately thirty years ago, who applied the concepts of linear free energy relationships to biological activity. While the 'Hansch approach' clearly underpins much of the QSAR knowledge at our disposal today, it is equally clear that more precise chemical descriptors of biological activity will provide even more coherent insights. In this context, Lewis summarizes for us both the conceptual nature of this approach and its applicability to the life sciences, particularly pharmacology and toxicology. Our MO-QSAR knowledge for drugs is surprisingly extensive and covers many of the pharmacologically important drug classes, effectively witnessing the importance attached to this topic, both by medical chemists in the pharmaceutical industry and by academic scientists.

In many respects, science is cyclic in that early, exceptional discoveries are made and their full impact is not recognized (or applied) in other branches in science until many years later. There are several reasons for this, and in the area of drug metabolism the main reason appears to be the time lag involved in development of suitable analytical techniques. A good example of this phenomenon is the early conceptual development of stereochemistry and its subsequent application to drug metabolism studies, a topic which is generating much current interest, as extensively reviewed by Hutt in the final chapter of this volume. This contribution provides excellent coverage of enantioselective immunoassay and radioceptor assays with the main emphasis being on the chromatographic methods of enantiomeric resolution as they relate to both derivitization of xenobiotics with chiral reagents, and the recently developed chiral phases for HPLC, TLC and GC. Development of these techniques has provided the bioanalyst with powerful tools to resolve drug enantiomers and their metabolites in addition to providing valuable information on mechanistic aspects of enzyme action. The development of this technology has largely passed the stage of random choice of the analytical method and more chiral phases are becoming commercially available based on sound chemical principles, thus making the choice of a particular method much easier for the analytical xenobiochemist. Information gained from such enantiomeric analyses is proving crucial in the development of more specific and safer drugs—a concept which has not escaped the attention of the regulatory agencies involved with the introduction of new drug candidates into the clinic.

G Gordon Gibson
University of Surrey

Contributors to Volume 12

C. BÄÄRNHIELM   *AB Hässel, Mölndal, Sweden*

B. EDGAR   *AB Hässel, Mölndal, Sweden*

A. N. FISHER   *Fisons plc, Loughborough, UK*

R. S. GOLDSTEIN   *Smith, Kline and French, Philadelphia, USA*

K-J. HOFFMAN   *AB Hässel, Mölndal, Sweden*

J. B. HOOK   *Smith, Kline and French, Philadelphia, USA*

A. J. HUTT   *Brighton Polytechnic, Brighton, UK*

D. F. V. LEWIS   *University of Surrey, Guildford, UK*

N. E. PREECE   *University of London, London, UK*

C. G. REGÅRDH   *AB Hässel, Mölndal, Sweden*

J. B. TARLOFF   *Philadelphia College of Pharmacy and Science, Philadelphia, USA*

J. A. TIMBRELL   *University of London, London, UK*

CHAPTER 1

Xenobiotic biotransformation by the kidney: pharmacological and toxicological aspects

Joan B. Tarloff[1], Robin S. Goldstein[2] and Jerry B. Hook[2]

[1]Department of Pharmacology and Toxicology, Philadelphia College of Pharmacy and Science, 43rd Street at Woodland Avenue, Philadelphia, PA 19104, USA;

[2]Smith Kline & French Laboratories, Research and Development, 709 Swedeland Road, King of Prussia, PA19406-0939, USA

1. Introduction

Recent investigations have demonstrated that the kidney has a capacity for xenobiotic metabolism. For at least several xenobiotics, the kidney plays an important role in the formation of toxic intermediates. In contrast, the contribution of renal metabolism to the generation of pharmacologically inactive metabolites is unclear. The focus of this chapter is three-fold: 1. to review our current state of knowledge of enzyme systems catalyzing xenobiotic biotransformation in the kidney; 2. to discuss the contribution of xenobiotic metabolism in the kidney to the generation of pharmacologically active or inactive metabolites, and 3. to discuss the role of intrarenal xenobiotic metabolism in the bioactivation of protoxicants.

2. Balance between enzymatic activation and detoxification

For most xenobiotics, metabolic processes are not one-step events but occur via multiple competing and sequential pathways. Formation of inactive metabolites is only one possible result of these pathways. The metabolism of xenobiotics to active and/or inactive products represents both bioactivation and/or detoxification processes, respectively. The relative rates of these reactions may determine, to a large extent, the response of an organ to xenobiotic exposure. Clearly, alterations in the relative activities of bioactivation and detoxification pathways could affect the generation of pharmacologically active and/or toxic metabolites, and therefore the therapeutic and/or injurious effects produced. In general, bioactivation reactions are catalyzed by cytochrome P450-dependent mixed function oxidases, whereas detoxification reactions are catalyzed by mixed function oxidases, non-oxidative cytosolic enzymes, and enzymes involved in conjugation (glucuronidases, sulphotransferases and glutathione transferases) and hydration (epoxide hydrase). However, there are exceptions to these generalities which will be discussed below.

3. Enzymes responsible for xenobiotic metabolism

Three major classes of enzymes involved in xenobiotic metabolism include:
1. cytochrome P450-dependent mixed function oxidases (Phase I reactions);
2. enzymes involved in conjugation reactions (glucuronidation, sulphation and glutathione conjugation, Phase II reactions); and 3. enzymes that do not belong to either of the first two groups.

Cytochrome P450-dependent mixed function oxidases (Phase I metabolism)

Mixed function oxidase concentrations and intrarenal localization

The specific activities of renal mixed function oxidases vary widely with species. In general, renal cytochrome P450 concentration is about 10 per cent of hepatic cytochrome P450 (Table 1). For example, rabbit hepatocytes contain 1.3 nmol cytochrome P450/mg protein (Zenser *et al.*, 1978) compared to rabbit renal proximal tubules, which contain 0.15 nmol cytochrome P450/mg protein (Endou, 1983). Renal NADPH-cytochrome P450 reductase activity is also about 10 per cent of hepatic activity in rabbits (Table 1) (Zenser *et al.*, 1978; Endou, 1983).

Low cytochrome P450 concentration in the kidney compared to that of the liver has led to the suggestion that the kidney plays a relatively small role in overall xenobiotic metabolism. However, with certain substrates, metabolic activity of renal cytochrome P450 may exceed that of the liver. For example, chloroform metabolism (measured as covalent binding or CO_2 production) by

Table 1. Concentration of cytochrome P450 mixed function oxidase components in renal tissue of various species. Values were compiled from Kluwe *et al.* (1978); Rush *et al.* (1983 a); Smith *et al.* (1986), Lake *et al.* (1973); Uotila *et al.* (1978).

Species	Cyt.P450[a]	NADPH cyt. c(P450) reductase[b]	Cyt b_5[a]
ICR mouse			
male	0.29 ± 0.06	32.3 ± 3.9	0.29 ± 0.04
female	0.06 ± 0.01	33.2 ± 7.2	0.15 ± 0.02
Wistar rat			
male	0.10 ± 0.01	48.8 ± 2.4	0.05 ± 0.01
female	0.13 ± 0.01	35.6 ± 5.6	0.07 ± 0.01
Rabbit	0.12 ± 0.01	8.6 ± 1.70	0.17 ± 0.01
Hamster	0.25 ± 0.01	60.4 ± 12.2	0.18 ± 0.01
Guinea-pig	0.13 ± 0.05	37.9 ± 13.4	0.11 ± 0.03

[a] nmol/mg protein
[b] nmol cytochrome c reduced/min/mg protein

renal microsomes from male mice is about half that observed with hepatic microsomes when expressed in terms of total protein. However, when chloroform metabolism is expressed as a function of cytochrome P450 concentration, renal activity is two-fold higher than hepatic activity (Smith and Hook, 1984).

Renal cytochrome P450 concentration and activity in male and female rats (Litterst *et al.*, 1977; Bachur *et al.*, 1979) and rabbits (Litterst *et al.*, 1977) is not different (Table 1). However, male mice have considerably higher renal cytochrome P450 concentrations and catalytic activities than female mice (Table 1) (Krijsheld and Gram, 1984; Smith *et al.*, 1984; Hawke and Welch, 1985), although these sex differences appear to be strain-dependent (Bachur *et al.*, 1979).

Mixed function oxidase activity is not distributed uniformly throughout the kidney. Cytochrome P450 and NADPH-cytochrome P450 reductase are in highest concentrations in the renal cortex; the concentration of each enzyme declines within the outer and inner medulla of rats (Fowler *et al.*, 1977) and rabbits (Zenser *et al.*, 1978; Endou, 1983). Within the renal cortex the greater activity of cytochrome P450 is localized in the proximal tubules; distal tubules have negligible cytochrome P450 activity (Endou, 1983; Cojocel *et al.*, 1983).

Morphologically, the proximal tubule is divided into three segments in rats (Maunsbach, 1966) and rabbits (Woodhall *et al.*, 1978). The S1 segment is the initial 1−1.5 mm of the proximal convoluted tubule, the S2 segment is a transitional 1−2 mm segment comprising the terminal proximal convoluted tubule and the initial proximal straight tubule, and the S3 segment is the terminal 1−2 mm of the proximal straight tubule extending from the corticomedullary junction through the outer medulla (Woodhall *et al.*, 1978). In rabbits, the S2 segment is the portion most active in organic anion secretion (e.g. para-aminohippurate) (Woodhall *et al.*, 1978) while the S1 segment is the portion most active in organic cation secretion (e.g. procainamide) (McKinney, 1982). In microdissected rabbit proximal tubules, cytochrome P450 concentration is two or three times higher in the S2 segment than in the S1 or S3 segments while the distal and cortical collecting tubules do not contain measurable cytochrome P450 (Endou, 1983). NADPH-cytochrome P450 reductase also is in highest concentration in the proximal tubule, primarily the S2 and S3 segments. In contrast to the lack of cytochrome P450 in the rest of the nephron, NADPH-cytochrome P450 reductase also is in the distal tubule and medullary structures (Endou, 1983).

In rabbit kidney, smooth endoplasmic reticulum (SER), the site of mixed function oxidase activity, is located primarily in the S3 segment and is absent in S1 and S2 segments (Rush *et al.*, 1983 a). There is generally a close correlation between induction of renal cytochrome P450 concentration and activity and proliferation of SER. Following pretreatment of rabbits with phenobarbital, there is an increase in SER in only S3 segments (Rush *et al.*, 1983 a). In rats, proliferation of SER in S3 segments results following pretreatment with β-naphthoflavone polybrominated biphenyls β-naphthoflavone (β-NF), polybrominated biphenyls (PBBs) (Rush *et al.*, 1986), 2,3,7,8-tetrachlorodibenzo-p-dioxin (TCDD) (Fowler, 1972), dieldrin (Fowler *et al.*, 1977), but not phenobarbital.

Multiplicity of renal cytochrome P450 isozymes

Multiple forms of cytochrome P450 have been identified in both hepatic and renal tissue. Current evidence suggests that hepatic cytochromes P450 consist of at least twelve isozymes coded for by at least eight distinct genes (Table 2) (Nebert and Gonzalez, 1987; Nebert *et al.*, 1987). Identification, characterization and nomenclature of cytochromes P450 are still evolving. In particular, establishing identity of hepatic and renal cytochrome P450 isozymes or among cytochrome P450 isozymes present in various species can be done with certainty only following complete amino acid, mRNA or cDNA sequence analysis. Low concentrations of cytochrome P450 isozymes present in kidney, as well as inherent difficulties in obtaining pure preparations for production of monoclonal antibodies, have hindered complete classification of both hepatic and renal cytochromes P450.

In rats, at least five isozymes of renal cytochrome P450 have been separated following gel chromatography of microsomal preparations (Imaoka and Funae, 1986). One isozyme, designated $P450_{K-5}$, has relatively low ethoxycoumarin deethylation and benzphetamine demethylation activities but high activity for lauric acid hydroxylation (Imaoka and Funae, 1986). Cytochrome $P450_{K-5}$ has catalytic properties and molecular weight similar to phenobarbital-inducible renal cytochrome P450a purified from rabbit kidney (Masters *et al.*, 1980) but bears a distinct amino-terminal sequence dissimilar to any rat hepatic P450s yet characterized (Imaoka and Funae, 1986; Nebert *et al.*, 1987). Another cytochrome P450 isozyme, designated $P450_{C-M/F}$,

Table 2. Suggested nomenclature for cytochrome P450 isozymes identified in rat, rabbit and mouse liver. From Nebert *et al.*, (1987), Nebert and Gonzalez (1987), Gonzalez (1989).

Family, subfamily and gene designation	Previous nomenclatures
P450I (Polycyclic aromatic compound-inducible)	
P450IA1	rat c, mouse P1, rabbit form 6
P450IA2	rat d, mouse P3, rabbit form 4
P450II (major)	
P450IIA subfamily	
P450IIA1	rat a
P450IIB subfamily (phenobarbital-inducible)	
P450IIB1	rat b, rabbit form 2
P450IIB2	rat e
P450IIC subfamily	
P450IIC1	rabbit PBc1
P450IIC2	rabbit PBc2, k
P450IIC3	rabbit PBc3, 3b
P450IIC4	rabbit PBc4, 1–8
P450IIC5	rabbit form 1
P450IIC6	rat PB1
P450IIC7	rat f
P450IID subfamily	
P450IID1	rat db1
P450IID2	rat db2
P450IIE subfamily (ethanol-inducible)	
P450IIE1	rat j, rabbit form 3a
P450III (steroid-inducible)	
P450IIIA1	rat pcn1
P450IIIA2	rat pcn2
P450IV (peroxisome proliferator-inducible)	
P450IVA1	rat LAw

present in both rat liver and kidney, catalyzes estrogen 2α- and 16α-hydroxylation (Sugita *et al.*, 1988). Complete amino acid sequences for cytochromes $P450_{K-5}$ and $P450_{C-M/F}$ have not been determined as yet, so that assignment of these isozymes into existing P450 families has not been made (Gonzalez, 1989). In rat kidneys, enzymes corresponding to, or mRNA coding for, hepatic cytochromes P450IA1, IIC2, IID1, IID2, IIE1, and IVA1 (Table 2) have been identified (Omiecinski, 1986; Foster *et al.*, 1986; Simmons and Kasper, 1989; Gonzalez, 1989). In contrast, activities associated with hepatic isozymes IIB1, IIB2, IIC1, and IIC3 (Table 2) are not expressed in rat kidney nor are their mRNAs detected (Omiecinski, 1986; Gonzalez, 1989).

Isozymes of cytochromes P450 in rabbit kidney are expressed somewhat differently than in rat kidney. Based on staining properties and autoradiography, rabbit kidney contains at least four major cytochromes P450 (Table 2): forms 2(P450IIB1), 3(P450IIE1), 4(P450IA2), and 6(P450IA1) (Johnson *et al.*, 1979; Liem *et al.*, 1980; Dees *et al.*, 1980). An ethanol-inducible cytochrome P450, originally designated form 3a and immunologically identical to one form of rat cytochrome P450j, is present in rabbit kidney, although at extremely low concentrations in kidney compared to liver or lung (Ueng *et al.*, 1987).

The ability to induce renal cytochrome P450 activity varies widely among species (Table 3). Rat renal mixed function oxidases are induced by polycyclic aromatic hydrocarbons (3-methylcholanthrene (3-MC) or β-NF) but not by phenobarbital, consistent with absence of the P450II subfamily (Table 2) in kidneys of rats. In contrast, rabbit renal mixed function oxidases are induced by both polycyclic aromatic hydrocarbons and phenobarbital (Rush *et al.*, 1983 a, 1983 c). Renal cytochrome P450 is induced by polycyclic aromatic hydrocarbons in most species; renal cytochrome P450 is induced by phenobarbital in hamsters and rabbits but not in guinea pigs, rats or mice (Rush *et al.*, 1983 c; Smith *et al*, 1986).

The ability to inhibit renal cytochrome P450 activity also varies among species. For example, α-naphthoflavone (α-NF), a relatively selective inhibitor of 3-MC-inducible cytochromes P450, inhibits renal cytochrome P450 activity in rabbits and rats pretreated with β-NF and PBBs but not phenobarbital (Rush *et al.*, 1983 c). Metyrapone, a relatively selective inhibitor of phenobarbital-inducible cytochromes P450, does not inhibit renal cytochrome P450 activity in rats, consistent with lack of phenobarbital-inducible renal cytochrome P450 in this species (Rush *et al.*, 1983 c). In contrast, metyrapone inhibits rabbit

Table 3. Induction of renal mixed function oxidase activities.[a] Values were compiled using data from Kluwe *et al.*, (1978); Rush *et al.*, (1983 a); Kuo *et al.*, (1982 a); Lake *et al.* (1973); Smith *et al.* (1986).

Inducer	Species	Phenobarbital-inducible		3-MC , β-NF-inducible	
		BPND	ECOD	EROD	BP
Phenobarbital	mouse				0.9
	rat	ND	0.9	0.8	1.2
	rabbit	5.6	14.0	1.2	
	hamster	1.8	1.1	1.0	1.3
	guinea pig	ND	0.7	1.0	1.0
	mini-pig	3.9		9.5	
3-MC	mouse				2.9
	rat				200
β-NF	rat	ND		80	
	rabbit	1.0		120	
	hamster	0.8	0.9	15	2.5
	guinea-pig	ND	0.7	5.7	5.7
TCDD	mouse				55.6
	rat		23.3		60.4
PCD/PBB	mouse				2.1
	rat		6.4		
	hamster	0.9	0.8	0.7	1.5
	guinea-pig	ND	1.3	13.2	10.3

[a] Data are presented as the ratio of induced/control activity (moles product formed/min/mg protein) for the following mixed function oxidase activities: benzphetamine N-demethylation (BPND), ethoxycoumarin-O-deethylation (ECOD), ethoxyresorufin O-deethylation (EROD), and benzo(a)pyrene hydroxylation (BP). ND = non-detectable activity.

renal cytochrome P450 following β-NF, PBB or phenobarbital induction (Rush *et al.*, 1983 a, 1983 c). Inhibition of renal β-NF-inducible cytochrome P450 by metyrapone is unexpected, since β-NF does not induce cytochromes P450IIB1 or IIB2, isozymes induced by phenobarbital and inhibited by metyrapone. Thus, the effects of inhibitors of cytochrome P450 are not as clearly defined in kidney as in liver. Complicating the interpretation of inhibitor data is the observation that SKF-525A and piperonyl butoxide, inhibitors of phenobarbital-induced hepatic cytochrome P450, reduce the renal cortical accumulation of phenobarbital in rats and rabbits (Kuo *et al.*, 1982 b). Thus, inhibitors may have multiple effects on renal metabolism by altering transport, intracellular binding at non-catalytic sites, and cytochrome P450-dependent biotransformation.

In summary, the activities of renal cytochrome P450 mixed function oxidases are low in renal homogenates compared to liver. However, since renal cytochrome P450 appears to be localized in S2 and S3 segments, renal cytochrome P450 may have high cell-specific activity. The capability to concentrate xenobiotics within the proximal tubular epithelium via organic anion and cation transport pathways, coupled with the relatively high concentration of cytochrome P450, predisposes this nephron segment to toxic injury due to mixed function oxidase-dependent metabolic bioactivation. At least several xenobiotics suspected of undergoing bioactivation by cytochrome P450-dependent mixed function oxidase reactions produce selective injury to the renal proximal tubules, the site of highest monooxygenase activity.

Conjugation reactions (Phase II metabolism)

Uridine diphosphate (UDP) glucuronyl transferase

a. INTRARENAL LOCALIZATION OF UDP-GLUCURONYL TRANSFERASES
UDP-glucuronyl transferase activity is not uniformly distributed throughout renal tissue but follows the gradient established for mixed function oxidase activity, i.e. highest activity in cortex and lowest in medulla (Fowler *et al.*, 1977). Although mixed function oxidase activity is not detectable in the medulla, measurable p-nitrophenol glucuronyl transferase activity is present in rat kidney medulla (Fowler *et al.*, 1977). In rat kidney, UDP-glucuronyl transferase activity is found in both proximal and distal tubules, with glucuronidation capacity of the distal tubule about 50 per cent that of proximal tubules (Cojocel *et al.*, 1983). Glucuronyl transferase activity may be limited by the availability of cosubstrate, UDP-glucuronic acid. UDP-glucuronic acid concentration in rabbit kidney cortex is twice as high as in medulla (Hjelle *et al.*, 1986).

For most substrates, renal glucuronidation represents a minor metabolic pathway. For example, isolated renal cells, largely originating from the proximal tubule, produce only 5 per cent as much acetaminophen-glucuronide as hepatocytes (Jones *et al.*, 1979). Glucuronidation of ortho-aminophenol by rat renal homogenates is only 30 per cent of liver activity. (Hanninen and Aitio, 1968). However, for some substrates, renal glucuronyl transferase activity may be comparable or even higher than that of liver. For example, hepatocytes and renal cells show similar rates of 7-hydroxycoumarin glucuronidation (Fry and Perry, 1981). Renal homogenates produce 2–2.5 times as much glucuronide conjugate of 4-methylumbelliferone and para-nitrophenol as hepatic tissue (Aitio and Parkki, 1978; Kuo *et al.*, 1981).

Hepatic glucuronide conjugation is sex-dependent in rats; males form considerably more glucuronide conjugates than females. This difference is dependent on steroid hormones; testosterone enhances glucuronidation in females while oestradiol reduces glucuronidation in males (Mandel, 1971). These sex-related differences are not apparent in humans (Mandel, 1971). Renal glucuronyl transferase activity is also sex-dependent but in the opposite direction, i.e. microsomes from female rats form considerably more of the glucuronide conjugates of 1-naphthol and 4-nitrophenol than microsomes prepared from male rat kidneys (Rush *et al.*, 1983 b). Increased glucuronidation in female renal microsomes appears to be related to a higher V_{max} for females (1.5 nmol/min/mg protein vs 0.22 nmol/min/mg protein in males) with no effect on K_m (0.23 mM in males vs 0.28 mM in females) (Rush, 1983 b).

b. MULTIPLE UDP-GLUCURONYL TRANSFERASE ISOZYMES

UDP-glucuronyl transferases from male rat liver have been partially purified and characterized with respect to substrate specificity (Table 4) (Bock *et al.*, 1979; Bock *et al.*, 1980; Burchell, 1981; Falany and Tephly, 1983). At least four distinct hepatic UDP-glucuronyl transferase isozymes have been characterized:

1. UDP-glucuronyltransferase form A, probably identical to UDP-GT1, catalyzes the glucuronidation of planar substrates such as 2-aminobenzoate, 2-aminophenol, 4-methylumbelliferone, 1-naphthol, 4-nitrophenol, N-hydroxy-2-naphthylamine and 3-hydroxybenzo(a)pyrene, as well as non-planar compounds including morphine and testosterone;
2. UDP-glucuronyl transferase form B utilizes bilirubin and morphine as substrates;
3. UDP-glucuronyl transferase form C utilizes oestrone and 4-nitrophenol as substrates;
4 UDP-glucuronyl transferase form D, probably identical to UDP-GT2, catalyzes the glucuronidation of compounds where the substituent at the para position is non-planar and bulky, such as chloramphenicol, 4-hydroxybiphenyl and morphine.

Rat kidney microsomes catalyze glucuronidation of 1-naphthol, 4-nitrophenol, phenol, bilirubin, benzo(a)pyrene-3,6-quinol and β-oestradiol but not testosterone, fenoterol or morphine (Koster *et al.*, 1986; Coughtrie *et al.*, 1987). Two distinct renal polypeptides are resolved by immunoblot analysis: a major polypeptide of molecular weight 55 000 Da and a minor polypeptide

Table 4. Substrate specificities of highly purified isozymes of rat liver UDP-glucuronyl transferases. Data were obtained from Falany and Tephly (1983) reprinted with permission of authors and Academic Press.

Substrate	Specific activity (units/mg protein)[a]		
	PNP-UDPGT	17-OH UDPGT	3-OH UDPGT
4-Nitrophenol	5733	1650	ND[b]
4-Methylumbelliferone	1129	ND	ND
1-Naphthol	4331	1120	ND
Morphine	ND	ND	ND
Testosterone	ND	190	ND
β-oestradiol	ND	64	ND
Androsterone	ND	ND	560
Etiocholanolone	ND	ND	851

[a] One unit of activity represents 1 nmol substrate conjugated/min.
[b] ND = no detectable activity. Limits of detection are as follows: steroid substrates was 0.5–1.0 units/mg protein; 4-nitrophenol, 15 units/mg protein; 4-methylumbelliferone, 2 units/mg protein; and morphine, 1 unit/mg protein.

of molecular weight 54 000 Da (Coughtrie *et al.*, 1987). These isozymes display activity with planar phenols (UDPGT form A (GT1) substrates) and bilirubin (UDPGT form B) (Coughtrie *et al.*, 1987). A polypeptide with molecular weight of 56 000 Da, inducible by 3-MC and active with 4-nitrophenol, 4-methylumbelliferone and 1-naphthol, is present in rat liver and kidney (Koster *et al.*, 1986). Bilirubin glucuronyl transferase activity specifically is induced by clofibrate in both liver and kidney (Koster *et al.*, 1986), but immunological comparisons of liver and kidney bilirubin glucuronyl transferases have not been determined. Messenger RNA coding for two UDP-glucuronyl transferase isozymes has been detected in rat kidney, although at very low concentrations (Mackenzie, 1987). Interestingly, mRNA for a UDPGT isozyme catalyzing glucuronidation of steroids, including testosterone and β-oestradiol, is present in rat kidney (Mackenzie, 1987; Coughtrie *et al.*, 1987) although β-oestradiol, but not testosterone, undergoes glucuronide conjugation in renal tissue (Coughtrie *et al.*, 1987). Rat renal tissue also contains an MRNA coding for a UDPGT isozyme active with UDPGT form D (GT2) substrates including chloramphenicol, 4-hydroxy-biphenyl and 4-methylumbelliferone (Mackenzie 1987), although UDPGT form D activity is not detectable in rat kidney (Tarloff *et al.*, 1987).

Species differences in renal glucuronyl transferase activities exist; human kidneys have high glucuronyl transferase activity toward 4-hydroxybiphenyl and morphine (Bock *et al.*, 1980), both of which are UDPGT form D substrates. Rabbit kidneys also have high glucuronyl transferase activity toward 4-hydroxybiphenyl and low, but detectable activity toward chloramphenicol (Hjelle *et al.*, 1986). Additionally, rabbit kidneys glucuronidate oestrone, diethylstilboestrol and acetaminophen (paracetamol) (Hjelle *et al.*, 1986), UDPGT forms C and D substrates.

Conflicting results have been reported regarding the inducibility of UDP-GT1 activity in renal tissue following 3-MC pretreatment, with some investigators reporting a stimulation of activity (Aitio *et al.*, 1972; Jones *et al.*, 1979) and others reporting no effect (Hanninen and Aitio, 1968; Aitio, 1973; Rush and Hook, 1984). Several other compounds have been found to increase renal and hepatic GT1 activity: cincophen induces both hepatic and renal GT1 and UDP-glucose dehydrogenase (Hanninen and Aitio, 1968); trans-stilbene oxide (Kuo *et al.*, 1981; Rush and Hook, 1984), TCDD (Fowler *et al.*, 1977; Aitio and Parkki, 1978), Aroclor 1254 (Bock *et al.*, 1980), and β-NF (Rush and Hook, 1984) all increase renal and hepatic GT1 activity. Salicylate specifically increases the activity of rat renal GT1 with no effect on hepatic glucuronyl transferase activities (Hanninen and Aitio, 1968).

In summary, for most substrates, the activities of renal UDP-glucuronyl transferases are low in renal homogenates compared to liver. Renal UDP glucuronyl transferases seem to be present in highest concentrations in proximal tubular cells, also the site of highest cytochrome P450 activity. For substances that attain high concentrations within renal proximal tubular cells and are substrates for glucuronyl transferases, glucuronidation may be a route of xenobiotic metabolism. Additionally, intrarenal formation of N-glucuronides perhaps due to UDP-glucuronyl transferases present in the distal nephron, may be important for urinary bladder carcinogens.

Sulphotransferases

Formation of sulphate esters is an important detoxification step, since sulphate conjugates are highly polar and rapidly excreted in urine or bile. The endogenous sulphate pool is limited and may be depleted by extensive sulphate conjugation.

Renal tissue contains sulphotransferase activity but the formation of sulphate conjugates by renal tissue is markedly lower than that of the liver (Tarloff *et al.*, 1987).The concentrations of both sulphotransferases and 3'-phosphoadenosine 5'-phosphosulphate (PAPS) are highest in renal cortex and decline through the medulla (Hjelle *et al.*, 1986). Cortical PAPS concentration in rabbit kidney is one-tenth of cortical UDP-glucuronic acid concentration (Hjelle *et al.*, 1986).

Rat renal tissue can synthesize sulphate conjugates of acetaminophen (Jones *et al.*, 1979; Tarloff *et al.*, unpublished observations) and 7-hydroxycoumarin (Fry and Perry, 1981). Renal sulphotransferase activity is not increased by pretreatment with 3-MC (Jones *et al.*, 1979) or PBBs (Fry and Perry, 1981). The contribution of sulphotransferases to renal xenobiotic metabolism has not been fully explored.

Glutathione conjugation and mercapturate synthesis

In a complex series of reactions, electrophilic substrates are conjugated with glutathione (γ-glutamyl-cysteinylglycine), sequentially degraded to the cysteine conjugate and excreted as the N-acetyl-cysteine (mercapturic acid) conjugate (Figure 1). Xenobiotic substrates that form glutathione conjugates include alkyl and aryl halides, epoxides and alkenes.

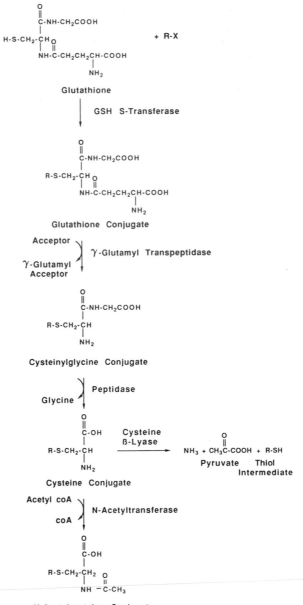

Figure 1. Glutathione conjugation and mercapturic acid biosynthesis. RX = substrate for glutathione S-transferases; CoA = coenzyme A.

a. GLUTATHIONE S-TRANSFERASES

The initial step in glutathione conjugation of xenobiotics is catalyzed by a family of soluble enzymes, glutathione (GSH) S-transferases. In rat liver, microsomal GSH-S-transferases have been identified; microsomal GSH-S transferase activity is lacking in rat kidney (Morgenstern *et al.*, 1984). Substrates for GSH-S-transferases include halogenated aromatic compounds, epoxides, halogenated alkyl and aralkyl groups, and α,β-unsaturated compounds (Reed and Beatty, 1980). Endogenous substrates for GSH-S-transferases include oestrogen, prostaglandin A and 15-keto-prostaglandins (Reed and Beatty, 1980; Kaplowitz, 1980).

Glutathione S-transferases account for about 10 per cent of total cytoplasmic protein in hepatocytes. Substrates react with glutathione by 1. substitution reactions, such as halogen replacement by the thioether group of glutathione, and 2. addition reactions, such as glutathione attacking an epoxide or α,β-unsaturated site (Kaplowitz, 1980). The transferase enzyme facilitates the conjugation reaction by lowering the pK_a (9.3) of glutathione resulting in ionization ($GSH \rightarrow GS^- + H^+$) which promotes interaction with enzyme-bound substrates through nucleophilic-electrophilic interactions (Kaplowitz, 1980).

GSH-S-transferases have been purified from rat kidney; activity corresponds to at least three distinct proteins. One renal transferase is identical to hepatic transferase B (ligandin), a second renal transferase is active in the conjugation of trans-4-phenylbut-3-en-2-one (α,β-unsaturated transferase activity displayed by hepatic GSH-S-transferases), while the third renal transferase is active with p-nitrobenzyl chloride and does not correspond to any identified hepatic transferase (Hales *et al.*, 1978). Hepatic GSH-S-transferases A and C have low renal activity (with 1,2-dichloro-4-nitrobenzene as the substrate) and transferases AA, B, and E (with methyl iodide as the substrate) are relatively active in the kidney (Chasseaud, 1980).

Total renal GSH-S-transferase activity, expressed per gram of wet tissue, is considerably less than hepatic activity (Hales *et al.*, 1978). Isolated renal cells or proximal tubules synthesize glutathione conjugates of acetaminophen (Jones *et al.*, 1979; Moldeus *et al.*, 1978) and 7-ethoxycoumarin (Fry and Perry, 1981). GSH-S-transferase activity towards 1-chloro-2,4-dinitrobenzene (α,β-unsaturated) is present exclusively and to an equal extent in rabbit proximal convoluted and proximal straight tubule (Fine *et al.*, 1978).

For hepatic GSH-S-transferases, there is close correlation between induction of conjugation activity and induction of mixed function oxidase activity. The classical inducing agents, phenobarbital and 3-MC, both increase the activities of rat hepatic GSH-alkyl-, aryl- aralkyl-, and epoxide-transferases (Kaplowitz *et al.*, 1975; Clifton *et al.*, 1975). A more complex picture emerges for renal GSH-S-transferase. Although phenobarbital fails to induce cytochrome P450-dependent mixed function oxidase activity in rat kidney, phenobarbital does specifically increase GSH-S-aralkyl transferase. GSH-S-alkyl, aryl-, and epoxide-transferase activities are not induced by phenobarbital treatment of rats. 3-MC induces renal GSH-S-aryl and aralkyl-transferase activities but not GSH-S-alkyl- or epoxide-transferases (Clifton *et al.*, 1975; Chasseaud, 1980). Trans-stilbene oxide increases rat hepatic and renal GSH-aryl-S-transferase (1-chloro-2,4-dinitrobenzene) but not epoxide-S-transferase (1,2-epoxy-3-(p-nitrophenyl)propane) activity (Kuo *et al.*, 1981).

Sex differences are apparent in the hepatic GSH-S-transferase activities in rats. Male rats have higher hepatic transferase activities than females (Kaplowitz *et al.*, 1975). Sex differences exist in renal GSH-S-transferases as well, but generally in the opposite direction. Specifically, for renal aralkyl, epoxide, and alkyl transferase activities, male rats have lower conjugation rates than females. In contrast, male rats have slightly higher renal GSH-S-aryl-transferase activity than females (Clifton *et al.*, 1975).

Comparative differences in renal and hepatic GSH-S-transferase activity depend upon the substrate in question. For example, renal GSH-S-aryl-transferase activity in both male and female rats is less than 5 per cent of the corresponding hepatic activity (Kaplowitz *et al.*, 1975; Clifton *et al.*, 1975). In male rats, renal GSH-S-transferase activities as a percentage of hepatic activities are: aryl-transferase, 3 per cent; aralkyl transferase, 17 per cent; epoxide transferase, 68 per cent; and alkyl transferase, 92 per cent. For female rats, renal GSH-S-transferase activities as a percentage of hepatic activities are: aryl transferase, 5 per cent; aralkyl transferase, 67 per cent; epoxide transferase, 138 per cent; and alkyl transferase, 121 per cent (Kaplowitz *et al.*, 1975; Clifton *et al.*, 1975).

b. MERCAPTURIC ACID SYNTHESIS

While the kidney may be active in the formation of glutathione conjugates, another important role of the kidney is in the degradation of preformed glutathione conjugates into the corresponding mercapturic acid. The kidney contains an enzyme, γ-glutamyl transpeptidase, capable of cleaving the γ-glutamyl linkage of glutathione to produce the cysteinylglycine conjugate (Figure 1). γ-Glutamyl transpeptidase is concentrated within the brush border of renal proximal tubules, hydrolyzing substrates within the tubular lumen (Meister and Tate, 1976). The cysteinylglycine conjugate formed by the action of γ-glutamyl transpeptidase is a substrate for numerous peptidases (Figure 1), including aminopeptidase M, located within the brush border of proximal tubules (Rankin *et al.*, 1980; McIntyre and Curthoys, 1980). These peptidases will cleave the glycine-cysteine linkage, producing the cysteinyl conjugate of the xenobiotic (Figure 1). The xenobiotic-cysteine conjugate may be excreted or, more likely, be absorbed and converted to the corresponding mercapturic acid by the action of microsomal N-acetyltransferase (Figure 1) (Green and Elce, 1975). The three enzymes primarily involved in mercapturic acid synthesis are concentrated within the outer stripe of the medulla in rat kidney (Orrenius *et al.*, 1983). N-Acetylation is rate-limiting for excretion of mercapturic acids (Orrenius *et al.*, 1983; Newton *et al.*, 1986). Microsomal cysteine S-conjugate N-acetyltransferase is active with thioethers of L-cysteine and analogues such as O-benzyl-L-serine. Catalytic efficiency is a function of the lipophilicity of the sulphur substituent (Duffel and Jakoby, 1982).

The role of the kidney in mercapturic acid synthesis has been investigated in studies using hepatocytes and isolated renal proximal tubule cells incubated with acetaminophen. Hepatocytes produce primarily glutathione-S-acetaminophen with little detectable cysteine or N-acetylcysteine conjugates (Jones *et al.*, 1979). Renal cells produce very little glutathione-S-acetaminophen but, rather, produce almost exclusively the N-acetylcysteine conjugate of acetaminophen (Jones *et al.*, 1979). If glutathione-S-acetaminophen produced by hepatocytes is added to medium containing isolated renal cells, the N-acetylcysteine-acetaminophen conjugate quickly accumulates intracellularly (Orrenius *et al.*, 1983). Finally, when phenyl-alanylglycine, an inhibitor of cysteinylglycine dipeptidase, is included in the renal cell incubation medium, the cysteinylglycine-acetaminophen conjugate accumulates and N-acetylcysteine-acetaminophen is not detected (Orrenius *et al.*, 1983). Isolated perfused rat kidneys excrete perfused acetaminophen or acetaminophen-S-glutathione as the mercapturic acid conjugate (Newton *et al.*, 1982; Newton *et al.*, 1986). Thus, kidneys can form N-acetyl-cysteine-acetaminophen de novo from acetaminophen, or from the hepatic metabolite, glutathione-S-acetaminophen. Hepatocytes contain very little γ-glutamyl transpeptidase, the first enzyme in the reaction scheme. Once the glutathione conjugate is formed within the hepatocyte it cannot undergo further metabolism and is released into the medium (or bile *in vivo*). Mercap-turic acids are highly polar and will be readily excreted into urine. Movement of mercapturic acid conjugate from proximal tubular cell to tubular lumen may occur via probenecid-sensitive organic anion secretion (Newton *et al.*, 1986). Thus, further processing of glutathione conjugates to mercapturic acids represents a detoxification pathway for potentially reactive compounds. The kidney also contains a poorly characterized enzyme that can deacetylate N-acetylcysteine conjugates, reforming the cysteine conjugate (Duffel and Jakoby, 1982).

c. CYSTEINE CONJUGATE β-LYASE

Glutathione conjugation generally functions as a detoxification pathway. However, compounds may undergo bioactivation following glutathione con-jugation. The kidney contains an enzyme, cysteine conjugate β-lyase, that is capable of cleaving the β-carbon bond between cysteine and sulphur, forming ammonia, pyruvate and a reactive thiol intermediate (Figure 1) (Lash *et al.*, 1986). The cysteine conjugate β-lyase enzyme is inactive with aliphatic cysteine conjugates and requires compounds that bear a good leaving group on the β-carbon of cysteine (Stevens and Jakoby, 1983).

Immunocytochemical techniques have localized renal cytosolic cysteine con-jugate β-lyase in the proximal tubule of rat kidneys (McFarlane *et al.*, 1989; Jones *et al.*, 1989), the primary site of morphologic damage due to nephro-toxic cysteine conjugates. Cysteine conjugate β-lyase is present in outer mitochondrial membrane and cytosol in rat kidney (Lash *et al.*, 1986), and is virtually absent from brush border membranes (Stevens, 1985). Rat renal cysteine conjugate β-lyase proteins do not cross-react with antibody raised against rat liver enzyme (Stevens, 1985), suggesting that the enzymes in rat liver and kidney are different. Mitochondrial and cytosolic forms of the enzyme differ with respect to substrate specificity; mitochondrial cysteine conjugate β-lyase has higher affinity for S-(2-benzothiazolyl)-L-cysteine than does cytosolic enzyme (Lash *et al.*, 1986) whereas cytosolic and mitochondrial enzymes have similar affinities for S-1,2-dichlorovinyl-L-cysteine (DCVC) (Stevens, 1985) and S-(2-chloro-1,1,2-trifluoroethyl)-L-cysteine (Lash *et al.*, 1986). Mitochondrial and cytosolic cysteine conjugate β-lyase activities also differ with respect to inhibition: aminooxyacetic acid (AOA), a potent inhibitor of pyridoxal phosphate-dependent enzymes, inhibits mitochondrial cysteine conjugate β-lyase activity at a lower concentration ($K_i = 0.4\ \mu M$) than that required for inhibition of cytosolic enzyme activity ($K_i = 8\ \mu M$) (Lash *et al.*, 1986).

Cysteine conjugate β-lyase enzymes are pyridoxal phosphate-dependent enzymes and the catalytic mechanism involves a β-elimination reaction. Sequential proton abstraction from the α-carbon, β-elimination, and hydrolysis of the enzyme-bound eneamine intermediate yields an α-keto acid (usually pyruvate) and ammonia as well as a reactive thiol intermediate (Anders *et al.*, 1987). Thus, replacement of the α-hydrogen with a methyl group yields a substrate unable to complete the catalytic cycle. If metabolism via cysteine conjugate β-lyase is essential for nephrotoxicity, these methyl-substituted cysteine conjugates should not produce nephrotoxicity (Anders *et al.*, 1987). Indeed, an α-methyl analogue of DCVC, S-(1,2-dichlorovinyl)-DL-α-methylcysteine, does not produce nephrotoxicity *in vivo* or *in vitro* (Elfarra *et al.*, 1986 a and b, Anders *et al.*, 1987). Alternatively, cysteine analogues capable of interacting with cysteine conjugate β-lyase to generate a thiol intermediate should be nephrotoxic. Indeed, S-(1,2-dichlorovinyl)-L-homocysteine (DCVHC) produced marked nephrotoxicity in rats *in vivo*; this toxicity was attenuated when cysteine conjugate β-lyase activity was inhibited by AOA; and the α-methylanalogue, S-(1,2-dichlorovinyl)-DL-α-methylhomocysteine, was not nephrotoxic (Elfarra *et al.*, 1986 b).

The significance of cysteine conjugate β-lyase as an activator of protoxicants only recently has begun to be explored. Interestingly, mitochondrial cysteine conjugation β-lyase activity is present in the outer mitochondrial membrane in higher concentration than in the inner mitochondrial membrane (Lash *et al.*, 1986). Substrates for cysteine conjugate β-lyase are relatively polar molecules and would not be expected to penetrate mitochondrial membranes readily. Localization of cysteine conjugate β-lyase activity on outer mitochondrial membranes suggests that mitochondrial metabolism of potential toxicants may occur. Indeed, at least several cysteine conjugates are proposed to exert nephrotoxicity, at least in part, through alterations of mitochondrial function (Stonard and Parker, 1971a and 1971b; Parker, 1965;

Lash *et al.*, 1986). Those compounds that produce nephrotoxicity *in vivo* dependent on metabolism via cysteine conjugate β-lyase (e.g. DCVC, DCVHC) also inhibit respiration in intact mitochondria but not mitoplasts (inner mitochondrial membrane preparations) (Anders *et al.*, 1987; Elfarra *et al.*, 1987). These observations suggest that mitochondrial metabolism via cysteine conjugate β-lyase may contribute, at least in part, to nephrotoxicity induced by some cysteine conjugates.

Other enzymes involved in xenobiotic metabolism

There are pathways for xenobiotic metabolism in the kidney that cannot be classified as Phase I or II reactions. This section will discuss several alternative pathways of xenobiotic metabolism.

Epoxide hydrase (epoxide hydrolase)

Epoxides are highly reactive electrophiles that may interact with tissue macromolecules, leading ultimately to mutagenic and carcinogenic effects. Along with cytosolic GSH S-transferases, microsomal epoxide hydrase serves to detoxify epoxides. Epoxide hydrase catalyzes the conversion of aliphatic and aromatic epoxides to trans-hydrodiols (Anders, 1980).

Epoxide hydrase activity frequently is coupled to cytochrome P450 mixed function oxidase activity, as in the case of benzo(a)pyrene metabolism. Both enzyme activities are localized in the microsomal fraction of cells, making coordinated reactions likely. The initial steps in benzo(a)pyrene metabolism are cytochrome P450-dependent oxidations to benzo(a)pyrene-4,5-oxide and benzo(a)pyrene-7,8-oxide. Epoxide hydrase catalyzes the hydration of both reaction products, forming 4,5-dihydroxy-4,5-dihydrobenzo(a)pyrene, a non-toxic product, and 7,8-dihydroxy-7,8-dihydrobenzo(a)pyrene, thought to be the ultimate carcinogen (Schmassmann *et al.*, 1978). Thus, epoxide hydrase may serve to either detoxify or activate a protoxicant.

The kidney contains epoxide hydrase activity that is approximately 10 per cent of hepatic activity in rats, mice and hamsters (Oesch and Schmassmann, 1979). Hepatic epoxide hydrase activity is enhanced by pretreatment of rats with phenobarbital, 16α-cyanopregnenolone and trans-stilbene oxide, but is refractory to 3-MC or TCDD treatment (Aitio and Parkki, 1978; VanCantfort *et al.*, 1979; DePierre *et al.*, 1984). In rats, trans-stilbene oxide specifically increases renal epoxide hydrase activity with no change in cytochrome P450 aryl hydrocarbon hydroxylase activity (Kuo *et al.*, 1981; Schmassmann *et al.*, 1978), indicating that induction of epoxide hydrase and cytochrome P450 activities may be dissociated. Species differences exist in epoxide hydrase induction; epoxide hydrase activity is not induced by trans-stilbene oxide in mice and hamsters (Oesch and Schmassmann, 1979). Hepatic epoxide hydrase activity is slightly higher in male compared to female rats; sex differences are not apparent in renal epoxide hydrase activity (Oesch and Schmassmann, 1979).

Prostaglandin H synthetase

The enzymatic processes discussed above are localized primarily in the renal cortex and proximal tubule. It has long been recognized that the renal medulla and papilla are also targets for toxicity. Specifically, the chronic abuse of analgesics (phenacetin, aspirin, acetaminophen) and non-steroidal anti-inflammatory agents (NSAIDs) is associated with renal papillary necrosis (Duggin, 1980; Bach and Bridges, 1985). One mechanism by which these lesions occur is thought to involve xenobiotic cooxidation catalyzed by prostaglandin H synthetase.

Prostaglandin H synthetase is a haemoprotein involved in biosynthesis of prostaglandins, thromboxanes and prostacyclins. Two enzyme activities are involved in the conversion of arachidonic acid to PGH_2; fatty acid cyclooxygenase and prostaglandin hydroperoxidase (Figure 2). Fatty acid

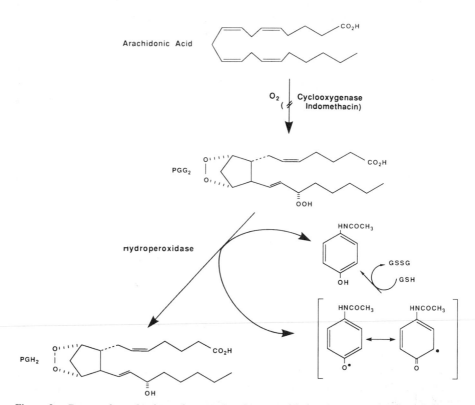

Figure 2. Proposed mechanism of acetaminophen cooxidation by prostaglandin synthetase. Adapted with permission from Moldeus *et al.* (1982).

cyclooxygenase catalyzes the initial bis-oxidation of unsaturated fatty acids, converting arachidonic acid to PGG_2. Two atoms of molecular oxygen are inserted into arachidonic acid to form a 15-hydroperoxy prostaglandin cyclic epoxide intermediate. Prostaglandin hydroperoxidase catalyzes the cleavage of the 15-hydroperoxy group and acts as an electron donor, reducing PGG_2 to PGH_2, a 15-hydroxy cyclic endoperoxide. Prostaglandin hydroperoxide is reduced, resulting in (co)oxidation of the xenobiotic (Figure 2). PGH_2 undergoes further biotransformation to produce prostaglandins and thromboxanes (Davis *et al.*, 1981). The two enzyme activities may be distinguished by several criteria: 1. substrate requirement (fatty acid cyclooxygenase specifically requires polyunsaturated fatty acids while prostaglandin hydroperoxidase activity is supported by cumene hydroperoxide or tert-butyl hydroperoxide); 2. inhibitors (aspirin and NSAIDs are specific inhibitors of fatty acid cyclooxygenase activity without affecting prostaglandin hydroperoxidase activity); 3. haem requirement (prostaglandin hydroperoxidase specifically requires a ferric haem component; fatty acid cyclooxygenase does not); 4. oxygen requirement (fatty acid cyclooxygenase requires oxygen whereas prostaglandin hydroperoxidase will function under anaerobic conditions), and 5. production of radical intermediates (fatty acid cyclooxygenase does not produce free radicals, prostaglandin hydroperoxidase does) (Davis *et al.*, 1981).

In rabbit kidney, prostaglandin H synthetase activity is not distributed uniformly but follows a concentration gradient opposite to that described for cytochrome P450 mixed function oxidase activity. Specifically, prostaglandin H synthetase activity is highest in inner medulla, intermediate in outer medulla and barely detectable in cortex (Zenser *et al.*, 1977; Zenser *et al.*, 1979). Within cells, prostaglandin H synthetase activity is localized in the endoplasmic reticulum and nuclear membrane (Rollins and Smith, 1980). Hepatocytes contain relatively low prostaglandin H synthetase activity (Eling *et al.*, 1983).

a. XENOBIOTIC COOXIDATION CATALYZED BY PROSTAGLANDIN H SYNTHETASE

Prostaglandin H synthetase from ram seminal vesicular microsomes metabolizes a variety of organic compounds by cooxidation (Marnett *et al.*, 1975). Xenobiotic substrates include phenylbutazone and acetaminophen (Eling *et al.*, 1983), compounds implicated in renal papillary necrosis. Other xenobiotic substrates for cooxidation include phenobarbital, sulindac sulphate, oxyphenylbutazone and benzo(a)pyrene (Eling *et al.*, 1983). One consequence of xenobiotic cooxidation is covalent binding of the activated xenobiotic metabolite to cellular macromolecules, DNA or RNA (Davis *et al.*, 1981).

Xenobiotic cooxidation is supported by the prostaglandin hydroperoxidase activity and may be independent of fattv acid cyclooxygenase activity of prostaglandin H synthetase (Figure 2). Fatty acid cyclooxygenase activity is necessary for xenobiotic cooxidation when arachidonic acid is a cosubstrate. Coincubation of acetaminophen and arachidonic acid with rabbit renal medullary microsomes results in covalent binding of radiolabel derived from acetaminophen to trichloroacetic acid-precipitable proteins. Inhibition of microsomal binding occurs with *in vitro* addition of, or *in vivo* pretreatment with, aspirin (Zenser *et al.*, 1983). Glutathione also inhibits covalent binding of radiolabel from acetaminophen during arachidonic acid-stimulated cooxidation, consistent with generation of an electrophilic intermediate by cooxidation (Zenser *et al.*, 1983). When 15-HPETE (a substrate for prostaglandin hydroperoxidase that does not require prior metabolism by fatty acid cyclooxygenase) and acetaminophen are coincubated with medullary microsomes, covalent binding of radiolabel from acetaminophen still occurs but is no longer inhibited by aspirin. Covalent binding also occurs in aspirin-treated microsomes when 15-HPETE is supplied (Zenser *et al.*, 1983). Thus, acetaminophen cooxidation and the resultant covalent binding require prostaglandin peroxidase activity but do not necessarily depend on cyclooxygenase activity.

A major criticism of the cooxidation theory of analgesic-induced renal papillary necrosis is the observation that most analgesics are inhibitors of fatty acid cyclooxygenase (Flower, 1974). Although some degree of cyclooxygenase inhibition may occur with analgesics, endogenous lipid peroxides may serve as cosubstrates for prostaglandin hydroperoxidase (Mohandas *et al.*, 1981; Zenser and Davis, 1984). Thus, the ability of analgesics to inhibit cyclooxygenase activity does not preclude their activation via the separate prostaglandin hydroperoxidase activity.

Xenobiotics that undergo cooxidation include compounds known to produce renal and bladder cancer, such as N-[4-(5-nitro-2-furyl)-2-thiazolyl]-formamide(FANFT) (Zenser *et al.*, 1980a), benzidine (Zenser *et al.*, 1980b), and 2-amino-4-(5-nitro-2-furyl)thiazole formamide (Mattammal *et al.*, 1981). Reactive intermediates produced by cooxidation may be conjugated with glucuronic acid, catalyzed by medullary UDP-glucuronyl transferases (Fowler *et al.*, 1977). Generally, conjugation would serve to detoxify a reactive intermediate. However, N-glucuronides, as produced from some procarcinogens, are unstable at acidic pH. In the urinary bladder, these conjugates may be hydrolyzed to release the free aryl hydroxylamines, which are capable of covalent binding to tissue macromolecules (Davis *et al.*, 1981).

Prostaglandin H synthetase catalyzed xenobiotic cooxidation may represent a mechanism whereby compounds produce specific medullary or papillary damage. In addition, renal cooxidation may account for bioactivation of some bladder carcinogens. Cooxidation produces reactive intermediates that are thought to ultimately produce tissue damage. It is possible that antioxidants or scavenger radicals (glutathione, N-acetyl cystine) may prevent this type of tissue damage (Davis *et al.*, 1981).

4. Pharmacological consequences of renal xenobiotic metabolism

The ability of the kidney to generate pharmacologically active metabolites has long been appreciated in the case of vitamin D, where renal mitochondrial mixed function oxidases metabolize 25-hydroxyvitamin D_3 (25-hydroxycholecalciferol) to 1,25-dihydroxyvitamin D_3, the biologically active form of vitamin D (Tepperman, 1973). Other examples of xenobiotics that may be pharmacologically activated or inactivated by renal metabolism are discussed in the following sections.

Renal metabolism in the generation of pharmacologically inactive metabolites

Lower activities of enzymes catalyzing xenobiotic metabolism in kidney compared to liver has led to the suggestion that renal metabolism is of little significance in the formation of pharmacologically inactive metabolites. For the most part, this assumption is probably correct. However, at least a few drugs are metabolized to inactive agents in the kidney. The relative importance of these biotransformations to the pharmacodynamics of these drugs, however, is not entirely clear.

Digoxin

Renal elimination represents the major pathway for removal of digoxin from plasma (Koren, 1987). Simultaneous determination of inulin and digoxin clearances in humans (correcting for protein binding of digoxin) indicates digoxin clearance ratios (clearance of digoxin/clearance of inulin) ranging from 1.46 to 1.94 (Steiness, 1974). Digoxin/inulin clearance ratios greater than unity suggest that net tubular secretion of digoxin occurs. However, recent evidence suggests that apparent digoxin secretion may be accounted for, at least in part, by intrarenal metabolism.

Direct intrarenal metabolism of digoxin has been demonstrated in dogs using *in vivo* and *in vitro* techniques (Koren *et al.*, 1987). Following renal arterial injection of [^{3}H]-digoxin in dogs, urine contains radioactivity corresponding to authentic digoxin as well as a digoxin metabolite. The digoxin metabolite accounts for 14 per cent of digoxin radiolabel excreted by the ipsilateral kidney and 26 per cent of digoxin radiolabel excreted by the contralateral kidney (Koren *et al.*, 1987). A digoxin metabolite is formed *in vitro* by brush border but not by basolateral membrane vesicles (Koren *et al.*, 1987), and this metabolite has the same chromatographic mobility as the digoxin metabolite formed *in vivo*. The digoxin metabolite apparently cross-reacts with commercial radioimmunoassay antibodies used to detect digoxin (Koren *et al.*, 1987). Thus, digoxin measured by radioimmunoassay of urine probably represents a combination of parent compound and metabolite generated from renal metabolism. Therefore, the amount of 'digoxin' eliminated in urine may have been overestimated in previous studies, resulting in overestimation of digoxin clearance.

Apparent secretion of digoxin may be explained as follows (Figure 3). Digoxin enters renal tubular cells by passive diffusion across basolateral and/or luminal membranes. Within tubular cells, digoxin is biotransformed to a metabolite in the vicinity of the luminal membrane by an unidentified mechanism, although probably an enzymatic process since metabolite formation is protein-dependent (Koren *et al.*, 1987). The digoxin metabolite is less polar than the parent compound, and the enzymatic mechanism may involve cleavage of one or more carbohydrate moieties from the glycoside moiety (Koren *et al.*, 1987). This metabolite may subsequently diffuse into tubular urine or renal venous plasma. However, localization of metabolism at the brush border, as well as continuous removal of metabolite by urine flow, probably favours elimination in urine. The recent identification of intrarenal formation of a digoxin metabolite may serve to stimulate further investigation examining the contribution of renal metabolism to digoxin pharmacokinetics.

Clofibrate

Clofibrate, the ethyl ester of p-chlorophenoxyisobutyric acid (CPIB), is used in the treatment of familial hypercholesterolaemia (Brown and Goldstein, 1985). The pharmacologically active agent is CPIB; clofibrate is rapidly and

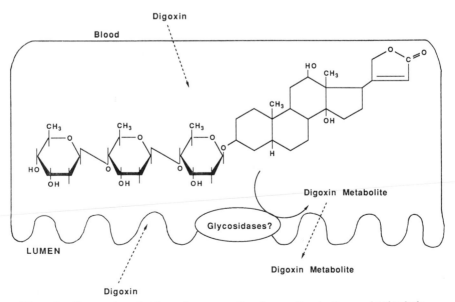

Figure 3.   Proposed mechanism of apparent digoxin secretion in the proximal tubule.

almost completely deesterified during transit across the intestinal epithelium (Thorp, 1962; Cayen *et al.*, 1977). CPIB is eliminated in the urine, with about 60 per cent of the administered dosage excreted as glucuronide conjugates (Brown and Goldstein, 1985). In humans and dogs, conjugated CPIB is virtually undetectable in plasma (Sedaghat and Ahrens, 1975; Cayen *et al.*, 1977). In rats, conjugated CPIB accounts for less than 5 per cent of plasma radioactivity between 3 and 24 hours following a single oral dose (Cayen *et al.*, 1977). In contrast, 47–73 per cent of urinary CPIB is present as glucuronide conjugates in humans, whereas conjugated CPIB accounts for 30 per cent of urinary CPIB in rats and about 16 per cent in dogs (Sedaghat and Ahrens, 1975; Cayen *et al.*, 1977). Biliary excretion represents a minor pathway of CPIB elimination: faecal excretion of conjugated and free CPIB accounts for less than 10 per cent administered clofibrate in humans, rats and dogs (Sedaghat and Ahrens, 1975; Cayen *et al.*, 1977).

High concentrations of conjugated CPIB in urine as compared to low or undetectable conjugated CPIB in plasma led to the suggestion that CPIB glucuronidation occurs within the kidneys. However, the ability of renal glucuronyl transferases to catalyse CPIB glucuronidation has not been investigated in detail. CPIB glucuronide is produced during incubation of CPIB with renal, but not hepatic, slices (J.M. Thorp, personal communication). Inability to detect glucuronide conjugates in plasma following CPIB administration or in liver slices during incubation with CPIB may be related to a relative inability of CPIB to penetrate hepatocytes. CPIB is not detectable in hepatocytes following perfusion of canine liver with 200 μg CPIB/ml (approximately 825 μmol CPIB/ml) for up to 4 hours (Platt and Thorp, 1966). In contrast, approximately 5 per cent of radiolabel derived from clofibrate is present in dog liver 3 hours following administration of 0.3 mmol clofibrate/kg (Cayen *et al.*, 1977). In comparison, serum contains approximately 6 per cent of radiolabel derived from clofibrate, and liver/serum ratio of radiolabel from clofibrate is approximately 0.85, suggesting that radiolabel from clofibrate does enter hepatocytes. Renal metabolism may play a role in the pharmacokinetics of CPIB, the active metabolite of clofibrate. However, further studies are required to establish the extent of renal vs hepatic glucuronidation of CPIB.

Renal metabolism and the generation of pharmacologically active intermediates

Metabolic reactions generally are considered as detoxification steps, leading to the production of compounds with less pharmacologic activity than the parent molecule. For at least some drugs, however, metabolism results in the generation of intermediates with equal or enhanced pharmacologic activity compared to the parent compound. In some cases, the formation of pharmacologically active metabolites significantly prolongs the therapeutic efficacy of a drug, as is the case for many benzodiazepines. In other cases, the parent compound may be pharmacologically inert, or at least less active than the active metabolite. In these instances, the parent compound may be considered to serve as a pro-drug, delivering a compound to be converted to an active intermediate via metabolic processes. For pro-drugs, the site of metabolic activation may be coincident with the site of pharmacologic action, enabling the pro-drug to serve as a method for targeting drug delivery. This section will discuss evidence supporting the concept of intrarenal metabolism as a mechanism to target drug delivery to the kidneys.

Vasodilators

Persistent renal hypoperfusion, as might occur with aortic or renal arterial stenosis, is associated with chronic hypertension. Improvement of renal perfusion would be expected to ameliorate the ensuing hypertension and various strategies have been pursued to produce selective renal vasodilators. Among the more promising compounds are dopamine and hydralazine derivatives coupled to γ-glutamyl moieties.

Dopamine is a well recognized vasodilator that, in low dosages (1–3 μg/kg/min in humans), increases renal blood flow and glomerular filtration rate and promotes natriuresis and diuresis. In higher dosages, dopamine activates adrenergic receptors, resulting in vasoconstriction and hypertension. In an effort to improve dopamine delivery to renal vascular receptors, investigators have synthesized L-γ-glutamyl-3,4-dihydroxy-phenylalanine (L-γ-glutamyl-DOPA). By sequential reactions with renal γ-glutamyl transpeptidase and aromatic L-amino acid decarboxylase, dopamine, the active vasodilator, may be generated in relatively high concentration within renal tubular cells (Wilk *et al.*, 1978). Indeed, following intravenous administration of L-γ-glutamyl-DOPA to anaesthetized rats, dopamine concentrations in mouse kidney were sixty-five times greater than in liver. In contrast, following L-DOPA administration, kidney dopamine concentrations were only fifteen-fold higher than in liver (Wilk *et al.*, 1978). Equimolar infusions of L-γ-glutamyl-DOPA and L-DOPA were not equipotent with respect to effects on renal plasma flow: L-γ-glutamyl-DOPA increased renal plasma flow approximately twice as much as L-DOPA (Wilk *et al.*, 1978). Thus, L-γ-glutamyl-DOPA is an effective and selective pro-drug that delivers dopamine, an active vasodilator, to the kidney. Generation of dopamine from the pro-drug relies on the relatively high renal concentration of γ-glutamyltranspeptidase compared to other organs, as well as on the ability of the kidney to accumulate γ-glutamyl compounds actively (Lash and Jones, 1984; Monks and Lau, 1987).

Rather than using a catecholamine as an antihypertensive agent, other investigators have designed an agent specifically to reduce renal vascular resistance and increase renal blood flow using a direct-acting vasodilator similar to hydralazine. Thus, investigators have coupled N-acetyl-L-γ-glutamate to 5-n-butyl,2-hydrazinopyridin (CGP 18137A). The resulting compound, CGP 22979A, is effective in reducing renal vascular resistance *in vivo* but not *in vitro* (Hofbauer *et al.*, 1985), suggesting that metabolism is required for vasodilation. Additionally, the threshold dosage of CGP 22979A for renal vasodilation is thirty-fold lower than the hypotensive threshold dosage (Hofbauer *et al.*, 1985), indicating selectivity for renal vasculature with minimal release of the active vasodilator to the systemic circulation. In spontaneously hypertensive rats, both hydralazine and CGP 18137A, the active drug formed from CGP 22979A, decrease mean arterial pressure and reflexly increase heart rate (Smits and Struyker-Boudier, 1985). In contrast, a dosage of CGP 22979A that maximally reduces renal vascular resistance has no effect on mean arterial blood pressure or heart rate (Smits and Struyker-Boudier, 1985). Additionally, CGP 22979A reduces renal vascular resistance selectively with no reduction in hind quarter or mesenteric resistances following infusions in spontaneously hypertensive rats (Smits and Struyker-Boudier, 1985). While acute administration of CGP 22979A is ineffective in reducing systemic blood pressure, preliminary studies indicate that chronic administration in spontaneously hypertensive rats leads to a chronic reduction of blood pressure (Smits and Struyker-Boudier, 1985). Thus, improvement of renal perfusion and/or perfusion pressure may ameliorate or attenuate hypertension in at least the spontaneously hypertensive rat. The relevance of selective renal vasodilators in the treatment of human hypertension remains to be demonstrated.

Mercaptopurine

Mercaptopurine is a well established chemotherapeutic agent used in the management of patients with leukaemias. Mercaptopurine is readily metabolized by xanthine oxidase (present in tissues such as liver, intestine, spleen, bone marrow and plasma) to an inactive product, 6-thiouric acid. For therapeutic efficacy, mercaptopurine usually is administered in large dosages over long periods of time, predisposing the liver and other tissues to cellular damage (Calabresi and Parks, 1985). The mechanism of antineoplastic activity relies on mercaptopurine-mediated inhibition of a number of enzymes involved in purine metabolism (Carrico and Sartorelli, 1977). The principal cytotoxic event limiting mercaptopurine therapy is bone-marrow suppression, and jaundice occurs in about 33 per cent of adult patients (Calabresi and Parks, 1985). Current therapeutic strategies revolve around conjugating mercaptopurine with moieties that can be cleaved within target tissues to release the mercaptopurine nucleotide (Calabresi and Parks, 1985).

   In an effort to target mercaptopurine for delivery to the kidney, mercaptopurine has been synthetically coupled to cysteine. This strategy takes advantage of the selective ability of the kidney to accumulate and metabolize cysteine conjugates. The prodrug, S-(6-purinyl)-L-cysteine (Figure 4), is rapidly converted to mercaptopurine *in vitro* by renal cortical homogenates, mitochondria, and microsomes (A. A. Elfarra, personal communication).

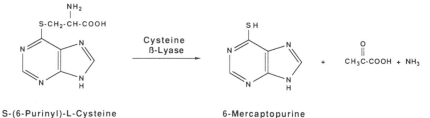

Figure 4. Proposed metabolism of S-(6-purinyl)-L-cysteine, a pro-drug of mercaptopurine.

Metabolism of S-(6-purinyl)-L-cysteine to mercaptopurine is inhibited *in vitro* by coincubation of renal homogenates with aminoxyacetic acid, a cysteine β-lyase inhibitor. Thus, C-S cleavage of S-(purinyl)-L-cysteine cata-lysed by cysteine β-lyase is essential for formation of mercaptopurine from the pro-drug. Following *in vivo* administration of S-(purinyl)-L-cysteine to rats, mercaptopurine is detectable in both liver and kidney, although mercapto-purine concentration in kidney is about two-fold greater than in liver. Renal mercaptopurine concentration is about 2500 times greater than that of plasma (A. A. Elfarra, personal communication). Thus, coupling mercaptopurine to cysteine appears to be an effective strategy to deliver the drug preferentially to the kidney. The use of a cysteine conjugate is a chemical strategy that takes advantage of the kidney's ability to accumulate and process cysteine conju-gates selectively via cysteine β-lyase-catalysed reactions. This approach may enable treatment of renal carcinomas with chemotherapy as an alternative to current treatment of nephrectomy (A. A. Elfarra, personal communication).

5. Toxicological aspects of renal xenobiotic metabolism

While xenobiotic metabolism may serve to detoxify reactive intermediates, some metabolic reactions may actually activate a protoxicant. Generation of a toxicant may occur *in situ* in the kidney following intracellular accumulation of either parent compound or metabolite formed in extrarenal tissue. This section will discuss several examples of xenobiotics that are activated to toxicants by renal metabolism.

Nephrotoxic metabolites generated within the kidney

Reactive intermediates are likely to bind covalently to tissue macromolecules in close proximity to the site of their formation. It is unlikely that a highly reactive and unstable species could be transported in blood or bile to the site of toxicity. Some nephrotoxicants produce highly selective damage, injuring exclusively the proximal straight tubule or renal medulla. The presence of spe-cific enzyme systems of xenobiotic metabolism in such discrete areas of the kidney suggests that the kidneys are involved in bioactivation of protoxicants.

Chloroform

An example of a chemical that is metabolically activated within the kidney is chloroform (Smith and Hook, 1984; Smith and Hook, 1983). Chloroform ($CHCl_3$) is a common organic solvent that has been used widely in the chemical industry. Chloroform has been associated with hepatic and renal injury in humans and experimental animals. Renal necrosis due to chloroform is sex- and species-specific. For example, male mice develop primarily renal necrosis whereas female mice develop primarily hepatic necrosis following chloroform administration (Smith *et al.*, 1983).

It has been suggested that tissue injury by chloroform is probably not due to $CHCl_3$ per se, but is produced by a $CHCl_3$ metabolite. The initial step leading to $CHCl_3$-induced tissue injury is believed to be cytochrome P450-dependent biotransformation of $CHCl_3$ to a reactive intermediate, phosgene ($COCl_2$) (Figure 5). Formation of $COCl_2$ may occur via oxidative dechlorination involving oxidation of the C-H bond of $CHCl_3$, producing the trichloromethanol (CCl_3-OH) intermediate, a highly unstable species that would spontaneously dechlorinate to $COCl_2$ (Figure 5). Phosgene is a highly reactive intermediate that may subsequently react with intracellular macromolecules to induce cell damage (Figure 5).

Since kidneys have relatively low xenobiotic-metabolizing enzyme activities,

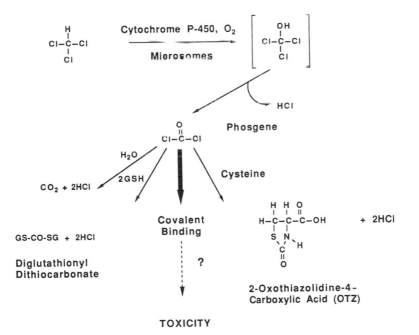

Figure 5. Metabolic pathways and proposed mechanism of nephrotoxicity of $CHCl_3$. Reprinted from Lock (1987) with permission of Kluwer Academic Publishers.

chemically induced nephrotoxicity has been assumed to be produced by toxic intermediates generated in the liver and transported to the kidney. If a single hepatic metabolite of $CHCl_3$ produced both kidney and liver injury, species, strain and sex differences in susceptibility to $CHCl_3$ nephro- and hepato-toxicity would be expected to be the same. However, species, strain and sex differences in susceptibility to $CHCl_3$ nephrotoxicity are not consistent with those of $CHCl_3$ hepatotoxicity. Additionally, several modulators of tissue xenobiotic-metabolizing activities alter $CHCl_3$ nephrotoxicity and hepato-toxicity differently. Since $CHCl_3$-induced kidney injury does not parallel liver damage, it is unlikely that hepatic metabolism of $CHCl_3$ is responsible for renal toxicity.

The concept that kidney injury is produced by a $CHCl_3$ metabolite gener-ated in the kidney has been demonstrated directly using *in vitro* techniques. In order to avoid hepatic metabolism of $CHCl_3$, renal cortical slices from naive animals were incubated with $CHCl_3$ *in vitro* (Smith and Hook, 1984). Under these conditions, the only site of metabolism of $CHCl_3$ is the kidney. *In vitro* exposure to $CHCl_3$ produced toxicity in kidney slices from male but not from female mice (Smith and Hook, 1984). Furthermore, $^{14}CHCl_3$ was metabolized to $^{14}CO_2$ and covalently bound radioactivity by male, but not female, renal cortical microsomes. The *in vitro* metabolism of $CHCl_3$ by male but not female renal slices is consistent with reduced susceptibility of female mice to *in vivo* $CHCl_3$ nephrotoxicity (Smith *et al.*, 1984; Smith *et al.*, 1983). Metab-olism required oxygen, an NADPH regenerating system, was dependent on incubation time, microsomal protein concentration, and substrate concentra-tion and was inhibited by carbon monoxide (Figure 5) (Smith and Hook, 1984). The negligible degree of $CHCl_3$ metabolism and toxicity in female mice is consistent with lower renal cytochrome P450 concentration and activity in female vs male mice (Table 1) (Smith and Hook, 1984). Pretreatment of rabbits with phenobarbital, a renal cytochrome P450 inducer in this species, enhanced the toxic response of renal cortical slices to chloroform *in vitro* (Bailie *et al.*, 1984).

$CDCl_3$ is metabolized by the liver to phosgene ($COCl_2$) at approximately half the rate of $CHCl_3$ metabolism to $COCl_2$. $CDCl_3$ is also less hepatotoxic than $CHCl_3$. Since the $C-D$ bond is stronger than the $C-H$ bond, these data suggest that cleavage of the $C-H$ bond is the rate-limiting step in the activation of $CHCl_3$. $CDCl_3$ is also less toxic to the kidney than $CHCl_3$ (Ahmadizedeh *et al.*, 1981; Branchflower *et al.*, 1984). This deuterium isotope effect on $CHCl_3$-induced nephrotoxicity suggests that the kidney metabolizes $CHCl_3$ in the same manner as the liver, e. g. by oxidation to $COCl_2$. Indeed, rabbit renal cortical microsomes incubated in media supple-mented with L-cysteine metabolized $^{14}CHCl_3$ to radioactive phosgene-cysteine 2-oxothiazolidine-4-carboxylic acid (Figure 5) (Bailie *et al.*, 1984). These *in vitro* data collectively support the hypothesis that mouse and rabbit kidneys biotransform chloroform to a nephrotoxic metabolite ($COCl_2$).

Acetaminophen

Large overdoses of acetaminophen may produce massive centrilobular hepatic necrosis and acute renal failure in humans and experimental animals. Acetaminophen-induced nephrotoxicity (proximal tubule necrosis) in laboratory animals is species-dependent. Large dosages of acetaminophen do not produce detectable histopathological changes in kidney of mice or rabbits, but do produce renal proximal tubular necrosis in male rats (Mitchell *et al.*, 1977; Hennis *et al.*, 1981; McMurtry *et al.*, 1978; Newton *et al.*, 1983b; Tarloff *et al.*, 1989).

Metabolism of acetaminophen by microsomal cytochrome P450 to a reactive, arylating intermediate is thought to be an obligatory biochemical event in acetaminophen-induced hepatic necrosis (Figure 6) (Mitchell *et al.*, 1973). Similarly, acetaminophen-induced renal tubular necrosis is also thought to occur following metabolic activation. However, the exact mechanism of renal metabolic activation is not entirely clear.

Administration of nephrotoxic dosages of acetaminophen to male rats results in covalent binding to renal proteins (Mitchell *et al.*, 1977; McMurtry *et al.*, 1978). Acetaminophen can be metabolically activated by rat renal cortical microsomes via an NADPH-dependent, cytochrome P450-mediated process (McMurtry *et al.*, 1978; Newton *et al.*, 1983 a; Newton *et al.*, 1983 b). However, renal cortical concentrations of cytochrome P450 are approximately one-tenth of that in liver, yet *in vivo* arylation of hepatic and renal macromolecules by acetaminophen is almost identical (McMurtry *et al.*, 1978), suggesting that some mechanism in addition to cytochrome P450 activation may be involved in acetaminophen nephrotoxicity.

An alternative mechanism to cytochrome P450 dependent activation of acetaminophen is enzymatic deacetylation to para-aminophenol (PAP) (Figure 6). PAP is a potent, selective nephrotoxicant that damages the latter third of the proximal tubule (Calder *et al.*, 1979). Both acetaminophen and PAP deplete renal cortical reduced glutathione concentrations and arylate renal macromolecules (McMurtry *et al.*, 1978; Crowe *et al.*, 1979). The functional and histopathological lesions produced by PAP are indistinguishable from the renal lesions produced by acetaminophen administration (Newton *et al.*, 1983 b). PAP has been identified as a urinary metabolite of acetaminophen in both hamster (Gemborys and Mudge, 1981) and Fischer-344 (F-344) rat (Newton *et al.*, 1983 b). In the renal cortex, acetaminophen deacetylation occurs primarily in the cytosolic fraction (Newton *et al.*, 1983 b). Similarly, metabolic activation of acetaminophen to an arylating intermediate is dependent on the presence of a cytosolic deacetylase (Newton *et al.*, 1983 a). Furthermore, both PAP and bis-(para-nitrophenyl) phosphate (a carboxyesterase/amidase inhibitor) inhibit the covalent binding of acetaminophen to renal macromolecules (Newton *et al.*, 1983 a). Further evidence that acetaminophen binds to renal macromolecules subsequent to

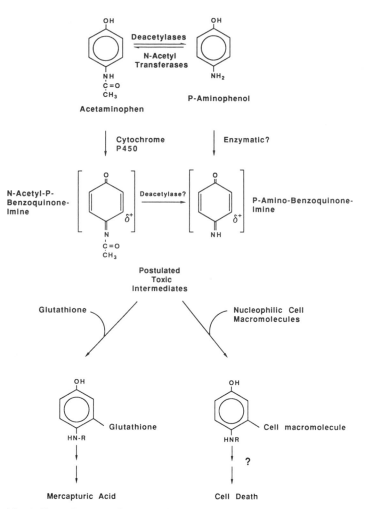

Figure 6. Metabolic pathways and proposed mechanism of nephrotoxicity of acetaminophen. R = H or COCH₃.

deacetylation and metabolic activation to PAP was demonstrated by the covalent binding of [ring-^{14}C]-acetaminophen but not [acetyl-^{14}C] acetaminophen to renal proteins (Newton *et al.*, 1983 a).

Acetaminophen-induced nephrotoxicity cannot be ascribed solely to PAP, however. Mouse renal cortical slices and homogenates catalyze acetaminophen deacetylation to PAP *in vitro* (Carpenter and Mudge, 1981), but mice are not susceptible to acetaminophen nephrotoxicity *in vivo* (McMurtry *et al.*, 1978). Furthermore, 2-month-old F-344 and Sprague-Dawley (SD) rats are equally susceptible to nephrotoxicity induced by PAP, but 2-month-old SD rats are not susceptible to acetaminophen-induced nephrotoxicity (Tarloff *et al.*, 1989). It is possible that reduced susceptibility of mice and 2-month-old

SD rats to PAP nephrotoxicity may be related to a reduced ability to bioactivate PAP to a reactive intermediate or increased ability to metabolize PAP to non-toxic products. However, covalent binding of radiolabel from PAP to renal proteins *in vitro* is similar in renal tissue from F-344 and SD rats (Newton *et al.*, 1983 a; Calder *et al.*, 1979), suggesting that kidneys from SD and F-344 rats are equally able to bioactivate PAP to a reactive intermediate, at least *in vitro*. In contrast, covalent binding of radiolabel derived from acetaminophen to renal proteins *in vivo* is about four times greater in F-344 compared to SD rats (Newton *et al.*, 1985). Similar amounts of PAP are excreted by F-344 and SD rats following acetaminophen administration *in vivo* and by isolated perfused kidneys *in vitro*, and formation of PAP from acetaminophen by renal cortical cytosol is similar in both strains of rats (Newton *et al.*, 1983 b). Thus, differences in susceptibility to nephrotoxicity induced by PAP cannot explain differences in susceptibility to acetaminophen nephrotoxicity between F-344 and SD rats.

Acetaminophen activation by renal cortical tissue may occur by two mechanisms. One mechanism is dependent upon microsomal cytochrome P450 as indicated by the requirement for NADPH. Another mechanism is dependent upon deacetylation of acetaminophen and subsequent metabolic activation of PAP. Formation of a reactive intermediate from each pathway, by implication, indicates that both mechanisms may be involved in the pathogenesis of acetaminophen-induced renal cortical necrosis (Figure 6).

Non-nephrotoxic metabolites generated in extrarenal tissues with subsequent intrarenal conversion to nephrotoxicants

In certain instances, xenobiotics may be metabolized in extrarenal tissue, e.g. liver, to products that may be substrates for renal enzymes. These non-nephrotoxic metabolites are converted to toxic intermediates and produce kidney damage *in situ*. For instance, nephrotoxicity produced by hexachloro-1,3-butadiene (HCBD) appears to occur via sequential hepatic and renal metabolism.

Hexachloro-1,3-butadiene

Hexachloro-1,3-butadiene (HCBD) is a widespread environmental pollutant that is a relatively potent nephrotoxicant in rats, mice, and other mammalian species. The kidneys appear to be the primary target of HCBD toxicity. In rats, HCBD produces selective necrosis in the S3 segment of the proximal tubule, resulting in a distinct band of damage in the outer stripe of the outer medulla (Harleman and Seinen, 1979; Lock and Ishmael, 1979; Lock *et al.*, 1982). Sex differences are apparent in HCBD nephrotoxicity: female rats are more susceptible to renal damage following HCBD than are male rats

(Harleman and Seinen, 1979; Hook *et al.*, 1983). Sex differences are species-dependent, however, as male and female mice are equally susceptible to HCBD (Lock *et al.*, 1984).

HCBD-induced alterations in renal function include decreased urinary concentrating ability (Harleman and Seinen, 1979; Lock and Ishmael, 1979; Berndt and Mehendale, 1979; Davis *et al.*, 1980), glucosuria and proteinuria (Lock and Ishmael, 1979; Berndt and Mehendale, 1979; Nash *et al.*, 1984), increased urinary excretion of alkaline phosphatase, alanine aminopeptidase, γ-glutamyltransferase, and N-acetyl-β-glucosaminidase (Lock and Ishmael, 1979; Nash *et al.*, 1984), and reduced renal clearances of inulin, urea, para-aminohippurate and tetraethylammonium (Lock and Ishmael, 1979; Davis *et al.*, 1980). A time-dependent loss of renal, but not hepatic, cytochrome P450 is observed during the first 12 hours following HCBD administration to rats (Wolf *et al.*, 1984). Neither cytochrome b_5 nor NADPH-cytochrome P450-reductase are significantly affected. The metabolism of several cytochrome P450 substrates is decreased in HCBD-treated female rats and male mice.

In adult male rats, HCBD causes depletion of hepatic but not renal GSH content, whereas, in female rats, significant depletion of GSH occurs in the kidney at much lower doses than in the liver (Kluwe *et al.*, 1981; Hook *et al.*, 1983; Lock and Ishmael, 1981). A systemically administered dose of HCBD is extensively metabolized; it appears that the majority of metabolites may originate from hepatic GSH conjugation with HCBD (Figure 7) (Lock and Ishmael, 1985). GSH depletion may be due to GSH conjugation with a reactive HCBD metabolite (such as an epoxide) generated via cytochrome P450-dependent metabolism, or glutathione S-transferase-mediated conjugation of HCBD directly with GSH. Several lines of evidence suggest that HCBD bioactivation is independent of cytochrome P450: 1. treatment of rats *in vivo* with inhibitors and inducers of hepatic and/or renal mixed function oxidases has little effect on HCBD nephrotoxicity (Lock and Ishmael, 1981; Hook *et al.*, 1982); 2. *in vivo* pretreatment with glutathione or cysteine does not protect against HCBD nephrotoxicity (Berndt and Mehendale, 1979; Davis *et al.*, 1980); 3. formation of a GSH conjugate of HCBD *in vivo* in rat liver microsomes occurs in the presence of N_2 and CO and in the absence of NADPH (Wolf *et al.*, 1984). This suggests that the reaction is a substitution of the halogen catalyzed by GSH-S-transferase, rather than by cytochrome P450 (Figure 7). Interestingly, HCBD conjugation in rat liver appears to occur via microsomal rather than cytosolic GSH S-transferases: the rate of pentachloro-butadienyl (PCBD)-GSH formation by hepatic microsomal fraction is about twice that of cytosol (Wolf *et al.*, 1984).

HCBD-GSH is the major HCBD metabolite present in rat bile (Nash *et al.*, 1984). Cannulation of the bile duct in HCBD-treated animals prevents nephrotoxicity, whereas administration of lyophilized bile produces renal necrosis similar to that caused by HCBD (Nash *et al.*, 1984). Administration of synthesized HCBD-GSH, the cysteine conjugate of HCBD (HCBD-CYS),

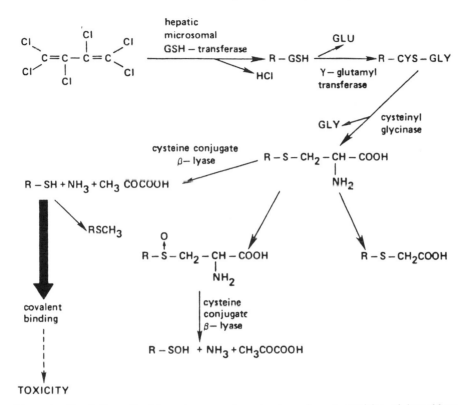

Figure 7. Metabolic pathways and proposed mechanism of nephrotoxicity of hexachloro-butadiene. R – hexachloro butadiene moiety of the glutathione adduct; GLU = glutamate; CYS = cysteine; GLY = glycine. Reprinted from Lock (1987) with permission of Kluwer Academic Publishers.

or the mercapturate conjugate (HCBD-NAC) produces selective damage to the S3 segment of the proximal tubule (Nash *et al.*, 1984; Lock and Ishmael, 1985; Lock *et al.*, 1984; Jaffe, *et al.*, 1983). These data suggest a glutathione-derived metabolite of HCBD mediates nephrotoxicity (Nash *et al.*, 1984).

Thus, HCBD undergoes conjugation in the liver with elimination via bile. Further metabolism occurs in bile, where a cysteinyl-glycine conjugate of HCBD has been identified, probably following cleavage by γ-glutamyl-transferase (Lock, 1987). Reabsorption of these conjugates allows them to reach the kidneys in amounts sufficient to cause toxicity. Renal susceptibility to HCBD metabolites is probably related to the kidney's ability to accumulate organic anions, since probenecid produces protection against HCBD-induced nephrotoxicity (Lock and Ishmael, 1985). PCBD-NAC is deacetylated by rat kidney cytosol to PCBD-CYS which subsequently undergoes covalent binding of radiolabel to renal proteins (Lock, 1987). Covalent binding of radiolabel from PCBD-NAC occurs *in vivo* and is prevented by probenecid (Lock and Ishmael, 1985). Thus, covalent binding and, by implication, nephrotoxicity are dependent on further renal metabolism and bioactivation of PCBD-CYS within renal proximal tubular cells. Cysteine conjugate β-lyase may be involved in bioactivation of HCBD metabolites. PCBD-CYS, but not PCBD-NAC, is a substrate for rat renal cysteine conjugate β-lyase (Green and Odum, 1985). Products of this reaction include pyruvate, ammonia, and a reactive intermediate that inhibits organic anion and cation transport in renal cortical slices (Green and Odum, 1985; Lock 1987). The reactive intermediate may react with 1. glutathione, thereby accounting for depletion of renal GSH in male kidneys (Kluwe *et al.*, 1981; Hook *et al.*, 1983; Lock *et al.*, 1984); 2. protein, via covalent binding (Lock and Ishmael, 1985; Reichert *et al.*, 1985), and/or 3. DNA, where PCBD-CYS is mutagenic in the Ames *Salmonella typhimurium* bacterial assay (Green and Odum, 1985).

6. Conclusions: the significance of renal xenobiotic metabolism

It is apparent that the kidney possesses the enzymatic machinery necessary to catalyse xenobiotic metabolism. The activities of renal cytochrome P450-dependent mixed function oxidases are low in renal homogenates when compared to liver. However, since mixed function oxidases appear to be concentrated within the S2 and S3 segments of proximal tubules, it is likely that these cells have high specific activities of cytochromes P450. This may render the cortex vulnerable to compounds requiring cytochrome P450-mediated systems for activation. In addition, phase II conjugative enzymes are localized in the proximal tubule. Phase I and II enzymes in the renal proximal tubule may contribute to the formation of pharmacologically inactive metabolites for xenobiotics that are concentrated within this nephron segment. In the inner medulla and papilla, prostaglandin H synthetase may bioactivate xenobiotics via cooxidation during synthesis of prostaglandins. This pathway may be of particular importance in the metabolism of bladder carcinogens. In addition, prostaglandin H synthetase may contribute to the aetiology of papillary necrosis resulting from chronic analgesic abuse. A clearer understanding of the contribution of renal xenobiotic metabolism to pharmacology and toxicology will require more complete information concerning the various enzymes involved in renal xenobiotic metabolism, including the precise localization of such enzymes along the nephron and a thorough understanding of how those enzymes may be modulated.

References

Ahmadizadeh, M., Kuo, C.-H. and Hook, J. B. (1981), *J. Toxicol. Environ. Health*, **8**, 105.
Aitio, A. (1973), *Life Sci.*, **13**, 1705.
Aitio, A. and Parkki, M. G. (1978), *Toxicol. Appl. Pharmacol.*, **44**, 107.
Aitio, A., Vainio, H. and Hanninen, O. (1972), *FEBS Lett.*, **24**, 237.

Anders, M. W. (1980), *Kidney Int.*, **18**, 636.
Anders, M. W., Elfarra, A. A. and Lash, L. H. (1987), *Arch. Toxicol.*, **60**, 103.
Bach, P. H. and Bridges, J. W. (1985), *CRC Crit. Rev. Toxicol.*, **15.**, 217.
Bachur, N. R., Gordon, S. L., Gee, M. V. and Kon, H. (1979), *Proc. Nat. Acad. Sci. (U.S.A.)*, **76**, 954.
Bailie, M. B., Smith, J. H., Newton, J. F. and Hook, J. B. (1984), *Toxicol. Appl. Pharmacol.*, **74**, 285.
Berndt, W. O. and Mehendale, H. M. (1979), *Toxicol.*, **14**, 55.
Bock, K. W., Josting, D., Lilienblum, W. and Pfeil, H. (1979). *Eur. J. Biochem.*, **98**, 19.
Bock, K. W., Clausbruch, U. C. V., Kaufmann, R., Lilienblum, W., Oesch, F., Pfeil, H. and Platt, K. L. (1980), *Biochem. Pharmacol.*, **29**, 495.
Branchflower, R. V., Nunn, D. S., Highet, R. H , Smith, J. H., Hook, J. B. and Pohl, L. R. (1984), *Toxicol. Appl. Pharmacol.*, **72**, 159.
Brown, M. S. and Goldstein, J. L., (1985), in *The Pharmacological Basis of Therapeutics* (A. G. Gilman, L. S. Goodman, T. W. Rall and F. Murad, eds), p. 827, Macmillan Publishing Company, New York.
Burchell, B. (1981), in *Reviews in Biochemical Toxicology* (E. Hodgson, J. R. Bend and R. M. Philpot, eds), Vol. 3, p. 1, Elsevier/North Holland, New York.
Calabresi, P. and Parks, R. E. (1985), in *The Pharmacological Basis of Therapeutics* (A. G. Gilman, L. S. Goodman, T. W. Rall and F. Murad, eds), p. 1240, Macmillan Publishing Company, New York.
Calder, I. C., Yong, A. C., Woods, R. A., Crown, C. A., Ham, K. N. and Tange, J. D. (1979), *Chem.-Biol. Interact.*, **27**, 245.
Carpenter, H. M. and Mudge, G. H. (1981), *J. Pharmacol. Exp. Ther.*, **218**, 161.
Carrico, C. K. and Sartorelli, A. C. (1977), *Cancer Res.*, **37**, 1868.
Cayen, M. N., Ferdinandi, E. S., Greselin, E., Robinson, W. T. and Dvornik, D. (1977), *J. Pharmacol. Exp. Ther.*, **200**, 33.
Chasseaud, L. F. (1980), in *Extrahepatic Metabolism of Drugs and Other Foreign Compounds* (T. E. Gram, ed.), p. 427, Spectrum Publications, New York.
Clifton, G., Kaplowitz, N., Wallin, J. D. and Kuhlenkamp, J. (1975), *Biochem. J.*, **150**, 259
Cojocel, C., Maita, K., Pasino, D. A., Kuo, C-H. and Hook, J. B. (1983), *Life Sci.*, **33**, 855.
Coughtrie, M. W. J., Burchell, B. and Bend, J. R. (1987), *Biochem. Pharmacol.*, **36**, 245.
Crowe, C. A., Yong, A. C., Calder, I. C., Ham, K. N. and Tange, J. D. (1979), *Chem.-Biol. Interact.*, **27**, 235.
Davis, B. B., Mattammal, M. B. and Zenser, T. V. (1981), *Nephron*, **27**, 187.
Davis, M. E., Berndt, W. O. and Mehendale, H. M. (1980), *Toxicology*, **16**, 179.
Dees, J. H., Coe, L. D., Yasukochi, Y. and Masters, B. S. S. (1980), *Science*, **208**, 1473.
DePierre, J. W., Seidegard, J., Morgenstern, R., Balk, L., Meijer, J., Astrom, A., Norelius, I. and Ernster, L. (1984), *Xenobiotica*, **14**, 295.
Duffel M. W. and Jakoby, W. B. (1982), *Molec. Pharmacol.*, **21**, 444.
Duggin, G. G. (1980), *Kidney Int.*, **18**, 553.
Elfarra, A. A., Jakobson, I. and Anders, M. W. (1986 a), *Biochem. Pharmacol.*, **35**, 283.
Elfarra, A. A., Lash, L. H. and Anders, M. W. (1986 b), *Proc. Nat. Acad. Sci. (U.S.A.)*, **83**, 2667.
Elfarra, A. A., Lash, L. H. and Anders, M. W. (1987), *Mol. Pharmacol.*, **31**, 208.
Eling, T., Boyd, J., Reed, G., Mason, R. and Sivarajah, K. (1983), *Drug Metab. Rev.*, **14**, 1023.
Endou, H. (1983), *Jpn. J. Pharmacol.*, **33**, 423.

Falany, C. N. and Tephly, T. R. (1983), *Arch. Biochem. Biophys.*, **227**, 248.
Fine, L. G., Goldstein, E. J., Trizna, W., Rozmaryn, L. and Arias, I. M. (1978), *Proc. Soc. Exp. Biol. Med.*, **157**, 189.
Flower, R. J. (1974), *Pharmacol. Rev.*, **26**, 33.
Foster, J. R., Elcombe, C. R., Boobis, A. R., Davies, D. S., Sesardic, D., McQuade, J., Robson, R. T., Hayward, C. and Lock, E. A. (1986), *Biochem. Pharmacol.*, **35**, 4543.
Fowler, B. A. (1972), *Am. J. Pathol.*, **69**, 163.
Fowler, B. A., Hook, G. E. R. and Lucier, G. W. (1977), *J. Pharmacol. Exp. Ther.*, **203**, 712.
Fry, J. R. and Perry, N. K. (1981), *Biochem. Pharmacol.*, **30**, 1197.
Gemborys, M. W. and Mudge, G. H. (1981), *Drug Metab. Dispos.*, **9**, 340.
Gonzalez, F. W. (1989), *Pharmacol. Rev.*, **40**, 243.
Green, R. M. and Elce, J. S. (1975), *Biochem. J.*, **147**, 283.
Green T. and Odum, J. (1985), *Chem.-Biol. Interact.*, **54**, 15.
Hales, B. F., Jaeger, V. and Neims, A. H. (1978), *Biochem. J.*, **175**, 937.
Hanninen, O. and Aitio, A. (1968), *Biochem. Pharmacol.*, **17**, 2307.
Harleman, J. H. and Seinen, W. (1979), *Toxicol. Appl. Pharmacol.*, **47**, 1.
Hawke, R. L. and Welch, R. M. (1985), *Molec. Pharmacol.*, **27**, 283.
Hennis, H. L., Allen, R. C., Hennigar, G. R. and Simmons, M. A. (1981), *Electrophoresis*, **2**, 187.
Hjelle, J. T., Hazelton, G. A., Klaassen, C. D. and Hjelle, J. J. (1986), *J. Pharmacol. Exp. Ther.*, **236**, 150.
Hofbauer, K. G., Sonnenburg, C., Stalder, R., Criscione, L., Kraetz, J., Fuhrer, W. and Habicht, E. (1985), *J. Pharmacol. Exp. Ther.*, **232**, 838.
Hook, J. B., Rose, M. S. and Lock, E. A. (1982), *Toxicol. Appl. Pharmacol.*, **65**, 373.
Hook, J. B., Ishmael, J. and Lock, E. A. (1983), *Toxicol. Appl. Pharmacol.*, **67**, 121.
Imaoka, S. and Funae, Y. (1986), *Biochem. Biophys. Res. Commun.*, **141**, 711.
Jaffe, D. R., Hassall, C. D., Brendel, K. and Gandolfi, A. J. (1983), *J. Toxicol. Environ. Health*, **11**, 857.
Johnson, E. F., Schwab, G. E. and Muller-Eberhard, U. (1979), *Molec. Pharmacol.*, **15**, 708.
Jones, D. P., Sundby, G.-B., Ormstad, K. and Orrenius, S. (1979), *Biochem. Pharmacol.*, **28**, 929.
Jones, T. W., Qin, C., Schaeffer, V. H. and Stevens, J. L. (1989), *Molec. Pharmacol.*, **34**, 621.
Kaplowitz, N. (1980), *Am. J. Physiol.*, **239**, G439.
Kaplowitz, N., Kuhlenkamp, J. and Clifton, G. (1975), *Biochem. J.*, **146**, 351.
Kluwe, W. M., McCormack, K. M. and Hook, J. B. (1978), *J. Pharmacol. Exp. Ther.*, **207**, 566.
Kluwe, W. M., McNish, R., Smithson, K. and Hook, J. B. (1981), *Biochem. Pharmacol.*, **30**, 2265.
Koren, G. (1987), *Clin. Pharmacokinetics*, **13**, 334.
Koren, G., Klein, J. and Silverman, M. (1987), *Can. J. Physiol. Pharmacol.*, **65**, 2500.
Koster, A. S. J., Schrimer, G. and Bock, K. W. (1986), *Biochem. Pharmacol.*, **35**, 3971.
Krijsheld, K. R. and Gram, T. E. (1984), *Biochem. Pharmacol.*, **33**, 1951.
Kuo, C.-H., Hook, J. B. and Bernstein, J. (1981), *Toxicology*, **22**, 149.
Kuo, C.-H., Braselton, W. E. and Hook, J. B. (1982 a), *Toxicol. Appl. Pharmacol.*, **64**, 244.
Kuo, C.-H., Rush, G. F. and Hook, J. B. (1982 b), *J. Pharmacol. Exp. Ther.*, **220**, 547.
Lake, B. G., Hopkins, R., Chakraborty, J., Bridges, J. W. and Parke, D. V. W. (1973), *Drug Metab. Dispos.*, **1**, 342.

Lash, L. H. and Jones, D. P. (1984), *J. Biol. Chem.*, **259**, 14508.
Lash, L. H., Elfarra, A. A. and Anders, M. W. (1986), *J. Biol. Chem.*, **261**, 5930.
Liem, H. H., Muller-Eberhard, U. and Johnson, E. F. (1980), *Molec. Pharmacol.*, **18**, 565.
Litterst, C. L., Mimnaugh, E. G. and Gram, T. E. (1977), *Biochem. Pharmacol.*, **26**, 749.
Lock, E. A. (1987), in *Nephrotoxicity in the Experimental and Clinical Situation*, Part 1 (Developments in Nephrology Series) (P. H. Bach and E. A. Lock eds), p. 429, Martinus Nijhoff, Lancaster.
Lock, E. A. and Ishmael, J. (1979), *Arch. Toxicol.*, **43**, 47.
Lock, E. A. and Ishmael, J. (1981), *Toxicol., Appl. Pharmacol.*, **57**, 79.
Lock, E. A. and Ishmael, J. (1985), *Toxicol. Appl., Pharmacol*, **81**, 32.
Lock, E. A., Ishmael, J. and Pratt, I. S. (1982), *J. Appl. Toxicol.*, **2**, 315.
Lock, E. A., Ishmael, J. and Hook, J. B. (1984), *Toxicol Appl. Pharmacol.*, **72**, 484.
Mackenzie, P. I. (1987), *J. Biol. Chem.*, **262**, 9744.
Mandel, H. G. (1971), in *Fundamentals of Drug Metabolism and Drug Disposition* (B. N. LaDu, H. G. Mandel and E. L. Way, eds.), p. 149, Williams & Wilkins, Baltimore.
Marnett, L., Wlodawer, P. and Samuelsson, B. (1975), *J. Biol. Chem.*, **250**, 8510.
Masters, B. S. S., Yasukochi, Y., Okita, R. T., Parkhill, L. K., Taniguchi, H. and Dees, J. H. (1980), in *Microsomes, Drug Oxidations, and Chemical Carcinogenesis* (M. J. Coon, A. H. Conney, R. W. Estabrook, H. V. Gelboin, J. R. Gillette and P. J. O'Brien, eds.) Vol. 2, p. 709, Academic Press, New York.
Mattammal, M. B., Zenser, T. V. and Davis, B. B. (1981), *Cancer Res.*, **41**, 4961.
Maunsbach, A. B. (1966), *J. Ultrastruct. Res.*, **16**, 239.
McFarlane, M., Foster, J. R., Gibson, G. G., King, L. J. and Lock, E. A. (1989), *Toxicol. Appl. Pharmacol.*, **98**, 185.
McIntyre, T. M. and Curthoys, N. P. (1980), *Int. J. Biochem.*, **12**, 545.
McKinney, T. D. (1982), *Am. J. Physiol.*, **243**, F404.
McMurtry, R. J., Snodgrass, W. R. and Mitchell, J. R. (1978), *Toxicol. Appl. Pharmacol.*, **46**, 87.
Meister, A. and Tate, S. S. (1976), *Ann. Rev. Biochem.*, **45**, 559.
Mitchell, J. R., Jollow, D. J., Potter, W. Z., Davis, D. C., Gillette, J. R. and Brodie, B. B. (1973), *J. Pharmacol. Exp. Ther.*, **187**, 185.
Mitchell, J. R., McMurtry, R. J., Statham, C. N. and Nelson, S. D. (1977), *Am. J. Med.*, **62**, 518.
Mohandas, J., Duggin, G. G., Horvath, J. S. and Tiller, D. J. (1981), *Res. Commun. Chem. Pathol. Pharmacol.*, **34**, 69.
Moldeus, P., Andersson, B., Rahimtula, A. and Berggren, M. (1982), *Biochem. Pharmacol.*, **31**, 1363.
Moldeus, P., Jones, D. P., Ormstad, K. and Orrenius, S. (1978), *Biochem. Biophys. Res. Commun.*, **83**, 195.
Monks, T. J. and Lau, S. S. (1987), *Drug Metab. Dispos.*, **15**, 437.
Morgenstern, R., Lundqvist, G., Andersson, G., Balk, L. and DePierre, J. W. (1984), *Biochem. Pharmacol.*, **33**, 3609.
Nash, J. A., King, L. J., Lock, E. A. and Green, T. (1984), *Toxicol. Appl. Pharmacol.*, **73**, 1984.
Nebert, D. W. and Gonzalez, F. J. (1987), *Ann. Rev. Biochem.*, **56**, 945.
Nebert, D. W., Adesnik, M., Coon, M. J., Estabrook, R. W., Gonzalez, F. J., Guengerich, F. P., Gunsalus, I. C., Johnson, E. F., Kemper, B., Levin, W., Phillips, I. R., Sato, R. and Waterman, M. R. (1987), *DNA* **6**, 1.
Newton, J. F., Braselton, W. E., Kuo, C.-H., Kluwe, W. M., Gemborys, M. W., Mudge, G. H. and Hook, J. B. (1982), *J. Pharmacol. Exp. Ther.*, **221**, 76.

Newton, J. F., Bailie, M. B. and Hook, J., B. (1983 a), *Toxicol. Appl. Pharmacol.*, **70**, 433.

Newton, J. F., Yoshimoto, J., Bernstein, J., Rush, G. F. and Hook, J. B. (1983 b), *Toxicol. Appl. Pharmacol.*, **69**, 291.

Newton, J. F., Pasino, D. A. and Hook, J. B. (1985), *Toxicol. Appl. Pharmacol.*, **78**, 39.

Newton, J. F., Hoefle, D., Gemborys, M. W., Mudge, G. H. and Hook, J. B. (1986), *J. Pharmacol. Exp. Ther.*, **237**, 519.

Oesch, F. and Schmassmann, H. (1979), *Biochem. Pharmacol.*, **28**, 171.

Omiecinski, C. J. (1986), *Nucleic Acids Res.*, **14**, 1525.

Orrenius, S., Ormstad, K., Thor, H. and Jewell, S. A. (1983), *Fed. Proc.*, **42**, 3177.

Parker, V. H. (1965), *Food Cosmet. Toxicol.*, **3**, 75.

Platt, D. S. and Thorp, J. M. (1966), *Biochem. Pharmacol.*, **15**, 915.

Rankin, B. B., McIntyre, T. M. and Curthoys, N. P. (1980), *Biochem. Biophys. Res. Commun.*, **96**, 991.

Reed, D. W. and Beatty, P. W. (1980), in *Reviews of Biochemical Toxicology* (E. Hodgson, J. R. Bend and R. M. Philpot, eds.), vol. 2, p. 213, Elsevier/ North-Holland, New York.

Reichert, D., Schutz, S. and Metzler, M. (1985), *Biochem. Pharmacol.*, **34**, 499.

Rollins, T. and Smith, W. (1980), *J. Biol. Chem.*, **255**, 4872.

Rush, G. F. and Hook, J. B. (1984), *Life Sci.*, **35**, 145.

Rush, G. F., Maita, K., Sleight, S. D. and Hook, J. B. (1983 a), *Proc. Soc. Exp. Biol. Med.*, **172**, 430.

Rush, G. F., Newton, J. F. and Hook, J. B. (1983 b), *J. Pharmacol. Exp. Ther.*, **227**, 658.

Rush, G. F., Wilson, D. M. and Hook, J. B. (1983 c), *Fund. Appl. Toxicol.*, **3**, 161.

Rush, G. F., Pratt, I. S., Lock, E. A. and Hook, J. B. (1986), *Fund Appl. Toxicol.*, **6**, 307.

Schmassmann, H., Sparrow, A., Platt, K. and Oesch, F. (1978), *Biochem. Pharmacol.*, **27**, 2237.

Sedaghat, A. and Ahrens, E. H. (1975), *Eur. J. Clin. Invest.*, **5**, 177.

Simmons, D. L. and Kasper, C. B. (1989), *Arch. Biochem. Biophys.*, **271**, 10.

Smith, J. H. and Hook, J. B. (1983), *Toxicol Appl. Pharmacol.*, **70**, 480.

Smith, J. H. and Hook, J. B. (1984), *Toxicol. Appl. Pharmacol.*, **73**, 511.

Smith, J. H., Maita, K., Sleight, S. D. and Hook, J. B. (1983), *Toxicol. Appl. Pharmacol.*, **70**, 467.

Smith, J. H., Maita, K., Sleight, S. D. and Hook, J. B. (1984), *Toxicology*, **30**, 305.

Smith, J. H., Rush, G. F. and Hook, J. B. (1986), *Toxicology*, **38**, 209.

Smit, J. F. M. and Struyker-Boudier, H. A. J. (1985), *J. Pharmacol. Exp. Ther.*, **232**, 845.

Steiness, E. (1974), *Circulation*, **50**, 103.

Stevens, J. L. (1985), *Biochem. Biophys. Res. Commun.*, **129**, 499.

Stevens, J. and Jakoby, W. B. (1983), *Molec. Pharmacol.*, **23**, 761.

Stonard, M. D. and Parker, V. H. (1971 a), *Biochem. Pharmacol.*, **20**, 2417.

Stonard, M. D. and Parker, V. H. (1971 b), *Biochem. Pharmacol.*, **20**, 2429.

Sugita, O., Nagashima, K., Sassa, S. and Kappas, A. (1988), *Biochem. Biophys. Res. Commun.*, **150**, 925.

Tarloff, J. B., Goldstein, R. S. and Hook, J. B. (1987), in *Nephrotoxicity in the Experimental and Clinical Situation* (P. H. Bach and E. A. Lock, eds.), Part 1, p. 371, Martinus Nijhoff, Lancaster.

Tarloff, J. B., Goldstein, R. S., Morgan, D. G. and Hook, J. B. (1989), *Fund. Appl. Toxicol.*, **12**, 78.

Tepperman, J. (1973), *Metabolic and Endocrine Physiology*, p. 229, Year Book Medical Publishers, Chicago.

Thorp, J. M., (1962) *Lancet*, **1**, 1323.
Ueng, T.-H., Friedman, F. K., Miller, H., Park, S. S., Gelboin, H. V. and Alvares, A. P. (1987), *Biochem. Pharmacol.*, **36**, 2689.
Uotila, P., Parkki, M. G. and Aitio, A. (1978), *Toxicol. Appl. Pharmacol.*, **46**, 671.
VanCantfort, J., Manil, L., Gielin, J. E., Glatt, H. R. and Oesch, F. (1979), *Biochem. Pharmacol.*, **28**, 455.
Wilk, S., Mizoguchi, H. and Orlowski, M. (1978), *J. Pharmacol. Exp. Ther.*, **206**, 227.
Wolf, C. R., Berry, P. N., Nash, J. A., Green, T. and Lock, E. A. (1984), *J. Pharmacol. Exp. Ther.*, **228**, 202.
Woodhall, P. B., Tisher, C. C., Simonton, C. A. and Robinson, R. R. (1978), *J. Clin. Invest.*, **51**, 1320.
Zenser, T. V. and Davis, B. B. (1984), *Fund. Appl. Toxicol.*, **4**, 922.
Zenser, T. V., Levitt, M. and Davis, B. (1977), *Prostaglandins*, **13**, 143
Zenser, T. V., Mattammal, M. B. and Davis, B. B. (1978), *J. Pharmacol. Exp. Ther.*, **207**, 719.
Zenser, T. V., Mattammal, M. and Davis, B. (1979), *J. Pharmacol. Exp. Ther.*, **208**, 418
Zenser, T. V., Mattammal, M. and Davis, B. (1980 a), *Cancer Res.*, **40**, 114.
Zenser, T. V., Mattammal, M., Armbrecht, H. and Davis, B. (1980 b), *Cancer Res.*, **40**, 2839.
Zenser, T. V., Mattammal, M., Rapp, N. S. and Davis, B. B. (1983), *J. Lab. Clin. Med.*, **101**, 58.

CHAPTER 2

Pharmacokinetics and biotransformation of 1,4-dihydropyridine calcium antagonists

C. G. Regårdh, C. Bäärnhielm, B. Edgar and
K-J. Hoffmann

Cardiovascular Research Laboratories, AB Hässle, S-431 83 Mölndal,
Sweden

1. Introduction

The concept of drug-dependent calcium (Ca) antagonism was created in the 1960s by Fleckenstein on the basis of results from experiments with prenylamine and verapamil (Fleckenstein *et al.*, 1969). It was later shown that the drugs do not interfere with the calcium regulation involved in the contraction of the myofibrils of the myocardial cell but instead impede the passage of the calcium ions across the cell membrane. Because of this, the biochemical action of this class of drugs is described by names such as Ca-entry blockers, Ca-channel blockers and Ca-channel modulators. However, the term calcium antagonist seems widely accepted and will be used throughout this review.

There are several groups of chemical compounds that can be characterized as calcium antagonists. Some of these are non-specific in their action, whereas others possess a specific action on the calcium ion transport. Also, the specifically acting antagonists represent a heterogeneous group of compounds, in particular the phenylethylamines (verapamil), the benzodiazepines (diltiazem) and the 1,4-dihydropyridines (nifedipine) (Figure 1). Most of the development of new calcium antagonists during the last decade has primarily concerned

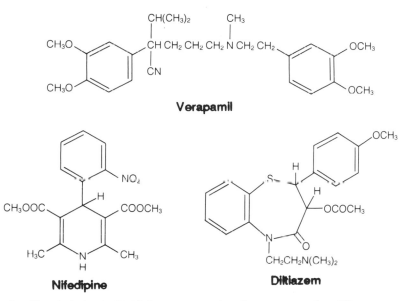

Figure 1. Chemical structures of drugs representing the prototypes for different groups of calcium antagonists.

cerned various derivatives of the dihydropyridine (DHP) structure while much less research has been directed towards the discovery and development of new phenylalkylamine and benzodiazepine derivatives. At present there are six DHPs approved by Health Authorities in various countries and according to the literature, there are several more to come within the next few years.

As shown in Figure 1, the specific calcium antagonists exhibit great differences in their chemical structures. The question as to whether these compounds have a common target molecule and/or receptor and the same mechanism of action might therefore be a field of future research.

Because of the structural heterogeneity among the calcium antagonists and the dominating interest in the DHPs, as regards the development of new drugs in this particular field, this review will only cover 1,4-dihydropyridine derivatives. The chemical structures of the selected DHPs covered by this review are shown in Figure 2. The criteria for inclusion is that data on metabolism and/or pharmacokinetics in humans are available.

Therapeutic indications/use

The DHPs are used for treatment of various cardiovascular disorders. Nifedipine, the prototype of these drugs, was originally introduced for the treatment of angina pectoris. The efficacy of these drugs in angina is probably related to their general ability to increase myocardial oxygen supply and decrease oxygen demand. In more recent years numerous studies have shown that the

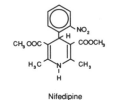

Nifedipine

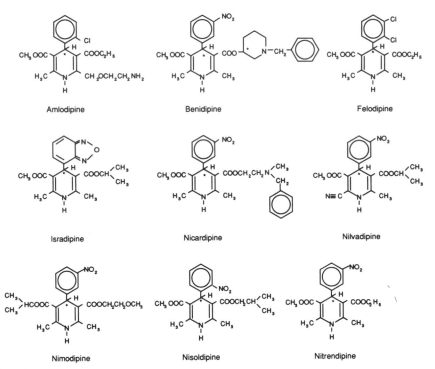

Amlodipine

Benidipine

Felodipine

Isradipine

Nicardipine

Nilvadipine

Nimodipine

Nisoldipine

Nitrendipine

Figure 2. Chemical structures of 1,4-dihydropyridines. The position of the chiral centre is indicated by *.

DHPs effectively reduce blood pressure during long-term treatment of essential and renal hypertension and some have now achieved prominent positions as valuable antihypertensive agents. One DHP, nimodipine, has been claimed to possess a preferential effect on brain blood vessels, as demonstrated by Harper *et al.* (1981) and Kazda and Towart (1982) among others.

Physicochemical properties

The 1,4-dihydropyridine derivatives are a class of calcium antagonists that exhibit closely related chemical structures. The most common variations in the structure are found in the ester functions. The substituent in the aromatic ring is usually either a nitro group or a chlorine in position 2 and/or 3 (Figure 2). Among the the DHPs covered by this review, nifedipine is the only one lacking a chiral centre. Eight of the drugs are used as racemates of two stereoisomers and one, benidipine, is a diastereomer with two asymmetric carbons. The majority of the drugs are neutral molecules within the normal physiological pH range, but three—amlodipine, benidipine and nicardipine—are weak bases. The pK_a for amlodipine is 8.7 and for nicardipine 7.2 which means that amlodipine exists primarily in its ionized form in plasma (pH = 7.4), while nicardipine is ionized to about 40 per cent. Amlodipine is used as the salt with maleic acid while the other two are hydrochlorides. The water solubility of these three compounds is increased by salt formation. The neutral drug molecules are extremely lipophilic and virtually insoluble in water. For example, the partition coefficient between toluene and water of felodipine is about 30 000 (Ahnoff, 1984) and its water solubility at $37°C$ is about 2.6 μmol/L (1 mg/L). The solubility of nifedipine is about ten times greater and that of nicardipine HCl about thirty times the value for felodipine (Higuchi and Shiobara, 1980 a). Because of their very low water solubility, particularly the neutral DHPs, considerable pharmaceutical development is necessary to achieve formulations with complete uptake from the gastrointestinal tract. This problem becomes an even greater challenge when the drug is formulated as a controlled release product as is the case for felodipine, nifedipine and nitrendipine.

2. *Animal pharmacokinetics*

Pharmacokinetic characteristics of the DHPs in various animal species are given in Table 1. The data for the different drugs are quite similar in the same species with the exception of the weak base amlodipine. Thus, oral doses are well absorbed and t_{max} is reached within 1 hour in both rats and dogs (amlodipine 3 hours). The majority of the substances are subjected to high first-pass elimination mainly in the liver and only amlodipine exhibits 100 per cent bioavailability in dogs (at the 2 mg/kg dose level). In the same species, however, the bioavailability increases in a dose dependent manner for benidipine from 2 to 17 per cent when the dose is increased from 1–10 mg/kg, and for nicardipine, from 9 to 34 per cent in the 2–10 mg/kg dose range. This is most likely due to saturation of drug metabolizing enzymes in the liver. The terminal half-life of the individual drugs generally varies between 1–2 hours in the rat (amlodipine 3 hours) and between 2–5 hours in the dog (amlodipine 30 hours). The longer $t_{1/2}$ of amlodipine in the dog is due to a lower systemic plasma clearance (11 ml/min/kg) associated with a larger volume of distribution (25 L/kg) compared to the corresponding parameters for other DHPs (CL_s 20–50 ml/min/kg, V_d 3–10 L/kg).

The systemic plasma clearance of the DHPs decreases in the order

Table 1. Pharmacokinetic characteristics of 1,4-dihydropyridines (DHPs) in different animal species.*

Drug	Species	Route of Administration	t_{max} (hours)	$t_{1/2}$ (hours)	V_{ss} (L/kg)	CL (ml/min/kg)	F	Reference
Amlodipine	rat	p.o.	3	3	25	11	100	Beresford et al. (1988 a)
	dog	i.v./p.o.		30				Beresford et al. (1985)
Benidipine	rat	i.v./p.o.	0.5	2–4	3–5	70–90[d]	3–26[d]	Kobayashi et al. (1988 b)
	dog	i.v./p.o.	0.25–2	2	3–5	30–50[d]	2–17[d]	
Felodipine	rat	i.v./p.o.	0.25	1.5	12	85	17	Bäärnhielm et al. (1986 b)
	dog	i.v./p.o.	0.5	4	8	20	20	
Nicardipine	rat	i.v./p.o.	0.5	0.25	1–4[d]	100–200[d]	22–58[d]	Higuchi and Shiobara (1980 a)
	dog	i.v./p.o.	1–2	0.5–1	1–4[d]	40	9–34[d]	
	monkey	i.v./p.o.	2	1	2	30	10	
Nilvadipine	mouse	i.v./p.o.	0.5	0.7–3	7	155	40	Tokuma et al. (1988)
	rat	i.v./p.o.	0.5	1.3–13[d]	7	94 (88)[f]	4 (30)[f]	
	rabbit	i.v./p.o.	0.7	4	7	46	2	
	dog	i.v./p.o.	0.8–5	5	4	15	40	
Nisoldipine	rat	i.v./p.o.	0.5	0.4–0.7		45	3	Ahr et al. (1988 a)
	dog	i.v./p.o.	1	2–4		36	12	
	monkey	p.o.	4	4				
Nitrendipine	rat	i.v./p.o.	0.5	1.5		17	12	Krause et al. (1988 a)
	dog	i.v./p.o.	0.8	1.5		22	29	

d = dose dependent; f = female rat

* Abbreviations used: t_{max} = time to reach maximum plasma concentration;

$t_{1/2}$ = half-life;

V_{ss} = volume of distribution at steady state;

CL = plasma clearance;

F = bioavailability.

mouse > rat > rabbit,dog,monkey > man as shown in studies with nicardipine, felodipine and nilvadipine (Higuchi and Shiobara, 1980 a,b; Bäärnhielm *et al.*, 1986 b; Tokuma *et al.*, 1988). This species difference correlates well with the rank order of the rate of metabolism in liver microsomal preparations.

3. Metabolism

The metabolism of dihydropyridine analogues has been studied extensively in animals and healthy volunteers. Available data are currently reviewed with the main emphasis on results in human studies and the references used if not otherwise stated are given in Table 2. The metabolites have been isolated from urine, as renal elimination of formed metabolites is of major importance with more than 60 per cent dose recovery for most DHPs in man as discussed below. The proportion of the radioactive dose found in urine is often lower in animals (Table 3).

A major part of the drug-related radioactivity excreted in faeces is secreted via the bile (Tokuma *et al.*, 1987 a; Sutfin *et al.*, 1987). Bile duct cannulated rats have also been used as a source of production of sufficient amounts of metabolites for identification. Further studies in rats have shown extensive enterohepatic circulation mainly of metabolites; for instance more than 40 per cent of felodipine metabolites secreted into bile were reabsorbed.

The biliary secretion of a radioactive intravenous dose of felodipine was recently studied in man by means of a multiple marker dilution principle with double lumen tubes in the stomach and intestine. During a period of 4.5 hours after administration, 3 to 9 per cent of the radioactive dose was recovered from intestinal aspirates. Less than 0.1 per cent was due to unchanged felodipine. These results indicate that biliary secretion is a minor route of elimination for felodipine and its metabolites in man (Sutfin *et al.*, 1989).

The identity of metabolites is based on cochromatography with synthetic references in various analytical systems, such as thin layer chromatography (TLC) and reverse-phase gradient liquid chromatography (LC) with radioisotope detection. Mass spectrometry (MS) is frequently used to generate spectroscopic evidence of unknown structures. Underivatized urinary metabolites of amlodipine have been separated by LC and introduced into the ion source of the MS instrument via a thermospray interface. Alternatively, isolated fractions are measured by direct probe insertion MS. This technique has been used for nicardipine and high resolution MS has been successfully applied in the case of nimodipine. Prior to analysis by gas chromatography (GC) combined with MS, derivatization of polar acidic metabolites in most cases is accomplished by methylation with diazomethane. Lactonization of hydroxy acid derivatives (e.g. benidipine), is performed prior to GC-MS by heating acidified samples according to a method developed by Weidolf and Hoffmann (1984). Amino groups, potentially formed by reduction of the nitro group, are

Table 2. Metabolic studies on 1,4-dihydropyridines (DHPs).

DHPs	Species[1]	Route of administration	Sample[2]	Number of identified metabolites	References
Amlodipine	H, D, R, M	i.v./oral	U	18	Beresford et al. (1988 b) Beresford et al. (1989) Stopher et al. (1988)
Benidipine	D, R	oral	B, U	13	Kobayashi et al. (1988 c)
Felodipine	H, D, R, M	oral	U	15	Hoffmann and Andersson (1987) Weidolf et al. (1984) Hoffmann and Weidolf (1985) Bäärnhielm et al. (1986 a)
Isradipine	H	oral	P	6	Jean and Laplanche (1988)
Nicardipine	H, D, R	oral	U	12	Rush et al. (1986) Graham et al. (1985) Higuchi et al. (1977)
Nifedipine	H	sublingual, rectal, oral	P, U	3	Raemsch and Sommer (1983)
Nilvadipine	D, R	i.v./oral	B, U	9	Terashita et al. (1987)
Nimodipine	D, Mo, R	oral	B, U	18	Scherling and Karl (1988) Meyer et al. (1983 b)
Nisoldipine	H, D, Mo, R	oral	B, P, U	18	Scherling et al., 1988
Nitrendipine	H, R	oral	U	9	Meyer et al. (1983 a) Kann et al. (1984)

[1] H (healthy men), D (dog), Mo (monkey), R (rat) and M (mouse)
[2] B (bile), P (plasma) and U (urine)

Table 3. Excretion of total radioactivity in various animal species after administration of different 1,4-dihydropyridines (DHPs).

Drug	Species	Route of administration	Collection period (hours)	% Administered dose			Total dose recovered (%)	References
				Urine	Faeces	Bile		
Amlodipine	rat	i.v./p.o.	72	33–38	58–60		91–98	Beresford et al. (1988 a)
	dog	i.v./p.o.	168	38–51	38–49		85–91	
Benidipine	rat	p.o.	72	19	74	34 (50)e	93	Kobayashi et al. (1988 a)
	dog	p.o.	72	25	66		91	
Felodipine	mouse	p.o.	72	53	32		85	Weidolf et al. (1984)
	rat	i.v./p.o.	168	42–49*	49–57*	50 (40)e	99*	Sufin et al. (1987)
	dog	i.v./p.o.	72	48–51*	44*		92–98*	
Nicardipine	rat	i.v./p.o.	72	24	67–74	65	91–97	Higuchi et al. (1977)
	dog	i.v./p.o.	48	23–29	68–71		94–97	
Nifedipine	rat	i.v./p.o.	48	50–70d	30–50d	50 e	>90	von Duhm et al. (1972)
	dog	p.o.	72	10–20	70–85			
Nilvadipine	rat	i.v./p.o.	72	21–24	70–80	75	97–103	Tokuma et al. (1987 a)
	dog	i.v./p.o.	72	56–61	34–36		93–97	
Nimodipine	rat	i.v./p.o.	48	20	77–84	74 (43)e	>98	Maruhn et al. (1985)
	dog	i.v./p.o.	216	18–25	77–82		>98	Suwelack and Weber (1985)
Nisoldipine	monkey	p.o.	240	41–53	51–59		>98	Ahr et al. (1988 a)
	rat	i.v./p.o.	24	29–42	60–75	72 (43)e	>94	
	dog	i.v./p.o.	24	36–39	55–59		>94	
	monkey	p.o.	24	77	14		>94	
	swine		24	39	55		>94	
Nitrendipine	rat	i.v./p.o.	24	35–46	50–65	75 (49)e		Krause et al. (1988 a)
	dog	i.v./p.o.	24	32–44	43–64			

e = enterohepatic circulation of metabolites. In brackets is reabsorbed radioactivity in per cent of the amount excreted in bile; d = dose dependent; * = unpublished data.

reacted with trifluoroacetic acid anhydride. Felodipine metabolites are trimethylsilylated followed by transesterification with diazomethane, where deuterated derivatives and chemical ionization add complementary structural information. Due to the isotope cluster of the chlorine substituent(s) in the phenyl ring of amlodipine and felodipine, mass spectra of metabolites contain doublet peaks thus enhancing the confidence with which small amounts of unknown metabolites can be identified. Metabolites of nilvadipine and nisoldipine have been further characterized by ^{1}H-NMR spectroscopy.

A classification of metabolic pathways involved in the biotransformation of DHPs is shown in Figure 3. Due to a common structural feature of these drugs (the 4-phenyl substituted 1,4-dihydropyridine dicarboxylate system), similar reactions are observed for some functional groups like aliphatic hydroxylation whereas other reactions are more specifically dependent on a particular substituent present in the molecule. The principal pathways reported in the literature (Table 2) will be discussed as follows:

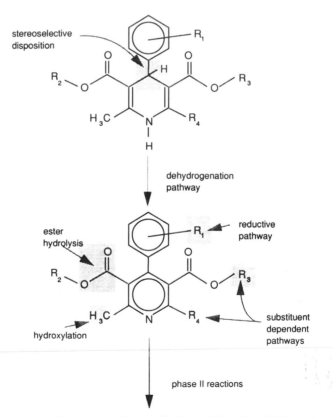

Figure 3. Common metabolic pathways for 1,4-dihydropyridines. In addition, minor amounts of primary metabolites with an intact dihydropyridine ring may directly undergo phase II reactions.

1. dehydrogenation of the 1,4-DHP system;
2. ester hydrolysis;
3. aliphatic hydroxylation;
4. substituent dependent pathways;
5. phase II reactions;
6. reduction of the nitro group (if present);
7. decarboxylation.

The relative importance of these reactions seems to decline in the order listed. The combination of these seven principal metabolic steps with potential consecutive reactions of primary metabolites, e.g. glucuronidation, will generate a large number of possible structures to challenge the analytical chemist.

Dehydrogenation

Dehydrogenation of the 1,4-DHP system to the corresponding pyridine is consistently reported as a primary metabolic step. This reaction entails deactivation of the parent drug in terms of pharmacological activity (Triggle, 1982). The pyridine metabolite is present in plasma and further metabolism to more polar products is required prior to renal elimination. However, dehydrogenation occurs not only *in vivo* but the 1,4-DHP ring system is also readily oxidized under various analytical conditions, for instance in the GC injector port and column (Ahnoff, 1984). This leads to analytical problems in avoiding artefactual data. Furthermore, the pyridine metabolite can be detected in plasma samples spiked with nifedipine and stored at room temperature for several hours. Results from *in vitro* studies with felodipine (Bäärnhielm *et al.*, 1984) and nilvadipine (Niwa *et al.*, 1988 b) support the assumption of almost quantitative *in vivo* conversion by dehydrogenation of these compounds before sequential metabolism of this key metabolite.

The relative rate of microsomal oxidation is mainly dependent on the substituents in the aromatic ring and seems not to be affected by small changes in the ester substituents (Bäärnhielm and Westerlund, 1986; Böcker and Guengerich, 1986). The oxidation rate increased with increasing steric bulk, lipophilicity and electron withdrawal of the substituents in the 2' position. Interestingly, the large ester substituents in the nicardipine and benidipine molecule appear to render the 1,4-DHP system less susceptible to oxidation and alternative metabolic reactions are observed as discussed below.

The oxidation of the DHPs to their corresponding pyridines is a major metabolic and inactivation pathway of this class of drugs. Evidence for the involvement of cytochrome P-450 in this oxidation process has been found in different induction and inhibition studies with liver microsomes, (Augusto *et al.* 1982; Bäärnhielm *et al.*, 1984; Guengerich *et al.* 1986; Niwa *et al.* 1988 b). Furthermore, Guengerich *et al.* (1986) have characterized cytochrome P450 forms from rat and human liver microsomes involved in the oxidation of nifedipine. In rat, two specific isoenzymes $P450_{UT-A}$ and

P450$_{PCN-E}$, mainly present in the adult male rat, were identified as having significant roles in the oxidation reaction. This sex-related difference in enzyme activity might explain the observed higher metabolic rate of different DHPs in male compared to female rats (Bäärnhielm et al., 1986 a, Guengerich et al., 1986; Niwa et al., 1989). From reconstitution and immunochemical inhibition studies of the oxidation of nifedipine, a cytochrome P450 isoenzyme (cytochrome P450$_{NF}$), has been identified in human liver (Guengerich et al., 1986). This isoenzyme or related ones are probably also responsible for the oxidation of other DHPs. This human isoenzyme is different from the cytochrome P450-dependent debrisoquine hydroxylase but is involved in the metabolism of other compounds like testosterone, quinidine, cyclosporine and erythromycin. This might not necessarily lead to an interaction between ordinary doses of DHPs and these compounds but one should be aware of this possibility. Interactions with DHPs are dealt with in more detail in a separate section of this review. Another enzyme system (prostaglandin synthase) has also been shown to catalyse the dehydrogenation of felodipine (Bäärnhielm and Hansson, 1986).

The mechanism of dehydrogenation of the DHPs has gained much interest since it is a major metabolic step in their inactivation. Based on the results presented by Augusto et al. (1982), Bäärnhielm and Hansson (1986), Böcker and Guengerich (1986), Guengerich and Böcker (1988), a number of different mechanisms has been proposed for the oxidation of DHPs as outlined in Figure 4. The oxidation of the 4-arylsubstituted DHPs proceeds most likely via a stepwise electron transfer involving initial formation of a cation radical which after deprotonation (-H$^+$) forms a neutral radical (pathway a). The latter is then oxidized to the pyridinium cation which in aqueous medium is in equilibrium with the free base. It is less likely, but also possible, that the pyridinium cation can also be formed via loss of a hydrogen radical (-H$^•$) as indicated in pathway b. Whether or not the abstraction of the hydrogen atom in position 4 of the DHP ring is rate limiting remains to be completely clarified. No deuterium isotope effect has been observed in the dehydrogenation of felodipine in rat liver microsomes (Bäärnhielm and Westerlund, 1986) and labelled felodipine is additionally oxidized by the prostaglandin synthase system. When glutathione (GSH) is added to the latter system, no formation of the pyridine metabolite has been observed. Furthermore, the ratio of unlabelled to deuterated felodipine assayed by selected ion monitoring remained unchanged throughout the experiment, suggesting that the intermediate retained the deuterium in position 4 (Bäärnhielm and Hansson, 1986). With nifedipine, Guengerich and Böcker (1988) observed no significant kinetic hydrogen isotope effect in either inter- and intramolecular competition experiments. In contrast, Born and Hadley (1989) reported a significant kinetic isotope effect for the oxidation rate of nifedipine in rat liver microsomes and proposed pathway f, implying a direct loss of a hydrogen radical (-H$^•$). Although the loss of the hydrogen in position 4 may be rate limiting it does not necessarily need to be the first step. Most probably the loss of one electron

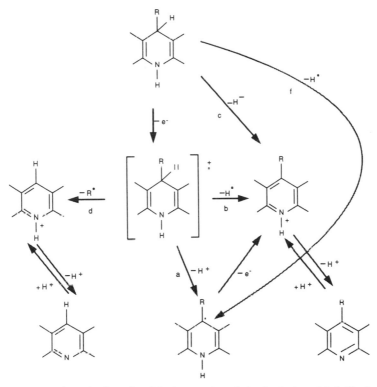

Figure 4. Proposed mechanisms for dehydrogenation of the 4-substituted 1,4-dihydropyridine 3,5-dicarboxylate system.

initiates the process. Interestingly, the direct two electron oxidation is most common for other NADPH-promoted reactions of cytochrome P450 (pathway c).

Alkyl-substituted DHPs in position 4 without calcium antagonistic properties are oxidized via pathway d (Figure 4) via the prosthetic haem of cytochrome P450 and subsequently inactivates the enzyme (Augusto *et al.*, 1982). Neither nifedipine nor felodipine are able to destroy cytochrome P450 by this mechanism, probably due to low radical stability of the phenyl group.

Despite the significance of the dehydrogenation reaction, some 1,4-dihydropyridine metabolites are found in urine collected from healthy volunteers after an oral dose of nicardipine. Furthermore, the existence of both DHP and pyridine metabolites suggests parallel pathways with possible interconversion by dehydrogenation at any stage. The 2-aminoethoxymethyl substituent in amlodipine does not influence the oxidation of the parent drug to its pyridine analogue as a principal route of metabolism in man. In dog and rat urine, however, some 1,4-dihydropyridine derivatives of amlodipine are observed where the long side-chain is altered by oxidative deamination, esters are hydrolysed and the 6-methyl group is hydroxylated as discussed below.

Ester hydrolysis

Oxidation of DHPs to corresponding pyridine derivatives results in metabolites of similar lipophilicity to the parent drugs. Formation of secondary metabolites by ester hydrolysis is therefore very crucial for forming more polar metabolites. With the exception of nifedipine, all DHPs in Figure 2 are non-symmetric with respect to ester functions, an important factor for vascular selectivity of these drugs as reported for felodipine by Berntsson *et al.* (1987). Except for nimodipine, the methyl ester group is present in all molecules and is often more resistant to hydrolysis than the other ester functions as can be seen by simply counting the number of reported metabolites containing the methyl ester. More specifically, the methyl ester group of a felodipine analogue has been shown to be more stable toward hydrolysis in human liver microsomes than the ethyl ester (Bäärnhielm *et al.*, 1988).

In general terms, the esters of various DHPs are fairly stable under acidic conditions and even the enzymatically mediated reaction seems to be slower than dehydrogenation. Mechanistically, esterases in blood and liver catalyse the reaction. The involvement of the liver cytochrome P450 enzyme system in this process has been suggested for nifedipine (Guengerich, 1987; Guengerich *et al.*, 1988). According to these latter authors, the reaction most likely proceeds via aliphatic hydroxylation as discussed below. Such cytochrome P450-dependent de-esterification is reportedly mediated by cytochrome $P450_{PB-B}$ and may also occur directly with other DHPs but the reaction will only be apparent if the concurrent dehydrogenation step is comparatively slow. Due to the stability of amlodipine in rat liver microsomes as regards aromatization, a small amount (~ 10 per cent in 30 min) of the formed DHP-5-acid metabolite is detectable (Beresford *et al.*, 1988 c). This reaction requires NADHP and is inhibited by carbon monoxide, which is indicative of the involvement of cytochrome P450 in ester hydrolysis. In this particular experiment, the ethyl ester of amlodipine was stable, probably due to the proposed local steric hindrance by the 2-aminoethoxymethyl side-chain. The DHP-5-acid is the only dihydropyridine containing metabolite of nisoldipine excreted in urine, whereas the corresponding metabolite of nimodipine is present only in plasma.

Hydrolysis of both ester functions is proposed for some calcium channel blockers and the resulting diacid in the form of hydroxylated pyridine is the major metabolite of benidipine in the dog. These pyridine-diacid metabolites, found in studies with amlodipine (dog), nimodipine (rat) and nitrendipine (rat), are highly polar compounds. They are difficult to analyse, as derivatization of the acids with diazomethane yields dimethyl esters indistinguishable from the methyl ester present in the the parent compound. Trimethylsilylation of the pyridine-diacid of felodipine in rat urine circumvents this latter problem.

Hydroxylation

Hydroxylation of the methyl groups in position 2 and 6 of the DHP pyridine ring is frequently encountered and is mediated by cytochrome P450 (Guengerich *et al.*, 1988). If this reaction precedes ester cleavage it will indirectly contribute to the hydrolysis of the neighbouring ester group. This process has been studied in detail in *in vitro* experiments with felodipine. Interestingly, the 2- or 6- methyl groups of the pyridine monoacids of felodipine are metabolically stable when incubated with liver microsomes. These results emphasize the likely sequence of events in the formation of hydroxy acids where the initial hydroxylation of the 2- or 6-methyl groups preferably takes place with intact ester functions still being present. Mechanistically, the formed hydroxyl acts as a nucleophile and attacks the ester carbonyl with subsequent lactone formation and concomitant elimination of an alcohol. Lactones (e.g. of felodipine) are relatively lipophilic metabolites which are found in plasma but not urine. It is of particular interest that the lactones of felodipine are preferentially metabolized further by ester hydrolysis rather than by ring opening. The equilibrium between the lactones and the corresponding hydroxy acids is dependent on pH and temperature (Weidolf and Hoffmann, 1984). Most likely, only the ring-opened hydroxy acids are renally cleared from plasma and are some of the major urinary metabolites of the DHPs. The primary 2- or 6-pyridine alcohol formed is occasionally further oxidized in small quantities to the corresponding carboxylic acid as reported for felodipine in the rat.

In addition to hydroxylation of the 2- and 6-methyl groups of the DHPs, other aliphatic carbons are oxygenated to a significant extent. Hydroxylation of the α-carbon in the alcohol part of the alkylesters will generate unstable intermediates spontaneously decomposing to the corresponding free carboxylic acids. The ethyl ester, encountered in amlodipine and felodipine, is hydroxylated in the β-position and the same metabolic pathway is observed for the isopropyl and isobutyl moieties of nilvadipine and nisoldipine, respectively.

Substituent dependent pathways

Substituent dependent pathways consist of various reactions encountered in drug metabolism. Oxidative O-demethylation of the methoxy ethyl ester of nimodipine generates the same type of hydroxy metabolite as described for felodipine, but formed by a different mechanism. This nimodipine metabolite is present as dihydropyridine only in rat urine and as its pyridine analogue in all animal species studied. Further oxidation of the alcohol will yield the corresponding carboxylic acid isolated from monkey urine.

The long side-chain of nicardipine is metabolized in several consecutive steps as outlined schematically below:

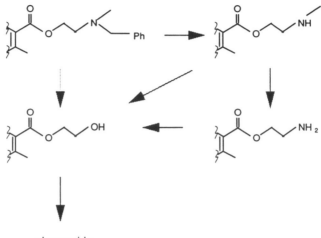

glucuronide

Arrows indicate possible routes via intermediates. Oxidative N-dealkylation yields the secondary and primary amine, which may undergo deamination to give the primary alcohol via reduction of an intermediary aldehyde. Alternatively, this important alcohol metabolite is generated by direct deamination, a reaction which will release benzylmethylamine as a secondary metabolite. The dihydropyridine and pyridine alcohol of nicardipine are predominantly excreted as glucoronides in urine and represent the major metabolites in man. N-debenzylation is reported as a prominent metabolic route for benidipine in rats and dogs.

The methyl group in position 2, present in most DHPs, is substituted by an aminoethoxy group in amlodipine and by a cyano group in nilvadipine. These substituents have significant influence on the metabolic fate of these drugs. Numerous amlodipine metabolites are formed by modification of this side-chain as depicted below. These are the principal pathways for the substituent which have been reported together with other metabolic modifications in the molecule, discussed above. The pyridine carboxylic acid formed by oxidative deamination is the major metabolite found in human urine.

The cyano group in nilvadipine confers considerable metabolic stability. The cyano moiety in two metabolites, in which the neighbouring group is a free carboxylic acid, is reported to be acid labile and is transformed to an amide. It is not known, however, whether these compounds are present as metabolites or formed as artefacts during purification.

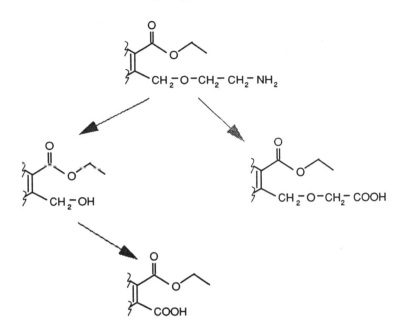

Conjugation

Conjugation of phase I metabolites of the DHPs with glucuronic acid and their renal elimination is not frequently described. After oral administration of nicardipine to volunteers the major urinary metabolites are the glucuronides of the 2 hydroxyethyl esters both in dihydropyridine and pyridine form. These metabolites account for approximately 36 per cent of the radioactivity excreted in the 0–8 hour post-dose period. All identified metabolites of felodipine in human urine are present both in free and conjugated forms. The major biotransformation product of nisoldipine in urine, plasma and bile (the dihydroxy pyridine monoacid), is excreted as a glucuronide.

Interestingly, all identified biliary metabolites of nimodipine in the rat are also detected as conjugates, but to a lesser extent in the dog. Some species variations may be involved in terms of phase 2 reactions with DHP metabolites. This is apparent with felodipine where conjugates in urine are less abundant in animals than in man.

Nitro reduction

Nitro reduction, a possible pathway in eight of the ten drugs shown in Figure 2, has been reported for benidipine, nicardipine, nilvadipine, nimodipine and nisoldipine. In all cases the primary aromatic amine has been isolated as a minor metabolite. Reduction of the nitro group in the unchanged DHPs or primary pyridine metabolite with remaining substituents intact has not been observed and is most likely because oxidative processes predominant. For example, the amine metabolite of nimodipine is eliminated as dihydroxy pyridine in animals. A minor biotransformation pathway for nisoldipine is the amino metabolite accounting at most for 1 and 0.1 per cent of the dose in rat and man, respectively. The formation of the δ-lactam nisoldipine metabolites is probably a chemical and not an enzymatic reaction.

Decarboxylation

Decarboxylation as a metabolic pathway for drugs is rarely described in the literature but has been observed for several of the DHPs. The loss of the 5-methoxycarbonyl function of amlodipine and isolation of this metabolite in its pyridine form has been reported in rats and this metabolite is found as a deaminated product in human urine. However, in a more recent report by Stopher *et al.* (1988), this human metabolite was not identified. Furthermore, metabolism by decarboxylation of the monoacid in position 3 of nicardipine yields minor metabolites. The debenzylated pyridine analogue of benidipine without the methoxycarbonyl group at C-5 is a major metabolite in rat urine but only a minor one in the dog.

In vitro studies with felodipine using liver microsomes from rat, dog and man revealed that both possible decarboxylated products as pyridine are formed in all species. Mechanistically this reaction is not well understood, but most likely the DHP ring structure of felodipine is required for this metabolic pathway to proceed. This assumption is based on the following observations: 1. no decarboxylation takes place after incubations with dehydro felodipine or the corresponding pyridine monoacids as substrates; 2. the dihydropyridine monoacids, although not being identified as metabolites of felodipine *per se*, are decarboxylated by the *in vitro* system.

In summary the complexity of the metabolic profiles of all DHPs, irrespective of the type of sample analysed, is a result of the profound variety of suitable sites for metabolic reactions and their high metabolic clearance in both animals and man. From the chemical viewpoint, the structural multiplicity is based on two different ester functions with various substituents and, furthermore, their lipophilic character makes them good substrates for metabolising enzymes. Apart from nitro reduction, all biotransformations occur in the DHP pyridine ring system or its substituents and a large number of metabolites are produced by some common metabolic reactions.

4. Human pharmacokinetics

Absorption

Gastrointestinal uptake

The uptake and bioavailability of orally administered DHPs have been studied quantitatively by using doses labelled with radioactive or stable isotopes of the drugs in question (Edgar *et al.*, 1985; Rush *et al.*, 1986; Mikus *et al.*, 1987; Tse and Jaffe, 1987; Beresford *et al.*, 1988 b). These studies have shown comparable urinary recoveries of radioactivity after i.v. and oral doses indicating complete absorption of the DHPs from the gastrointestinal tract. The use of controlled release formulations with a constant release rate for > 12 hours has further indicated that the absorption of the DHPs takes place over a large part of the intestine. Absorption from different segments of the small intestine of man has been studied for nicardipine by means of a perfusion technique (Delchier *et al.*, 1988). Complete absorption was found from both the jejunum and ileum. The effect of food on the absorption of nicardipine from these segments was too small to alter the pharmacokinetics of nicardipine.

Although absorption of the DHPs from the colon might be less than that from the small intestine as indicated for nitrendipine (Soons *et al.*, 1989), the absorption of nifedipine from the colorectal region is still sufficient to consider rectal administration as a useful dosing alternative in hypertensive emergencies (Kurosawa *et al.*, 1987).

As for the majority of other drugs, the rate of absorption of the DHPs is dependent on the type of formulation used. Following administration of a capsule, containing either a solution of the drug or a rapidly dissolving solid formulation, maximum concentration is usually attained during the first two hours after dosing (Table 4). The same is true for conventional tablet formulations whereas the time to reach peak concentration is substantially delayed for the controlled release (CR) formulations. This may occur first after 4–10 hours or the plasma concentration may reach a plateau and stay relatively constant over a considerable time after dosage.

Bioavailability

The fraction of orally given DHPs reaching the systemic circulation—the bioavailability (*F*)—varies considerably. Approximately 65 per cent of an oral dose of amlodipine is systemically available (Table 4). A relatively high bioavailablity around 50 per cent has also been reported for nifedipine in several studies whereas the other drugs have a bioavailability of 10–20 per cent. The deviation in bioavailability from 100 per cent is mainly an effect of first-pass elimination in the liver and/or the intestine (Waller *et al.*, 1984; Wang *et al.*, 1989) as experiments with radiolabelled doses of several of the DHPs have indicated complete uptake of these drugs from the gastrointestinal tract (von Horster *et al.*, 1972; Edgar *et al.*, 1985; Mikus *et al.*, 1987).

The rate of drug release in the intestine has some impact on the bioavailability of the dihydropyridines. Thus, if the *in vivo* release rate is made too slow, there is a risk of decreased bioavailability which might lead to loss of therapeutic effect. The reduction in bioavailability secondary to a diminished release rate may be a consequence of either a more pronounced first-pass effect or incomplete absorption from the gastrointestinal tract. According to

Table 4. Absorption characteristics of some 1,4-dihydropyridine calcium antagonists in young healthy subjects.

Drug	Formulation	Dose (mg)	t_{max} (hours)	C_{max} [nmol/(L/mg)]	F (%)	Effects of food	Effects of dose	References
Amlodipine	tabl	10, sd	7.6 ± 1.8	1.5	64			Faulkner et al. (1986)
	caps	15, sd			63			Beresford et al. (1988 b)
	tabl	2.5–10, sd	~6	1.2			↕	Williams and Cubeddu (1988)
Benidipine	tabl	16, sd	1.2 ± 0.5	1.3			↑	Maier-Lenz et al. (1988)
Felodipine	tabl	5, md	2.2 ± 1.0	1.2 ± 0.4	15 ± 9	↕	↕	Landahl et al. (1988)
	c.r.	10, md	3.0 ± 0.6	0.7 ± 0.3	~15	↕		Saltiel et al. (1988)
Isradipine	caps	10, sd	1.6 ± 0.6	2.5 ± 1.1	19 ± 7	↕		Schran et al. (1988)
Nicardipine	caps	10, md	1.0 ± 0.2	3.1 ± 0.8	19 ± 4	→	↑	Graham et al. (1984)
	caps	10, md			16 ± 6		↑	Wagner et al. (1987)
Nifedipine	caps	10, sd	0.8 ± 0.8	24 ± 12	43 ± 10	↕		Challenor et al. (1987 b)
	caps	10, sd	1.0 ± 0.9	23 ± 12	56 ± 25	↕		Reitberg et al. (1987)
	c.r.	20, sd	4.2 ± 0.7	3.8 ± 1.4	52 ± 13	↕	↑ > 12 mg	Kleinbloesem et al. (1984 b)
Nilvadipine	tabl	4, sd	1.5 ± 0.1	1.3 ± 0.5				Cheung et al. (1988)
	tabl	6, md	1.6 ± 0.8	1.4 ± 0.6				Cheung et al. (1989)
	tabl	2, sd	1.5 ± 0.8	1.9 ± 0.6		↕		Terakawa et al. (1987 a,b)
Nimodipine	tabl	60, sd	0.7	2.5	12 ± 5			van Harten et al. (1989)
	caps	60, sd	0.4	5.0	13 ± 4			van Harten et al. (1988 b)
Nisoldipine	tabl	10, md	2.0 ± 1.5	0.5 ± 0.4	3.9 ± 3.5			van Harten et al. (1988 c)
	sol	10, sd	0.4 ± 0.2	1.5 ± 1.4	3.7 ± 2.1			Soons et al. (1989)
	tabl	20, sd		0.6 ± 0.3				
Nitrendipine	c.r.	40, sd	10.7 ± 3.2[a]	0.2 ± 0.1	8.2 ± 1.6			Kann et al. (1984)
	tabl	20, sd	2.5 ± 1.2	1.1 ± 1.1	11.1 ± 4.5			
	tabl	5, md	1.8 ± 1.1	4.2 ± 2.8				
	tabl	30, sd			29 ± 17	↕		Raemsch and Sommer (1984)
	tabl	20, sd	2.3 ± 0.6	1.7 ± 1.0	20.0 ± 8			Mikus et al. (1987)

a = duration of plateau; sd = single dose; md = multiple dosing; tabl = tablet; caps = capsule; c.r. = controlled release.

Soons *et al.* (1989) the 25 per cent reduction in *F* for the Osmet® preparation of nitrendipine is probably due to release of drug in the lower part of the tract where its absorption is impaired. A similar reason probably lies behind the reduced *F*-value of a slow felodipine controlled release tablet in the study by Wingstrand *et al.* (1988). The loss of bioavailability thus may counteract the positive clinical effects of controlled release preparations of these very potent drugs, and optimizing the release rate is therefore very important. According to Soons *et al.* (1989) the dose should be released over a maximal time period of 12 hours to avoid loss of bioavailability of nitrendipine. Comparable bioavailability studies between the marketed controlled release formulation of felodipine and the conventional tablet have indicated a negligible loss of bioavailability of the former.

Interaction with food

Intake of food in association with oral administration of the DHPs has given somewhat conflicting results (Table 4). Often a concomitant meal affects the rate of absorption with a resultant altered C_{max} and t_{max} whereas the AUC and the bioavailability are very resistant to potential food effects. Based on available results, most DHPs independent of dosage form, can probably be administered irrespective of timing of food intake without producing changes in the therapeutic response.

Dose dependent absorption

Three of the DHPs, nicardipine, nilvadipine and benidipine, exhibit dose-dependent bioavailability due to a saturable first-pass elimination. As a result of this saturation effect, the bioavailability of nicardipine is increased from about 20 to 40 per cent when the oral dose is increased from 10 to 40 mg (Wagner *et al.*, 1987). For nilvadipine, there is a linear relationship between AUC and dose up to about 12 mg whereafter the relationship becomes non-linear, probably due to dose-dependent first-pass metabolism (Cheung *et al.*, 1988). The AUC of benidipine was found to increase three-fold upon an increase in the oral dose from 16 to 24 mg (Maier-Lenz *et al.*, 1988). Dose-dependent bioavailability is usually considered a disadvantage as changes in dosing may led to unpredictable plasma levels and untoward effects in the patient.

Distribution

Studies in which DHPs have been given intravenously have resulted in either bi- or triphasically declining plasma concentration vs time curves (Kleinbloesem *et al.*, 1984 b; Mikus *et al.*, 1987; Edgar *et al.*, 1985). The number of distinguishable phases depends to a great extent on the physico-chemical properties of the drug studied but dose, experimental design and sensitivity of the applied analytical method also have significant impact on the observed concentration–time profile. The relative contribution of the separate phases to the total area under the plasma or blood concentration–time curve determines whether a phase should be included or ignored in the pharmaco-kinetic evaluation of a drug. If the area is less than 10 per cent of the total area, the terminal phase can be ignored since this will impart negligible error in the pharmacokinetic results.

Observations of two or three discernible phases in the plasma concentra-tion–time curve probably have less to do with the physicochemical properties of the DHPs, which are fairly similar, but are more likely to be a result of the other three factors mentioned above. This has the consequence, for example, that reported half-lives, clearances and volumes of distribution might differ substantially between different studies of the same compound (Tables 5 and 6).

The initially available body space determined from intravenous doses (V_c) varies from 0.25 to 1.2 L/kg for the four dihydropyridines which have been studied in this respect so far (Table 5). The initial, transient distribution of these drugs into a volume which is about three to fifteen times the blood volume, indicates extremely rapid extravascular distribution since erythrocyte partitioning is virtually negligible. The further distribution is initially very rapid with reported half-lives varying from 4 to about 15 min for the different drugs studied (Table 5). The volume of distribution at steady state, V_{ss}, and the volume at pseudo-distribution equilibrium, V_z, differ significantly between the DHPs. Three have V_z values from 0.6 to 2 L/kg while values between 12 and 21 L/kg have been found for three others. The largest V_z volume (21 L) was found for amlodipine, the dihydropyridine with the highest degree of pro-tonization at physiological pH, suggesting that lipophilicity plays a minor role for the distribution of these drugs. The reported small volumes of distribution of nicardipine, nifedipine and nimodipine may be a result of not following plasma concentrations for sufficient time to detect a terminal third phase. This seems to be the case for nicardipine at least. For this drug, Graham *et al.* (1985) have reported a terminal-life about three times longer than the half-life given by Wagner *et al.* (1987), suggesting that the V_z value reported by the latter investigator was not determined from the terminal phase of the plasma concentration vs time curve.

The volume of distribution is primarily a proportionality factor relating plasma concentration to the amount of drug in the body but is also an indirect measure of the affinity of the drug to extravascular tissues. Thus, the higher the value of V_{ss} or V_z, the higher the tissue affinity. However, these param-eters give no information as to the localization of the drug to specific tissues. This requires animal studies and distribution studies have been carried out in various animal species by means of ^{14}C-labelled drugs. Unfortunately, how-ever, the results from these studies only provide data of total radioactivity, i.e. the sum of unchanged drug and metabolites. They are, therefore, of limited value as regards the distribution of DHPs to specific tissues.

Table 5. Distribution characteristics of 1,4-dihydropyridine calcium antagonists in man.

Drug	V_c L/kg	V_{ss} L/kg	V_Z L/kg	$t_{1/2\lambda 1}$ min	% bound plasma	% bound HSA	% bound AAG	C_b/C_p	References
Amlodipine		21.4 ± 4.4			98				Faulkner et al. (1986); Stopher et al. (1988)
Felodipine		10.3 ± 3.4	13.9 ± 4.1		99.6 ± 0.1			0.68	Landahl et al. (1988); Edgar et al. (1989); Edgar et al. (1985); Regårdh (unpublished)
Isradipine	0.6 ± 0.2			6.4 ± 2.3		97	83		Schran et al. (1988)
Nicardipine	0.4 ± 0.1	4.0 ± 1.9	1.7 ± 0.4	9.9 ± 6.4					Wagner et al. (1987)
	0.3 ± 0.1			14 ± 1.5					Graham et al. (1985)
Nifedipine	0.3 ± 0.1	0.8 ± 0.2		5.4 ± 1.8	99	89[a]	96[a]	0.71 ± 0.06	Urien et al. (1987); Otto and Lesko (1986); Kleinbloesem et al. (1984 b)
	0.3 ± 0.1	0.6 ± 0.2	2.3 ± 0.9	13	99.2 ± 0.8	97.0 ± 1.2	75.5 ± 3.5		Debbas et al. (1986); Raemsch and Sommer (1983)
Nilvadipine		1.9 ± 0.1			~99; 98.4 ± 0.2	97.9 ± 0.1	74.5 ± 2.3		Walley et al. (1987); Cheung et al. (1987)
Nimodipine			1.7		99				Niwa et al. (1987)
Nitrendipine	1.2 ± 0.5	6.4 ± 2.6	12.3 ± 5.4	4 ± 2	98			0.85 ± 0.03	Niwa et al. (1988 a); Raemsch et al. (1987)
	1.2 ± 0.6	5.4 ± 2.4							Soons et al. (1989); Mikus et al. (1987)
		5.8 ± 1.5							
Nisoldipine		1.6 ± 0.6			99.7				van Harten et al. (1988 a); Ahr et al. (1987); van Harten et al. (1988 b)
		4.1 ± 2.1							van Harten et al. (1988 c)

a = pH dependent; C_b = concentration in blood; C_p = plasma concentration; HSA = Human serum albumin; AAG = Alpha-1-Acid glycoprotein;
V_c = initially available body space
V_{ss} = volume of distribution at steady speed
V_Z = volume of distribution at pseudo distribution equilibrium
$t_{1/2\lambda 1}$ = distribution half-life

Table 6. Elimination characteristics of 1,4-dihydropyridine calcium antagonists in young healthy subjects

Drug	Dose (mg)	$t_{1/2}$ (hours)	CL (ml/min)	CL$_{oral}$ (L/min)	Recoveries Urine (%)	Recoveries Faeces (%)	Effect of dose	References
Amlodipine	10, sd, i.v.	34 ± 5	500 ± 100					Faulkner et al. (1986)
	5, sd, i.v.	35	490		59	23		Beresford et al. (1988b)
	5, sd, i.v.	31–37			62	23		Stopher et al. (1988)
	2.5–10, sd, p.o.						—	Williams and Cubeddo (1988)
Benidipine	16, sd, p.o.	0.5 ± 0.2					+	Maier-Lenz et al. (1988)
	24, sd, p.o.							
Felodipine	2.5, sd, i.v.	14 ± 8	820 ± 160		70 ± 5	11 ± 3		Edgar et al. (1985)
	27.5, sd, p.o.			7.8 ± 3.1				Edgar et al. (1987)
	0.5–3, sd, i.v.		1090 ± 150				—	Edgar et al. (1987)
	5–40, sd, p.o.			10.2 ± 1.9				Edgar et al. (1987)
Isradipine	2.5–10, md, p.o.	6.1 ± 2.1		5.3 ± 2.5				Clifton et al. (1988)
	5, md, p.o.	8.8 ± 7.1	720 ± 65		59 ± 5	26 ± 6		Tse and Jaffe (1987)
	ns							Schran et al. (1988)
Nicardipine	30, sd, p.o.	4.5 ± 3.0	580 ± 190		60	36		Rush et al. (1986)
	5, sd, i.v.	11.4 ± 0.9					+	Graham et al. (1985)
	30, md, p.o.	1.5 ± 0.7	938 ± 113	8.1 ± 2.2			+	Wagner et al. (1987)
	0.9, sd, i.v.							Wagner et al. (1987)

Drug	Dose (mg), regimen, route	$t_{1/2}$	$t_{1/2}$	CL	F	Reference
Nifedipine	1.0, sd, i.v.	1.7 ± 0.4		445 ± 90	58	Kleinbloesem et al. (1984b)
	3.5, sd, i.v.	3.2 ± 1.0		560 ± 120		Debbas et al. (1986)
	3.5, sd, i.v.	1.9 ± 0.4		450 ± 100		Waller et al. (1984)
	1.0, sd, i.v.	1.3 ± 0.6				Raemsch and Sommer (1983)
	4.6, sd, i.v.	1.5 ± 0.1		1070 ± 60		Walley et al. (1987)
	4.6–14.5, sd, i.v.				—	Walley et al. (1987)
	1.0, sd, i.v.				70–80	von Horster et al. (1972)
	10, sd, p.o.	5.0 ± 0.6			~15	Hoyo-Vadillo et al. (1989)
Nilvadipine	4–12, sd, p.o.	~10	7.0 ± 1.7			+ > 12 mg Cheung et al. (1987)
	2–6, sd, p.o.	11.0 ± 2.3	7.5 ± 0.9			Terakawa et al. (1987 a)
Nimodipine	2.0, sd, i.v.	0.9 ± 0.3		2070		Raemsch et al. (1987)
	40, md, p.o.	2.8 ± 0.5		600 ± 110		Kirch et al. (1984)
Nitrendipine	3.0, sd, i.v.	11.7 ± 5.4	15.2 ± 5.9	1470 ± 220		Soons et al. (1989)
	20, sd, p.o.	9.6 ± 6.0	13.6		50	Soons et al. (1989)
	20, sd, p.o.	15.3 ± 7.3			35	Kann et al. (1984)
	10, sd, p.o.	8.6 ± 4.2				Lasseter et al. (1984)
	2.0, sd, i.v.			1300 ± 250	88 ± 16	Mikus et al. (1987)
Nisoldipine	0.8, sd, i.v.	10.7 ± 2.4			82 ± 7	Scherling et al. (1988)
	2.4–9.6, sd, i.v.	4.0 ± 2.3		990 ± 160	14 ± 9.5	van Harten et al. (1988 c)
	0.37, sd, i.v.	9.7 ± 5.4		820 ± 180		van Harten et al. (1988 a)
	0.37, sd, i.v.			850 ± 300		van Harten et al. (1988)
	20, sd, p.o.		37 ± 38			van Harten et al. (1988)

ns = not stated; sd = single dose; md = multiple dose; CL$_{oral}$ = oral clearance value. $t_{1/2}$ and CL are defined in the footnote to table 1.

Placental transfer

Placental transfer of nimodipine, nisoldipine and nitrendipine has been studied in the rat using ^{14}C-labelled drug (Suwelack *et al.*, 1985; Maruhn *et al.*, 1985; Ahr *et al.*, 1988 b; Krause *et al.*, 1988 b). All three drugs and their metabolites were recovered in three to five times lower concentrations in the foetuses than in the maternal plasma. In the study by Ahr *et al.* (1988 b), the concentration of nitrendipine in amniotic fluid 1 hour after dosing was only 7.5 per cent of the total radioactivity and had decreased to 1 per cent at 24 hours. These data show that the placenta effectively shields the foetus from high loads of the investigated dihydropyridines and/or their metabolites.

Secretion in breast milk

Similar results to those of placental transfer have been obtained for the accumulation of radioactivity in breast milk following administration of ^{14}C-labelled doses of the above mentioned DHPs to lactating rats. The maximum concentration in milk was two to three times lower than the corresponding plasma concentration (Ahr *et al.*, 1988 b; Krause *et al.*, 1988 b). Nimodipine and/or its metabolites seems to be secreted into milk to a greater extent than the other two dihydropyridines. In the study by Maruhn *et al.* (1985), the concentration of radioactivity in breast milk of the rat exceeded the plasma concentration by a factor of two to five during the first 6 hours after dosing.

Passage across the blood–brain barrier

The transfer of the DHPs across the blood–brain barrier is reported in the same papers as the placental transport and accumulation in milk (see above). However, only total radioactivity in brain and cerebrospinal fluid (CSF) has been determined. The single pass uptake of radiolabelled isradipine in the brain has been studied after bolus injection of drug into the carotid artery of anaesthetized rats. The extraction from blood was greater than predicted from the unbound drug fraction but still related to the content of albumin, alpha$_1$-acid glycoprotein (AAG) and lipoproteins in the injection solution (Urien *et al.*, 1987).

A recent study in our laboratory has shown that felodipine rapidly equilibrates between CSF and plasma in the dog and that the concentration in CSF is approximately the same as the unbound fraction in plasma, i.e. the ratio between the felodipine concentrations in CSF and plasma is approximately 1 : 200. Approximately the same ratio was found for the radioactive metabolites which suggested that the plasma protein binding of these compounds is as high as that of felodipine itself (Mikulski, personal communication).

Protein binding

The dihydropyridines are extensively bound to plasma proteins. Reported values vary between 98 and 99.7 per cent depending on the particular drug (Table 5). Binding to different fractions of the plasma proteins has been reported for nicardipine, nifedipine, isradipine and nilvadipine. Uricn *et al.* (1985) found that nicardipine, like other basic lipophilic drugs, is extensively bound to the plasma lipoprotein fraction, VLDL, LDL and HDL, with a relatively low affinity and a very high number of binding sites. Similarly, the binding of nicardipine to AAG is high while binding to albumin is weaker. Nicardipine was found to bind to the same site on AAG as pindolol and imipramine.

The two neutral drugs nifedipine and nilvadipine are less extensively bound to AAG than the basic nicardipine (Otto and Lesko, 1986; Niwa *et al.*, 1987). Albumin and lipoproteins were the main nilvadipine binding proteins in plasma while, for nifedipine, albumin binding accounted for all the plasma binding although the authors did not exclude potential binding to other plasma proteins.

The concentration of DHPs has been found to be lower in erythrocytes than in plasma. Because of this, the levels of felodipine and nicardipine in whole blood are only about 70 per cent of those in plasma (Table 5). For nilvadipine, the ratio between the concentration in whole blood and plasma is 0.85.

Elimination

Mass balance studies with intravenous and oral doses of radioactively labelled DHPs have shown that 50 to 90 per cent of the given radioactivity is excreted by the kidneys in man and that the major part of the remaining fraction is recovered in faeces (Table 6). Insignificant (0.5 per cent), or even non-detectable amounts of unchanged DHPs have been reported in urine because of very high protein binding and the lipophilicity of the neutral molecules. However, ionization of the amlodipine molecule at normal urinary pH might be the explanation for its comparatively high renal excretion, 5–10 per cent, in unchanged form (Beresford *et al.*, 1988b; Stopher *et al.*, 1988).

As with urine, the unchanged fraction of the DHPs excreted in the stool is very small. Edgar *et al.* (1985) reported non-detectable amounts (<0.5 per cent) of a given intravenous felodipine dose to be excreted in unchanged form in the faeces. Tse and Jaffe (1987) recovered 5–10 per cent of unchanged isradipine in the stool following oral administration of 20 mg of the drug. It is unclear, however, whether this was due to incomplete gastrointestinal uptake or gastrointestinal and/or biliary secretion, although the authors stated that isradipine was completely metabolized prior to excretion because of the absence of intact drug in the urine.

The above findings show that the DHPs are predominantly eliminated by metabolism. The plasma clearance (CL) of ten individual drugs (Table 6), varies between 450 ml/min for nifedipine to about 2 L/min for nimodipine. The blood clearance, calculated from the ratios between the blood and plasma concentrations in Table 5, is 1.2–1.6 L/min for felodipine and

0.82–1.3 L/min for nicardipine. Assuming that the liver is the main organ for elimination of systemically available DHPs, the blood clearance value of felodipine characterizes this drug as a high clearance compound. Nicardipine, which has a dose-dependent first-pass elimination, appears to be a drug with intermediate clearance properties at high doses. The plasma clearance values of the remaining DHPs in Table 6 suggest that they either belong to the intermediate or high clearance class of drugs.

In addition to nicardipine, which might have a saturable metabolism, the clearance of two other DHPs, namely nifedipine and nimodipine, has been given widely differing values by different authors. The reason for this is not dose dependence but probably associated with the precision in the AUC determination. This depends on such factors as the analytical method for determining unchanged drug and the collection period for blood samples. If this period is too short, the result might be a substantial underestimation in AUC and an erroneously high clearance value. This could be the case in the nimodipine study by Raemsch *et al.* (1987) who reported CL and $t_{1/2}$ to be 2.1 L/min and 0.9 hours, respectively, compared with 0.6 L/min for CL and 2.8 hours for $t_{1/2}$ as found by Kirch *et al.* (1984). The longer $t_{1/2}$ in the latter study indicates that the plasma levels have been followed over a longer time period than in the study by Raemsch and as such, should increase the accuracy in the determination of AUC and CL.

The oral clearance values (CL_{oral}) given in Table 6 should equal intrinsic hepatic clearance provided the entire dose is taken up from the gastrointestinal tract and is metabolized only by the liver. The first requirement seems to be fulfilled by most of the DHPs as previously referred to. Furthermore, *in vitro* studies with subcellular fractions from different organs indicate that the major biotransformation of the DHPs is mediated by the liver (Higuchi and Shiobara, 1980 b; Bäärnhielm *et al.*, 1986 b; Niwa *et al.*, 1988 b). However, recent findings in rat and man have indicated substantial contribution of the intestine to the first-pass elimination of nifedipine and felodipine (Challenor *et al.*, 1987 c; Wang *et al.*, 1989; Regårdh *et al.*, 1989). Possibly the same is also true for other DHPs and therefore the oral clearance values given in Table 6 cannot be assumed, *a priori*, to represent intrinsic hepatic clearance.

The importance of being able to measure plasma or blood concentrations over a sufficient length of time after dosing to determine accurately the terminal half-life has already been discussed in some detail. It seems very likely that the short half-lives reported for some of the DHPs in Table 6 do not represent the true terminal values. Thus, some controversy exists in the reported $t_{1/2}$ value of nifedipine. In most studies with this drug, $t_{1/2}$ values have varied between 1.5 and 2 hours but recently Hoyo-Vadillo *et al.* (1989) have determined a terminal $t_{1/2}$ for the drug of about 5 hours. Further support for a terminal $t_{1/2}$ of nifedipine longer than the usually considered 1.5–2 hours has been given by Debbas *et al.* (1986) and by Waller *et al.* (1984).

Optical enantiomers

Apart from nifedipine, the carbon in position 4 of the dihydropyridine ring of all drugs in Figure 2 exhibit chirality due to asymmetric ester functions. Studies primarily by Japanese investigators have shown that the enantiomers of various DHPs differ in potency of their pharmacological effects as well as in the rates of metabolism.

Evidence of stereoselective vasodilating and hypotensive effects of nicardipine enantiomers have been obtained from studies in anaesthetized dogs, the (+)-enantiomer being three times more potent than (−)-nicardipine (Takenaka *et al.* 1982). Furthermore, it has been shown that the (−)-isomer of nimodipine is nearly twice as potent as the racemic mixture in inhibiting calcium-induced contractions of depolarized rabbit portal vein (Towart *et al.*, 1982). The (+)-enantiomer of nilvadipine is about 100 times more potent in relaxing potassium-induced contractions of isolated dog coronary arteries than (−)-nilvadipine (Niwa *et al.*, 1988 a).

Pharmacokinetic and metabolic studies with the two nilvadipine enantiomers have further indicated that the (+)- and (−)-forms are cleared with different rates. The intrinsic clearance determined from the V_{max}/K_m ratio for the oxidation of nilvadipine by human liver microsomes was twice as high for the (−)-enantiomer as for (+)-nilvadipine. This difference was mainly due to different K_m values while the V_{max} values of the enantiomers were essentially the same. The observation that the intrinsic clearance of (−)-nilvadipine is higher than for the corresponding (+)-isomer is consistent with the results from a study by Tokuma *et al.*, (1987 b). These authors found that the oral clearance in man of (+)-nilvadipine was lower than that of the (−)-form following administration of the racemic mixture. Binding to plasma proteins also seems to be affected by the stereochemical configuration of the nilvadipine molecule. Niwa *et al.* (1988 a) reported that the free fraction of nilvadipine in human plasma was 1.0 per cent for the (+)-enantiomer and 0.9 per cent for (−)-nilvadipine.

In a subsequent study by Niwa *et al.* (1989), the stereoselective metabolism of nilvadipine was found to be species dependent and also sex-related in the rat. Thus V_{max}/K_m for the oxidation of nilvadipine by male rat liver microsomes was 1.6 times greater for (+)-nilvadipine than for the oxidation of the (−)-enantiomer. The corresponding ratio for the female rat liver microsomes was 1.2. Dog liver microsomes, on the other hand, were found to metabolize the (−)-enantiomer approximately 40 per cent faster than the (+)-form.

These results agree reasonably with results from a recently completed study of the metabolism of R- and S-felodipine in liver microsomes from rat, dog and man. The intrinsic clearance of the more potent S-felodipine was two to three times lower than that of R-felodipine in human liver microsomes. There was no distinct difference between the oxidation of the two felodipine enantiomers by rat liver microsomes whereas dog liver microsomes oxidized the S-form more readily than the corresponding R-enantiomer (Eriksson *et al.*, 1989).

Genetic influence

Observations of wide interindividual differences in the disposition kinetics of nifedipine were the background for the study by Kleinbloesem *et al.* (1984 a) of frequency distribution histograms of kinetic and dynamic parameters following a single dose of 20 mg of this calcium antagonist to fifty-three healthy subjects. The histograms of AUC for nifedipine in plasma, the urinary excretion of a major secondary metabolite (the pyridine monoacid) and the effect on heart rate 5 to 6 hours after dosing led the authors to a conclusion of polymorphic disposition kinetics of nifedipine. One year previous to these findings, Idle and Sever (1983) had suggested that the disposition of nifedipine was related to the debrisoquine oxidation phenotype. However, this hypothesis could not be verified by studying nifedipine kinetics in extensive and poor metabolizers of debrisoquine (Lewis *et al.*, 1984). While this does not preclude the possibility of metabolic polymorphism via some cytochrome P450 isoenzyme other than debrisoquine hydroxylase, subsequent studies have failed to confirm genetic polymorphism of nifedipine.

Beerahee *et al.* (1987) found a slightly skewed unimodal distribution of the 12-hour plasma nifedipine concentrations in sixty-four hypertensive patients and no relationship between these concentrations and the debrisoquine hydroxylation phenotype. A skewed but unimodal distribution of AUC was recorded in fifty-nine young healthy males following a single dose of 10 mg nifedipine and the approach of using the AUC ratio between the parent drug and its primary metabolite, the nitropyridine, did not lead to bimodal distribution of the data. Furthermore, in this study there was no evidence of bimodality in the excretion of the major secondary metabolite (Renwick *et al.*, 1988). Schellens *et al.* (1988) came to the same conclusion that nifedipine disposition lacks bimodality by studying the AUC of nifedipine in 130 young healthy subjects concomitantly given single doses of 20 mg nifedipine, 50 mg sparteine and 100 mg phenytoin. The ratio of AUC for nifedipine and for its primary pyridine metabolite indicated potential bimodality. The problem with this ratio, however, is that the AUC of the metabolite reflects both formation and elimination since this metabolite is further transformed before being excreted in urine and faeces. Accordingly, it was not possible to determine whether the high AUC ratio in some subjects was due to reduced formation or increased metabolism of the primary metabolite. Hence, polymorphism via this route is theoretically possible although its clinical importance should be negligible as the metabolite is pharmacologically inactive. Schellens and associates concluded that the disposition of nifedipine is highly variable in a large population but that there was no evidence of polymorphism. According to these authors, a limited sample size probably led to the accidental observation of bimodality in the study by Kleinbloesem *et al.*, 1984.

Further support for the absence of polymorphic metabolism of the DHPs was obtained from a AUC frequency distribution histogram after oral administration of a solution of 10 mg felodipine to ninety-eight healthy male subjects. The histogram showed a unimodal but skewed distribution of the AUC with approximately a fivefold variation between the extreme values (Edgar, 1988).

Pharmacokinetic effects of various diseases and age

Results from pharmacokinetic studies with different DHPs in young healthy subjects have shown that the elimination properties of these drugs are consonant with those of medium or high clearance compounds. Furthermore, the elimination is mediated almost entirely by metabolism and negligible amounts are excreted unchanged by the kidneys. These properties suggest that factors affecting hepatic blood flow and/or enzyme activity may have a pronounced influence on the pharmacokinetics of this class of drug. Changes in renal function, on the other hand, should be of little importance unless the pharmacologically inactive metabolites (Triggle *et al.*, 1982), predominantly excreted in the urine in healthy subjects, reach such levels in the patient, that they interfere with the disposition of the parent drug. Accordingly, patients with impaired liver function, congestive heart failure and the elderly are those primarily at risk of having altered pharmacokinetics of the DHPs. All may have a reduced hepatic blood flow and those with liver disease and the elderly may also have a lower hepatic enzyme activity.

Effect of age

The influence of age on the pharmacokinetics of the DHPs has been studied to varying extents in six of the DHPs included in this review (Table 7). The consistent findings from these studies are higher plasma concentrations and lower clearances in the elderly than in the young healthy subjects. Furthermore, the half-life in the elderly is prolonged in three out of four studies. Bioavailability is essentially the same in the aged and in young subjects for felodipine and nifedipine, whereas it is increased for isradipine in the elderly. The protein binding of nifedipine is not affected by age.

The observed changes in the pharmacokinetics of felodipine and amlodipine in 70- to 80-year-old subjects were mainly a reduction in clearance by about 50 per cent and a twofold increase in the AUC and half-life compared with the corresponding values in young healthy individuals (Landahl *et al.*, 1988; Elliot *et al.*, 1988).

On the whole, the effects on the pharmacokinetics of the DHPs in the elderly can be explained by reduced hepatic blood flow. Such a change would have a direct influence on clearance of these high or medium clearance drugs

Table 7. The effect of impaired liver and kidney function and of age on pharmacokinetic parameters of different DHPs.

Drug	Liver dysfunction					Renal dysfunction					Age					References
	C_{max}	f	pb	CL	$t_{1/2}$	C_{max}	f	pb	CL	$t_{1/2}$	C_{max}	f	pb	CL	$t_{1/2}$	
Amlodipine						~				~	↑			→	↑	Laher et al. (1988) Elliott et al. (1988) Abernethy et al. (1988)
Felodipine	↑	~	→	→	~	↑	~	→	~	↑	↑	~		→	↑	Regårdh et al. (1989) Edgar et al. (1989) Landahl et al. (1988)
Isradipine	↑			→		~			~		↑	↑		→		Schran et al. (1988)
Nicardipine	↑		~	→	↑	↑			~		↑					Chellingsworth et al. (1988) D'Heygere et al. (1988) Dow and Graham (1986) Forette et al. (1985)
Nifedipine	↑	↑	→	→	↑	~	~	→	~	↑	↑	~	~	→	↑	Ene and Roberts (1987) Kleinbloesem et al. (1986) Kleinbloesem et al. (1985 a) Robertson et al. (1988)
Nimodipine						←										Kirch et al. (1984)
Nisoldipine	↑	↑		→	~	~	~	~	~							van Harten et al. (1988 b) Boelaert et al. (1988)
Nitrendipine	↑	↑	~	→	↑						↑			→	~	Dylewicz et al. (1987) Crome et al. (1988) Lettieri et al. (1987)

pb = protein binding

while the effect on f would be much less. Furthermore, the observed increases in $t_{1/2}$ agree with the reduced clearance ability in the elderly and suggest that age has little effect on the volume of distribution of these drugs. Even so, recent findings that the first-pass effect of felodipine might be due to some extent to metabolism in the gut wall indicate that the relationship between hepatic blood flow, bioavailability and disposition of the DHPs may be more complicated than discussed above (Landahl *et al.*, 1988).

The effect of age as a confounding factor stresses the importance of using age-matched controls whenever comparative pharmacokinetic studies on the effect of various diseases are performed with DHPs.

The age-related decrease in glomerular filtration rate which proceeds at a rate of approximately 1 per cent per year from the age of 30 years (Vestal, 1978) was found to significantly diminish the excretion rate of felodipine metabolites in the urine in healthy elderly subjects (Edgar, 1988).

Liver disease

The pharmacokinetic consequences of impaired liver function, diagnosed on the basis of clinical and biochemical data, and in most studies verified by biopsy samples of abnormal liver parenchyma, have been evaluated for six of the DHPs. The results from these studies have been very consistent as regards the effects on AUC and clearance, while some conflicting findings have been reported concerning bioavailability, degree of protein binding and half-life (Table 7).

In general terms, the effect of liver dysfunction has the same impact on plasma levels and clearance of DHPs as does advanced age. In comparison with healthy subjects, the increase in the peak plasma concentration in cirrhotic patients was 60 per cent for felodipine, 32 per cent for isradipine, 85 per cent for nicardipine, 110 per cent for nifedipine and 65 and 211 per cent for nitrendipine and nisoldipine, respectively. The increase in AUC of oral doses of DHPs due to impaired liver function was even greater than for the maximum concentration. Four to five times greater AUCs have been reported for nitrendipine, nisoldipine and nicardipine in cirrhotic patients than in healthy subjects (Lasseter *et al.*, 1984; van Harten *et al.*, 1988 b; D'Heygere *et al.*, 1988).

The main reasons for the pronounced effects of impaired liver function on the plasma levels of the DHPs are a reduction in clearance and in first-pass elimination. With nifedipine and felodipine, liver cirrhosis reduced clearance by approximately 50 per cent and almost doubled the systemic availability of nifedipine from 50 to 90 per cent while this parameter was unchanged for felodipine (Kleinbloesem *et al.*, 1986; Regårdh *et al.*, 1989). Maximal bioavailability, 100 per cent, was recorded for nifedipine in three patients with portacaval shunting. This surgery had no effect on the bioavailability of felodipine, which was about the same in two patients with liver by-pass as in the remaining patients and the control subjects. The negligible increase in the first-pass effect of felodipine in these patients was attributed to a major role of gut wall metabolism in the presystemic elimination of the DHP. Much less than maximal bioavailability in shunt operated patients has been reported for nisoldipine (van Harten *et al.*, 1988 b). In one patient the bioavailability, 16 per cent, was comparable with that in the non-shunted patients with impaired liver function. The other patient had an *f*-value of 36 per cent. These findings are in agreement with those by Regårdh *et al.* (1989), for felodipine but were explained by incomplete liver by-pass of the portal blood.

That the gastrointestinal tract may contribute to the first-pass elimination of the DHPs was documented in a recent study on felodipine in the rat (Wang *et al.*, 1989). Furthermore, Challenor *et al.*, (1987 c), found evidence of substantial extrahepatic metabolism of nifedipine in man by comparing the extraction ratio across the liver, the hepatic clearance and total clearance of the drug. Thus, although the liver appears to be the major organ for elimination of the DHPs, contribution by the gut and other organs to presystemic elimination and clearance of this class of drug cannot be ignored.

With both nifedipine and felodipine a doubling of the unbound drug fraction in plasma has been observed in patients with impaired liver function (Kleinbloesem *et al.*, 1986; Regårdh *et al.*, 1989). However, since the binding of these two drugs seems to be of the non-restrictive type, decreased binding is not a critical factor in the disposition of these DHPs. Furthermore, an altered free fraction does not affect the relationships between plasma concentration and effects on heart rate and blood pressure.

Since impaired liver function has a pronounced influence on the fraction of oral doses of DHPs reaching the systemic circulation, a reliable method for determining the degree of liver function would be invaluable. Unfortunately, such a method does not exist. Possibly antipyrine can be used as a marker for predicting the metabolic capacity of DHPs by the liver as a significant correlation has been observed between anitipyrine clearance and clearance of felodipine, isradipine and nitrendipine (Capewell *et al.* 1988; Dylewicz *et al.*, 1987; Schran *et al.*, 1988). At present, however, the only way of avoiding overdosing with DHPs in patients with liver disease seems to be commencement of treatment with low doses.

Kidney disease

Studies of the effect of impaired renal function on the pharmacokinetics of different DHPs have led with few exceptions to results consistent with the elimination characteristics in healthy subjects. Unforeseen results, for instance the increase in C_{max} for felodipine, nicardipine and nimodipine (Table 7), are possible effects of not using age-matched healthy individuals. The importance of including such controls is illustrated in the study by Edgar *et al.* (1989). The C_{max} was higher and $t_{1/2}$ longer in renal patients than in young healthy subjects, but when the same parameters were compared with those in hypertensive patients of comparable age, renal impairment was found to have no influence on C_{max} and $t_{1/2}$.

Amlodipine, which is the only DHP excreted unchanged in the urine of healthy subjects in appreciable amounts (5–10 per cent), would have the disposition properties most sensitive to changes in renal function among the DHPs. However, by comparing plasma levels and half-lives in healthy subjects with those in patients with varying degrees of renal dysfunction, Laher *et al.* (1988) and Doyle *et al.* (1989) came to the conclusion that dosage adjustment with amlodipine would not be necessary in renal impairment.

The most dramatic effects of renal dysfunction on DHP kinetics have been reported by Kirch *et al.* (1984) for nimodipine. Mean $t_{1/2}$ was increased from 2.0 hours in a group of young healthy subjects to 22.2 hours in patients with glomerular filtration rates (GFR) ranging between 3 and 63 ml/min. Similarly, the AUC was increased sevenfold in these patients. Based on these data, dosage adjustment was recommended for nimodipine when used in renal failure. However, six of twelve patients in the study were aged between 70 and 83 years and the difference in age between patients and controls may have contributed to the substantial difference in $t_{1/2}$ and AUC of the two groups.

Dow and Graham (1986) recommended adjustment of nicardipine dosage in renal patients based on a doubling in C_{max} and AUC values in renally impaired patients compared to healthy subjects. The age of the patients and controls was not given in this study. In another study with this drug, Clair *et al.* (1985) found no effect of kidney dysfunction on the plasma levels of nicardipine. Furthermore, there was no evidence of any increased antihypertensive effect in the renal patients and the authors concluded that nicardipine can be used in patients with advanced chronic renal failure without any change in dose or regimen.

The disposition of the DHPs is not influenced by haemodialysis as negligible amounts of these drugs are dialysable. The lipophilicity and protein binding of these drugs are too high and the extravascular distribution too extensive for transmembrane diffusion of unchanged drug into the dialysate in sufficient amounts. Even so, an increase in the unbound fraction of nifedipine from 4 to 6.5 per cent has been reported for nifedipine (Kleinbloesem *et al.*, 1985 a). For other DHPs studied, renal impairment has had negligible effect on this parameter (Table 7).

As the metabolites of the DHPs are excreted to a large extent via the kidneys, kidney function has a pronounced influence on the plasma levels and rate of elimination of these compounds. Edgar (1988) has shown a direct correlation between the renal clearance of the total pool of radioactive metabolites of felodipine and GFR. It can be assumed that patients with severely compromised renal function treated with various DHPs will have high blood levels of their corresponding metabolites. These metabolites, however, are devoid of calcium antagonistic activity (Triggle *et al.*, 1982) and their accumulation has not affected the beneficial therapeutic outcome of treating patients with severe renal dysfunction with various DHPs.

Table 8. Survey of mean pharmacokinetic data of felodipine in two different patient groups and in young healthy subjects.

	Congestive heart failure (Dunselman *et al.*, 1989)	Elderly hypertension (Landahl *et al.*, 1988)	Young healthy subjects (Landahl *et al.*, 1988)
Age (yrs)	62 ± 7	74 ± 5	26 ± 6
N	11	11	12
ABSORPTION			
C_{max} (nM)	38 ± 19	34 ± 14	12 ± 6
t_{max} (h)	1.8 ± 1.1	1.6 ± 0.9	2.2 ± 1.0
f (%)	29 ± 19	16 ± 6	15 ± 9
AUC (nM·h)	170 ± 91	175 ± 67	67 ± 24
ELIMINATION			
CL (ml·min^{-1})	527 ± 115	424 ± 172	934 ± 288
CL_{oral} (L·min^{-1})	4.6 ± 1.0	4.1 ± 1.8	10.3 ± 3.6
$t_{1/2\ z}$(h)	22.7 ± 11	27.5 ± 8.4	13.6 ± 4.9

A greater sensitivity of uraemic patients to the antihypertensive effect of various DHPs, even when no change in the pharmacokinetics has been observed, seems to be the most important finding from combined pharmacokinetic and pharmacodynamic studies in these patients. However, the enhanced blood pressure response in renal patients has not been sufficiently great to warrant recommendations of altered dose or regimen (Boelaert *et al.* 1988; van Harten *et al.*, 1989; Kleinbloesem *et al.*, 1985 a).

Heart failure

In severe cases of congestive heart failure, hypoperfusion of vital organs for the absorption and disposition of drugs is probably a reality. However, limited information about the pharmacokinetics of DHPs in heart failure patients has been published. Results from a recent study with felodipine in severely ill patients have indicated that these patients had higher plasma concentrations after oral dosing than young healthy subjects (Dunselman *et al.*, 1989). Mean AUC and clearance were comparable with the values observed in elderly hypertensive patients although there was a difference in mean age by 12 years (Table 8). Accordingly, felodipine treatment should be initiated with a low dose in heart failure patients. As the patients improve as a result of treatment, hepatic blood flow and clearance of the DHP may increase and necessitate a dosage increase.

Drug interactions

Because the DHPs are largely intended for lifelong treatment of various cardiovascular diseases, these compounds will frequently be prescribed together with a variety of other drugs. Accordingly, the potential for drug interactions with the DHPs appears relatively large. Interaction studies between DHPs and drugs selected on mechanistic grounds or because of narrow therapeutic indices or frequently combined with the DHPs, have also been undertaken to a relatively large extent.

Antipyrine

The influence on the biotransformation of antipyrine is often used as a marker for metabolic interference. The Ca-antagonists verapamil and diltiazem which differ significantly in structure from the DHPs, undergo N-demethylation similarly to antipyrine. These calcium antagonists significantly increase antipyrine clearance while, in contrast, no change is observed with nifedipine in healthy subjects (Bauer *et al.*, 1986; Dickinson *et al.*, 1988). Furthermore, repeated administration of 30 mg nicardipine three times daily to healthy subjects had no effect on antipyrine clearance and no effect on the urinary ratio of 6β-hydroxy-cortisol/17 hydroxy-corticosteroid.

Anticonvulsant drugs

Recently Capewell *et al.* (1988), reported substantially lower felodipine plasma levels in epileptic patients treated with carbamazepine, phenytoin or phenobarbitone—all well known inducers of the cytochrome P450 system (Perucca *et al.*, 1984). The anticonvulsant therapy led to a reduction in the bioavailability of felodipine from about 15 per cent in the control group to about 1 per cent in epileptic patients. It was further concluded that the bioavailability of other high clearance DHPs would be similarly reduced in patients with induced drug metabolizing enzymes.

Quinidine

Quinidine has been reported to inhibit competitively the metabolism of compounds hydroxylated by cytochrome $P450_{DB}$, the isoenzyme responsible for debrisoquine oxidation, without being subject to metabolic breakdown *per se*. However, quinidine is metabolized by the same cytochrome P450 isoenzyme ($P450_{NF}$) as nifedipine and interactions between these two drugs have been reported by several authors. Green *et al.* (1983) reported a case where decreased plasma concentrations of quinidine were observed when nifedipine was administered concomitantly. The plasma levels increased to normal when nifedipine was omitted. Possible explanations of this phenomenon are increased hepatic blood flow and systemic clearance or induction of cytochrome $P450_{NF}$ by this DHP. Oates *et al.* (1988), found a significant change in nifedipine pharmacokinetics in seven healthy males receiving concurrent quinidine therapy. The half-life for the Ca-antagonist was prolonged from 1.6 to 3.4 hours with no change in volume of distribution, suggesting an effect on metabolic clearance.

Cimetidine

An interaction leading to increased plasma concentrations of the DHPs is very common following coadministration of the histamine H_2-blocker cimetidine, an effective inhibitor of the cytochrome P450 system. Challenor *et al.* (1987 a) found increased mean C_{max} and AUC values of nifedipine during combined treatment with 400 mg cimetidine three times daily. Smith *et al.* (1987 a) made similar observations when nifedipine in therapeutic doses was combined with 800 mg cimetidine daily. The influence of the interaction on haemodynamic parameters was not evaluated in either of these studies. In further studies, cimetidine has been found to inhibit the metabolism of felodipine, increasing the plasma levels of the DHP by about 50 per cent (Janzon *et al.*, 1986), and to interact with nisoldipine metabolism to a similar extent. For the latter drug, cimetidine primarily increased bioavailability while clearance and $t_{1/2}$ remained essentially unchanged (van Haarten *et al.*, 1988 a). This interaction had no effect on measured haemodynamic parameters. Finally, cimetidine (200 mg twice daily and 400 mg at night) has been given together with a therapeutic dose of nitrendipine without altering the pharmacokinetics of the DHP. Thus, cimetidine seems to inhibit the metabolism of the majority of DHPs but the clinical consequences of this interaction have been studied to only a very limited extent. A potentiation of the hypotensive effect of nifedipine during concomitant cimetidine treatment has been reported by Kirch *et al.* (1983), while the antihypertensive effect of nisoldipine was essentially unchanged. Further dynamic interaction studies between the DHPs and cimetidine are needed to establish more firmly the clinical relevance of kinetic interactions between these drugs.

Digoxin

After the initial reports on the effect of verapamil and diltiazem on the pharmacokinetics and dynamics of digoxin (Piepho *et al.*, 1987) several studies have been undertaken to elucidate the potential influence of the DHPs on digoxin plasma concentrations in man. Beltz *et al.* (1981; 1983) found more than 40 per cent increase in the maximum digoxin serum concentration following a daily regimen of 30 mg nifedipine. Reports from at least five other laboratories, however, have failed to confirm the existence of such a pronounced interaction between nifedipine and digoxin. Pedersen *et al.* (1982) found no significant changes in renal clearance, distribution volume or half-life for digoxin during nifedipine coadministration. However, the DHP increased extrarenal clearance of digoxin by about 40 per cent. Kirch *et al.* (1986 a) reported 7–8 per cent increase in maximum digoxin plasma levels and 15 per cent increase in AUC of the glycoside following a three times daily regimen with 5, 10 and 20 mg nifedipine. A similar 15 per cent increase in digoxin serum levels was reported with nifedipine 20 mg twice daily (Kleinbloesem *et al.*, 1985 b). Mean serum concentrations of digoxin were not altered by 20 mg nifedipine three times daily in a study by Schwartz and Migliore (1984). Neither did coadministration of nifedipine lead to any change in the pharmacological effect of the cardiac glycoside. In a fifth study, no significant changes in digoxin pharmacokinetics were induced by concomitant nifedipine therapy (Koren *et al.*, 1986).

Thus the clinical significance of this interaction appears uncertain but the results of the last five studies indicate that this interaction probably has little relevance in the clinical situation. If an interaction still occurs, its full effects on the dynamics and plasma levels of digoxin will probably be seen within the first two weeks of treatment.

Interaction studies between other DHPs and digoxin have shown essentially similar results as for nifedipine. Nitrendipine coadministration (20 mg o.d.) resulted in an increase in digoxin AUC by about 15 per cent, but the effect on non-invasively measured haemodynamic parameters was unaltered compared with digoxin treatment alone (Kirch *et al.*, 1986 b). Felodipine in doses between 2.5 and 10 mg twice daily and nicardipine, 30 mg three times per day, when given to heart failure patients did not lead to any statistically significant changes in the steady-state AUC of digoxin and there was no effect on the 24-hour urinary excretion of the glycoside during coadministration of felodipine. The authors (Rehnquist *et al.*, 1987; Debruyne *et al.*, 1989) concluded that digoxin-induced side effects are unlikely to occur in association with felodipine or nicardipine therapy provided the patients' digoxin levels are normally monitored. Systolic time intervals and the trough plasma levels of digoxin were significantly altered in heart failure patients during concomitant nisoldipine therapy, 10 mg twice daily. According to the authors (Kirch *et al.*, 1986 c) the elevation in digoxin plasma levels due to nisoldipine could be clinically important in some patients.

Theophylline

Concomitant nifedipine therapy (20 mg b.i.d) caused non-significant changes in the AUC and clearance of intravenously administered theophylline. A small but significant increase in plasma theophylline levels was observed during the first hour which was attributed to a significant decrease in the volume of distribution. No statistically significant changes in nifedipine pharmacokinetics occurred in the presence of theophylline (Jackson *et al.*, 1986).

Beta-adrenoceptor antagonists

Administration of beta-adrenoceptor antagonists together with a DHP markedly increases the blood pressure-lowering effect of the calcium antagonist (Christensen *et al.*, 1982; Husted *et al.*, 1982; Saltiel *et al.*, 1988). This effect has been partly attributed to the blockade of baroreflex-mediated sympathetic stimulation in association with the fall of mean arterial pressure during calcium antagonist therapy (Guazzi *et al.*, 1977; Olivari *et al.*, 1979).

Because of this, beta-adrenoceptor antagonists and DHPs are frequently coadministered and several pharmacokinetic and pharmacodynamic studies have been performed in healthy subjects to evaluate possible interactions.

Kendall *et al.* (1984) found no pharmacokinetic interaction between nifedipine and the two beta₁-selective adrenoceptor antagonists, metoprolol and atenolol. These findings were subsequently confirmed by Rosenkranz *et al.* (1986) for the nifedipine-atenolol combination. These latter authors found a significantly more pronounced decrease in systolic and diastolic blood pressure for the combination as compared with either drug alone, whereas maximum plasma concentrations and terminal half-lives were not altered by their simultaneous administration.

In another study, nifedipine was found to have negligible influence on the pharmacokinetics of betaxolol which has similar disposition properties to atenolol but, unlike the latter, is almost completely available systemically (Vinceneux *et al.*, 1986). However, when three of the six subjects who participated in the betaxolol experiments changed to 80 mg propranolol twice daily in combination with 10 mg nifedipine twice daily, they responded with approximately doubled propranolol maximum concentrations as during monotherapy. Furthermore, the absorption rate was enhanced by the presence of nifedipine, as was the AUC. These three subjects differed from the remaining ones by having substantially higher plasma levels of propranolol during monotherapy suggesting that individual variability in propranolol kinetics is of importance for a potential pharmacokinetic interaction between propranolol and nifedipine and possibly other DHPs.

Smith *et al.* (1987 b) found that 10 mg felodipine twice daily increased the mean steady state C_{max} and AUC of coadministered metoprolol by 30 to 40 per cent. Although these changes were statistically significant the authors considered them unlikely to be of any clinical importance, particularly in view of the considerable interindividual variations in the pharmacokinetics of both drugs.

Acknowledgments

The expert editorial assistance by Mrs Lena Seger in the preparation of the manuscript is gratefully acknowledged.

References

Abernethy, D. R., Gutkowska, J. and Lambert, M. D. (1988), *Cardiovasc. Pharmacol.*, **12** (Suppl. 7), S67.

Ahnoff, M. (1984), *Pharm. Biomed. Anal.*, **2**, 519.

Ahr, H. J., Wingender, W. and Kuhlmann, J. (1987), in *Nisoldipine* (Hugenholz and Meyer, eds), pp. 59–66, Springer-Verlag, Heidelberg.

Ahr, H. J., Krause, H. P., Siefert, H. M., Suwelack, D. and Weber, H. (1988 a), *Arzneim.-Forsch*, **38**, 1093.

Ahr, J-K., Krause, H. P., Suwelack, D. and Weber, H. (1988 b), *Arzneim.-Forsch.*, **38**, 1099.

Augusto, O., Beilan, H. and Ortiz de Montellano, P. (1982), *J. Biochem.* **257**, 11288.
Bäärnhielm, C. and Hansson, G. (1986), *Biochem. Pharmacol.*, **35**, 1414.
Bäärnhielm, C. and Westerlund, C. (1986), *Chem-Biolog. Interact.*, **48**, 277.
Bäärnhielm, C., Skånberg, I. and Borg, K. O. (1984), *Xenobiotica*, **14**, 719.
Bäärnhielm, C., Backman, Å., Hoffmann, K.-J. and Weidolf, L. (1986 a), *Drug Metabol. Dispos.*, **14**, 613.
Bäärnhielm, C., Dahlbäck, H. and Skånberg, I. (1986 b), *Acta Pharmacol. Toxicol.*, **59**, 113.
Bäärnhielm, C., Mjörnstedt, S., Ahnoff, M. and Hoffmann, K.-J. (1988), IInd International ISSX Meeting, Japan, Abstract II-403-P14.
Bauer, L. A., Stenwall, M., Horn, J. R., Davis, R., Opheim, K. and Green, L. (1986), *Clin. Pharmacol. Therap.*, **40**, 239.
Beerahee, M., Wilkins, M. R., Jack, D. B., Beevers D. G. and Kendall, M. (1987), *Europ. J. Clin. Pharmacol.*, **32**, 347.
Beltz, G. G., Aust, P. E. and Munkes, R. (1981), *Lancet*, **1**, 844.
Beltz, G. G., Doering, W., Munkes, R. and Matthews, J. (1983), *Clin. Pharmacol. Therap.*, **33**, 410.
Beresford, A. P., Humphrey, M. J. and Stopher, D. A. (1985), *Br. J. Pharmacol.*, **85**, 333p.
Beresford, A. P., MacRae, P. V. and Stopher, D. A. (1988 a), *Xenobiotica*, **18**, 169.
Beresford, A. P., McGibney, D., Humphrey, M. J., MacRae, P. V. and Stopher, D.A. (1988 b), *Xenobiotica*, **18**, 245.
Beresford, A. P., MacRae, P. V., Alker, D. and Kobylecki, R. J. (1989), *Arzneim.-Forsch.*, **39**, 201.
Beresford, A. P., Smith, D. A. and Jezequel, S. G. (1988 c), Poster 1.30 presented at the 11th European Workshop on Drug Metabolism, Konstanz, F.R.G.
Berntsson, P., Johansson, E. and Westerlund, Ch. (1987), *J. Cardiovasc. Pharmacol.*, **10**(Suppl 1), S60.
Böcker, R. H. and Guengerich, F. P. (1986), *J. Medic. Chem.*, **29**, 1596.
Boelaert, J., Valcke, Y., Dammekens, H., de Vriese, G., Ahr, G., Schurgers, M., Daneels, R. and Bogaert, M. G. (1988), *Europ. J. Clin. Pharmacol.*, **34**, 207.
Born, J. L. and Hadley, W. M. (1989), *Chem. Res. Toxicol.*, **2**, 57.
Capewell, S., Freestone, S., Critchley, J. A. J. H., Pottage, T. and Prescott, L. F. (1988), *Lancet*, **111**, 480.
Challenor, V. F., Le Vie, J., Waller, D. G., Gruchy, B., Renwick, A. G. and George, C. F. (1987 a), *Br. J. Clin. Pharmacol.*, **23**, 112P.
Challenor, V. F., Waller, D. G., Gruchy, B. S., Renwick, A. G. and George, C. F. (1987 b), *Br. J. Clin. Pharmacol.*, **23**, 248.
Challenor, V. F., Waller, D. G., Renwick, A. G., Gruchy, B. S. and George, C. F. (1987 c), *Br. J. Clin. Pharmacol.*, **24**, 473.
Chellingsworth, M. C., Willis, J. V., Jack, D. B. and Kendall, M. J. (1988), *Am. J. Med.*, **84**(Suppl. 3B), 72.
Cheung, W. K., Tonelli, A., Gertsch, L., Nicolau, G., Look, Z. M. and Silber, B. M. (1987), *Pharmaceut. Res*, **4**(Suppl), Abstract PP-670, S-96.
Cheung, W. K., Woodward, D. L., Hibberd, S. K., Pearse, S., Desjardins, R. E., Yacobi, A. and Silber, B. M. (1988), *Int. J. Clin. Pharmacol. Res.*, **18**, 299.
Cheung, W. K., Sia, L. L., Hibberd, M., Pearse, S., Woodward, D. L., Desjardins, R. E., Bernstein, J., Yacobi, A. and Silber, B. M. (1989), *Drug Develop. Indust. Pharmacy*, **15**, 51.
Christensen, C. K., Lederballe Pedersen, O. and Mikkelsen, E. (1982), *Clin. Pharmacol. Therap.*, **32**, 572.
Clair, F., Bellet, M., Guerret, M., Druecke, T. and Grunfeld, J. P. (1985), *Curr. Therap. Res.* **38**, 74.
Clifton, G. D., Blouin, R. A., Dilea, C., Schran, H. F., Hassel, A. E., Gonasun, L. M. and Foster, T. S. (1988), *J. Clin. Pharmacol.*, **28**, 36.

Crome, P., Baksi, A., MacManon, D., Panditer-Gunawandena, N. D., Edwards, J. and Manky, J. (1988), *Br. J. Clin. Pharmacol.*, **26**, 323.

Debbas, N. M. G., Jackson, S. H. D., Shah, K., Abrams, S. M. L., Johnston, A. and Turner, P. (1986), *Br. J. Clin. Pharmacol.*, **21**, 385.

Debruyne, D., Commeau, P., Grollier, G., Huret, B., Scanu, P. and Maulin, M. (1989), *Int. J. Clin. Pharmacol. Res.*, **9**, 15.

Delchier, J. C., Guerret, M., Vidon, N., Dubray, C. and Lavene, D. (1988), *Europ. J. Clin. Pharmacol.*, **34**, 165.

D'Heygere, F., Ling, T., Waddell, G., Harlow, B., James, I. and McIntyre, N. (1988), *Br. J. Clin. Pharmacol.*, **25**, 96P.

Dickinson, T. H., Egan, J. M. and Abernethy, D. R. (1988), *Pharmacology*, **36**, 405.

Dow, R. J. and Graham, J. M. (1986), *Br. J. Clin. Pharmacol.*, **22**, 195S.

Doyle, G. D., Donohue, J., Carmody, M., Laher, M., Greb, H. and Volz, M. (1989), *Europ. J. Clin. Pharmacol.*, **36**, 205.

Dunselman, P. H. J. M., Edgar, B., Scaf, A. H. J., Kuntze, C. E. E. and Wesseling, H. (1989), *Br. J. Clin. Pharmacol.*, **28**, 45.

Dylewicz, P., Kirch, W., Santos, S. R., Hutt, H. J., König, M. and Ohnhaus, E. E. (1987), *Eur. J. Clin. Pharmacol.*, **32**, 563.

Edgar, B. (1988), Dissertation from Dept. Clin. Pharmacol, Sahlgrenska sjukhuset, Univ. of Göteborg, Göteborg, Sweden.

Edgar, B., Regårdh, C. G., Johnsson, G., Johansson, L., Lundberg, P. and Löfberg, I. (1985), *Clin. Pharmacol. Therap.*, **38**, 205.

Edgar, B., Regårdh, C. G., Lundborg, P., Romare, S., Nyberg, G. and Rönn, O. (1987), *Biopharmaceut. Drug Dispos.*, **8**, 235.

Edgar, B., Regårdh, C. G., Attman, P. O., Aurell, M., Herlitz, H. and Johnsson, G. (1989), *Br. J. Clin. Pharmacol.*, **27**, 67.

Elliott, H. L., Meredith, P. A., Reid, J. L. and Faulkner, J. K. (1988), *J. Cardiovas. Pharmacol.*, **12**(Suppl. 7), S64.

Ene, M. D. and Roberts, C. J. C. (1987), *J. Clin. Pharmacol.*, **27**, 1001.

Eriksson, U., Lundahl, J., Bäärnhielm, C. and Regårdh, C. G. (1989), Abstract, Third Europ. Symp. on *Foreign Comp. Metabol.*, ISSX, London, July 13–16.

Faulkner, J. K., McGibney, D., Chasseaud, L. F., Perry, J. L. and Taylor, I. W. (1986), *Br. J. Cardiovasc. Pharmacol.*, **22**, 21.

Fleckenstein, A., Tritthart, H., Fleckenstein, B., Herbst, A. and Grün, G. (1969). *Pflügers Archiv*, **307**, R25.

Forrette, F., Bellet, M., Henry, J. F., Henry, M. P., Poyand Salmeron, C., Bouchacourt, P. and Guerret, M. (1985), *Br. J. Clin. Pharmacol.*, **20**, 125S.

Graham, D. J. M., Dow, R. J., Freedman, D., Mroszczak, E. and Ling, T. (1984), *Postgrad. Med. J.*, **60**(Suppl. 4), 7.

Graham, D. J. M., Dow, R. J., Hall, D. J., Alexander, O. F., Mroszczak, E. J. and Freedman, D. (1985), *Br. J. Clin. Pharmacol.*, **20**, 23S.

Green, J. A., Clementi, W., Porter, C. and Stigelman, W. (1983), *Clin. Pharmacy*, **2**, 461.

Guazzi, M., Olivari, M. T., Polese, A., Fiorentini, C., Magrini, F. and Moruzzi, P. (1977), *Clin. Pharmacol. Therap.*, **22**, 528.

Guengerich, F. P. (1987), *J. Biol. Chem.*, **262**, 8459.

Guengerich, F. P. and Böckers, R. H. (1988), *J. Biol. Chem.*, **263**, 8168.

Guengerich, F. P., Martin, M. V., Beaune, P. H., Kremers, P., Wolff, T. and Waxman, D. (1986), *J. Biol. Chem.*, **261**, 5051.

Guengerich, F. P., Petersson, L. A. and Böckers, R. H. (1988), *J. Biol. Chem.*, **263**, 8176.

Harper, A. M., Craigen, L. and Kazda, S. (1981) *J. Cerebral Blood Flow Metabol.*, **3**, 349.

Higuchi, S. and Shiobara, Y. (1980 a), *Xenobiotica*, **10**, 447.

Higuchi, S. and Shiobara, Y. (1980 b), *Xenobiotica*, **10**, 889.
Higuchi, S., Sasaki, H., Shiobara, Y. and Sado, T. (1977), *Xenobiotica*, **7**, 469.
Hoffmann, K.-J. and Andersson, L. (1987), *Drugs*, **34**(Suppl 3), 43.
Hoffmann, K.-J. and Weidolf, L. (1985), *Biomedicas Mass Spectrometri*, **12**, 414.
Hoyo-Vadillo, C., Castanêda-Hernàndez, G., Herrera, J. E., Vidal-Gàrate. J., Salazar, L. A., Moreno-Ramos, A., Chàves, F., Tena, I. and Hong, E. (1989), *J. Clin. Pharmacol.*, **29**, 251.
Husted, S. E., Kraemmer-Nielsen, H., Christensen, C. K. and Lederballe-Pedersen, O. (1982), *Europ. J. Clin. Pharmacol.*, **22**, 101.
Idle, J. R. and Sever, P. S. (1983), *Br. Med. J.*, **286**, 1978.
Jackson, S. H. D., Shah, K., Debbas, N. M. G., Peverel-Cooper, C. A. and Turner, P. (1986), *Br. J. Clin. Pharmacol.*, **21**, 389.
Janzon, K., Edgar, B., Lundborg, P. and Regårdh, C. G. (1986), *Acta Pharmacol. Toxicol.*, **59**(Suppl. 5), 98, Abstract 258.
Jean, C. and Laplanche, R. (1988), *J. Chromatog.*, **428**, 61.
Kann, J., Krol, G. J., Raemsch, K. D., Burkholder, D. E. and Levitt, M. J. (1984), *J. Cardiovasc. Pharmacol.*, **6**, S 968.
Kazda, S. and Towart, R. (1982), *Acta Neurochirurg.*, **63**, 259.
Kendall, M. J., Jack, D. B., Laugher, S. J., Lobo, J. and Smith, R. S. (1984), *Br. J. Clin. Pharmacol.*, **18**, 331.
Kirch, W., Janisch, H. D., Heidemann, H., Rämsch, K. and Ohnhaus, E. E. (1983), *Dt. Med. Wschr.*, **108**, 1757.
Kirch, W., Rämsch, K. D., Dührsen, U. and Ohnhaus, E. E. (1984), *Int. J. Clin. Pharmacol. Res.*, **IV**, 381.
Kirch, W., Hutt, H. J., Dylewicz, P., Gräf, K. J. and Ohnhaus, E. E. (1986 a), *Clin. Pharmacol. Therap.*, **39**, 35.
Kirch, W., Logemann, H., Heidemann, S. R., Santos, E. E. and Ohnhaus, E. (1986 b), *Europ. J. Clin. Pharmacol.*, **31**, 391.
Kirch, W., Stenzel, J., Dylewicz, P., Hutt, H. J., Santos, S. R. and Ohnhaus, E. E. (1986 c), *Br. J. Clin. Pharmacol.*, **22**, 155.
Kleinbloesem, C. H., van Brummelen, P., Faber, H., Danhof, M., Vermeulen, N. P. E. and Breimer, D. D. (1984 a), *Biochem. Pharmacol.*, **33**, 3721.
Kleinbloesem, C. H., van Brummelen, P., van de Linde, J. A., Voogd, P. J. and Breimer, D. D. (1984 b), *Clin. Pharmacol. Therap.*, **35**, 742.
Kleinbloesem, C. H., van Brummelen, P., van Harten, J., Danhof, M. and Breimer, D. D. (1985 a), *Clin. Pharmacol. Therap.*, **37**, 563.
Kleinbloesem, C. H., van Brummelen, P., Hillers, J., Moolenaar, A. J. and Breimer, D. D. (1985 b), *Therap. Drug Monit.*, **7**, 372.
Kleinbloesem, C. H., van Harten, J., Wilson, J. P. H., Danhof, M., van Brummelen, P. and Breimer, D. D. (1986), *Clin. Pharmacol. Therap.*, **40**, 21.
Kobayashi, H., Ohishi, T., Nishiie, H., Kobayshi, S., Inoue, A., Oka, T. and Nakamizo, N. (1988 a), *Arzneim.-Forsch.*, **38**, 1742.
Kobayashi, H., Ohishi, T., Nishiie, H., Kobayshi, S., Inoue, A., Oka, T. and Nakamizo, N. (1988 b), *Arzneim.-Forsch.*, **38**, 1750.
Kobayashi, H., Okumura, S., Kosaka, Y., Kobayashi, S., Inoue, A., Oka, T and Nakamizo, N. (1988 c), *Arzneim.-Forsch.*, **38**, 1753.
Koren, G., Zylber-Katz, E., Granit, L. and Levy, M. (1986), *Int. J. Clin. Pharmacol., Therapy Toxicol.*, **24**, 39.
Krause, H. P., Ahr, H. J., Beermann, D., Siefert, H. M., Suwelack, D. and Weber, H. (1988 a), *Arzneim.-Forsch.*, **38**, 1593.
Krause, H. P., Ahr, H. J., Siefert, H. M., Steinke, W. and Suwelack, D. (1988 b), *Arzneim.-Forsch.*, **38**, 1599.
Kurosawa, S., Kurosawa, N., Owada, E., Matsuhashi, N. and Ito, K. (1987), *J. Int. Med. Res.*, **15**, 121.

Laher, M. S., Kelly, J. G., Doyle, G. D., Carmody, M., Donohue, J. F., Greb, H. and Volz, M. (1988), *J. Cardiovasc. Pharmacol.*, **12**(Suppl. 7), S60.

Landahl, S., Edgar, B., Gabrielsson, M., Larsson, M., Lernfelt, B., Lundborg, P. and Regårdh, C. G. (1988), *Clin. Pharmacokin.*, **14**, 374.

Lasseter, K. C., Shamblen, E. C., Murdoch, A. A., Burkholder, D. E., Krol, G. J., Taylor, R. J. and Vanov, S. K. (1984), *J. Cardiovasc. Pharmacol*, **6**, S977.

Lettieri, J., Krol, G., Yeh, S., Ryan, J., Jevin, A., McMahon, F. G., Burkholder, D. and Birkett, J. P. (1987), *J. Cardiovasc. Pharmacol.*, **9** (Suppl. 4), S142.

Lewis, R. V., Jackson, P. R. and Ramsay, L. E. (1984), *Br. J. Clin. Pharmacol*, **19**, 562P.

Maier-Lenz, H., Rode, H., Lenau, H., Thieme, G., Wölke, E., Kobayashi, H. and Kobayashi, S. (1988), *Arzneim.-Forsch*, **38**, 1757.

Maruhn, D., Siefert, H. M., Weber, H., Rämsch, K. and Suwelack, D. (1985), *Arzneim.-Forsch.*, **35**, 1781.

Meyer, H., Scherling, D. and Karl, W. (1983 a), *Arzneim-Forsch.*, **33**, 1528.

Meyer, H., Wehinger, E., Bossert, F. and Scherling, D. (1983 b), *Arzneim.-Forsch.*, **33**, 106.

Mikus, G., Fischer, C., Heuer, B., Langen, C. and Eichelbaum, M. (1987), *Br. J. Clin. Pharmacol.*, **24**, 561.

Niwa, T., Tokuma, Y. and Noguchi, H. (1987), *Res. Comm. Chem. Pathol. Pharmacol.*, **55**, 75.

Niwa, T., Tokuma, Y., Nakagawa, K., Noguchi, H., Yamazoe, Y. and Kato, R. (1988 a), *Res. Comm. Chem. Pathol. Pharmacol.*, **60**, 161.

Niwa, T., Tokuma, Y. and Noguchi, H. (1988 b), *Xenobiotica*, **18**, 217.

Niwa, T., Tokuma, Y., Nakagawa, K. and Noguchi, H. (1989), *Drug Metabol. Dispos. Biolog. Fate of Chemicals*, **17**, 64.

Olivari, M. T., Bartorelli, C., Polese, A., Fiorentini, C., Moruzzi, P. and Guazzi, M. D. (1979), *Circulation*, **59**, 1056.

Otto, J. and Lesko, L. J. (1986), *J. Pharmacy Pharmacol.*, **38**, 399.

Oates, N. S., Feher, M. D., Perry, H. E., Schmid, B. J., Sever, P. S. and Idle, J. R. (1988), *Br. J. Clin. Pharmacol.*, 675P.

Pedersen, K. E., Dorph-Pedersen, A., Hvidt, S., Klitgaard, N. A., Kjaer, K. and Nielsen-Kudsk, F. (1982), *Clin. Pharmacol. Therap.*, **32**, 562.

Piepho, R. W., Culbertson, V. L. and Rhodas, R. S. (1987), *Circulation*, **75**(Suppl V), V-181.

Perucca, E., Hedges, A., Makki, K. A., Ruprah, M., Wilson, J. F. and Richens, A. (1984), *Br. J. Clin. Pharmacol.*, **18**, 401.

Raemsch, K. D. and Sommer, J. (1984), in *Nitrendipine* (A. Scriabine, S. Vanov, K. Deck (eds), p. 409. Urban & Schwarzenberg Baltimore.

Raemsch, K. D. and Sommer, J. (1983), *Hypertension*, **5**(Suppl. II), 18.

Raemsch, K. D., Lücker, P. W. and Wetzelsberger, N. (1987), *Clin. Pharmacol. Therap.*, **41**, 216, (Abstr. PIIIA-10).

Regårdh, C. G., Edgar, B., Olsson, R., Kendall, M., Collste, P. and Shansky, C. (1989), *Europ. J. Clin. Pharmacol.*, **36**, 473.

Reitberg, D. P., Love, S. J., Quercia, G. T. and Zinny, M. A. (1987), *Clin. Pharmacol. Therap.*, **47**, 72.

Rehnquist, U., Billing, E., Moberg, L., Lundman, T. and Olsson, G. (1987), *Drugs*, **34**(Suppl. 3), 33.

Renwick, A. G., Robertson, D. R. C., Macklin, B., Challenor, V., Waller, D. G. and George, C. F. (1988), *Br. J. Clin. Pharmacol.*, **25**, 701.

Robertson, D. R. C., Waller, D. G., Renwick, A. G. and George, C. F. (1988), *Br. J. Clin. Pharmacol.*, **25**, 297.

Rosenkranz, B., Ledermann, H. and Frölich, J. C. (1986), *J. Cardiovasc. Pharmacol.*, **8**, 943.

Rush, W. R., Alexander, O., Hall, D. J., Cairncross, L., Dow, R. J. and Graham, D. J. G. (1986), *Xenobiotica*, **16**, 341.
Saltiel, E., Ellrodt, A. G., Monk, J. P. and Langley, M. S. (1988) *Drugs*, **36**, 387.
Schellens, J. H. M., Soons, P. A. and Breimer, D. D. (1988), *Biochem. Pharmacol.*, **37**, 2507.
Scherling, D. and Karl, W. (1988), Poster 3.50 presented at the 11th European Workshop on Drug Metabolism, Konstanz, F.R.G.
Scherling, D., Karl, W., Ahr, G., Ahr, H. J. and Wehinger, E. (1988), *Arzneim.-Forsch.*, **38**, 1105.
Schran, H. F., Jaffe, J. M. and Gonasun, L. M. (1988), *Am. J. Med.*, **84**(Suppl.3B), 80.
Schwartz, J. B. and Migliore, P. J. (1984), *Clin. Pharmacol. Therap.*, **36**, 19.
Smith, S. R., Kendall, M. J., Lobo, J., Beeraliee, A., Jack, D. B. and Wilkins, M. R. (1987 a), *Br. J. Clin. Pharmacol.*, **23**, 311.
Smith, S. R., Wilkins, M. R., Jack, D. B., Kendall, M. J. and Laugher, S. (1987 b), *Europ. J. Clin. Pharmacol.*, **31**, 575.
Soons, P. A., de Boer, A. G., van Brummelen, P. and Breimer, D. D. (1989), *Br. J. Clin. Pharmacol.*, **27**, 179.
Stopher, D. A., Beresford, A. P., MacRae, P. V. and Humphrey, M. J. (1988), *J. Cardiovasc. Pharmacol.*, **12**, (Suppl. 7), S 55.
Sutfin, T. A., Gabrielsson, M. and Regårdh, C. G. (1987), *Xenobiotica*, **17**, 1203.
Sutfin, T. A., Lind, T., Gabrielsson, M. and Regårdh, C. G. (1989), *Europ. J. Clin. Pharmacol.*, (accepted for publication).
Suwelack, D. and Weber, H. (1985), *Europ. J. Drug Metab. Pharmacokin.*, **10**, 231.
Suwelack, D., Weber, H. and Maruhn, D. (1985), *Arzneim.-Forsch.*, **35**, 1787.
Takenaka, T., Miyazaki, I., Asano, M., Higuchi, S. and Maeno, H. (1982), *Jap. J. Pharmacol.*, **32**, 665.
Terakawa, M., Tokuma, Y., Shishido, A. and Noguchi, H. (1987 a), *J. Clin. Pharmacol.*, **27**, 111.
Terakawa, M., Tokuma, Y., Shishido, A., Yasuda, K. and Noguchi, H. (1987 b), *J. Clin. Pharmacol.*, **27**, 293.
Terashita, S., Tokuma, Y., Fujiwara, T., Shiokawa, Y., Okumura, K. and Noguchi, H. (1987), *Xenobiotica*, **17**, 1415.
Tokuma, Y., Fujiwara, T. and Noguchi, H. (1987 a), *Xenobiotica*, **17**, 1341.
Tokuma, Y., Fujiwara, T. and Noguchi, H. (1987 b), *Res. Comm. Chem. Pathol. Pharmacol.*, **57**, 229.
Tokuma, T., Sekiguchi, M., Niwa, T. and Noguchi, H. (1988), *Xenobiotica*, **18**, 21.
Towart, R., Wehinger, E., Meyer, H. and Kazda, S. (1982), *Arzneim.-Forsch.*, **32**, 338.
Triggle, D. J. (1982), in *Calcium Blockers: Mechanism of Action and Clinical Applications* (S. F. Flaim and R. Zelis eds), p. 121, Urban and Schwarzenberg, Baltimor-Munich.
Tse, F. L. S. and Jaffe, J. M. (1987), *Europ. J. Clin. Pharmacol.*, **32**, 361.
Urien, S., Albengres, E., Comte, A., Kiechel, J.-R. and Tillement, J.-P. (1985), *J. Cardiovasc. Pharmacol.*, **7**, 891.
Urien, S., Pinquier, J.-L., Paquette, B., Chaumet-Riffaud, P., Kiechel, J.-R. and Tillement, J.-P. (1987), *J. Pharmacol. Exp. Therap.*, **242**, 349.
van Harten, J., van Brummelen, P., Lodewijks, M. Th. M., Danhof, M. and Breimer, D. D. (1988 a), *Clin. Pharmacol. Therap.*, **43**, 332.
van Harten, J., van Brummelen, P., Wilson, J. H. P., Lodewijks, M. Th. M. and Breimer, D. D. (1988 b), *Europ. J. Clin. Pharmacol.*, **34**, 387.
van Harten, J., van Brummelen, P., Zeegers, R. R. E. C. M., Danhof, M. and Breimer, D. D. (1988 c), *Br. J. Clin. Pharmacol.*, **25**, 709.

van Harten, J., Burggraaf, J., van Brummelen, P. and Breimer, D. D. (1989), *Clin. Pharmacokin.*, **16**, 55.

Vestal, R. E. (1978), *Drugs*, **16**, 358.

Vinceneux, P., Canal, M., Domart, Y., Roux, A., Cascio, B., Orfiamma, B., Larribaud, J., Flouvat, B. and Charbon, C. (1986), *Int. J. Clin. Pharmacol. Therap. Toxicol.*, **24**, 153.

von Duhm, B., Maul, H., Medenwald, K., Patzschke, K. and Wegner, L. A. (1972), *Arzneim.-Forsch.*, **22**, 42.

von Horster, F. A., Duhm, R., Maul, W., Medenwald, H., Patzschke, K. and Wegner, L. A. (1972), *Arzneim.-Forsch.*, **22**, 330.

Wagner, J., Ling, T. L., Mroszczak, E. J., Freedman, D., Wu, A., Huang, B., Massey, I. J. and Roe, R. R. (1987), *Biopharm. Drug Dispos.*, **8**, 133.

Waller, D. G., Renwick, A. G., Gruchy, B. S. and George, C. F. (1984), *Br. J. Clin. Pharmacol.*, **18**, 951.

Walley, T. J., Heagerty, A. M., Woods, K. L., Bing, R. F., Pohl, J. E. and Barnett, D. B. (1987) *Br. J. Clin. Pharmacol.*, **23**, 693.

Wang, S.-X., Sutfin, T., Bäärnhielm, C. and Regårdh, C. G. (1989), *J. Pharmacol. Exp. Ther.*, **250**, 632.

Weidolf, L. and Hoffmann, K.-J. (1984), *Acta Pharmaceut. Suecia*, **21**, 331.

Weidolf, L., Borg, K. O. and Hoffmann, K.-J. (1984), *Xenobiotica*, **14**, 657.

Williams, D. M. and Cubeddu, L. X. (1988), *J. Clin. Pharmacol.*, **28**, 990.

Wingstrand, K., Abrahamsson, B., Edgar, B. and Grind, M. (1988), Abstract. Int. Conf. *Pharmaceutical Sciences and Clinical Pharmacology*, Jerusalem, p. 81.

CHAPTER 3

Absorption across the nasal mucosa of animal species: compounds applied and mechanisms involved

A. N. Fisher

Fisons plc (Pharmaceutical Division), R & D Laboratories, Bakewell Road, Loughborough, Leicestershire LE11 0RH, England, UK

* Present address: Department of Pharmaceutical Sciences, School of Pharmacy, University of Nottingham, University Park, Nottingham NG7 2RD, England, UK

1. Introduction

The use of the nasal route for the systemic administration of compounds to man has recently received much attention (Chien and Chang, 1985, 1987). This interest has mainly been stimulated because of the potential of the route for the administration of peptides. These compounds include not only the known, therapeutically useful peptides such as insulin and calcitonin, but also the potential products of recombinant DNA technology.

The nasal administration of compounds for systemic effects is not new. Besides the long established intranasal use of tobacco snuff and cocaine there have, over many years, been occasional reports of compounds which have been systemically absorbed after intranasal administration to man. Early work included that of Blumgart (1922), who demonstrated the antidiuretic effect of intranasal pituitary extract in a case of diabetes insipidus; Cohen *et al.* (1930), who demonstrated the absorption of ragweed pollen after intranasal application; van Dellen *et al.* (1937), who demonstrated the absorption of mecholyl (acetyl-β-methylcholine chloride), and McKendry *et al.* (1954), who was one of several authors at that time reporting on the physiological and clinical effects of ACTH after intranasal application. There have been several reports of systemic side effects of compounds administered topically to the nose for local effects, including dexamethasone (Michels *et al.*, 1967 and Kimmerle and Rolla, 1985) or oxymetazoline (Soderman *et al.*, 1984). In the last few years the number of publications concerning nasal absorption in man has rapidly increased.

There is a recent large review, citing over 730 references, of many substances applied to the nose for both systemic and topical effects (Chien and Chang, 1987). These authors classified the compounds applied as hormones, amino acids and polypeptides, cardiovascular drugs, biological products, autonomic nervous system drugs, CNS stimulants, narcotics and antagonists, antimigraine drugs, antimicrobial agents, antiviral agents, histamines and antihistamines, vitamins and other nutrients, inorganic compounds and diagnostic drugs. This illustrates not only the large numbers of substances administered intranasally, but the range of types of compound.

Recent reports of compounds administered to the human nose have included: calcitonin (Pontiroli *et al.*, 1985 a, 1986 b; D'Agostino *et al.*, 1988; Tarquini *et al.*, 1988), levocabastine (Heykants *et al.*, 1985), budesonide (Edsbacker *et al.*, 1985), desmopressin (Vicente *et al.*, 1985; Harris *et al.*, 1986, 1987, 1988; Olanoff *et al.* 1987), α-human natriuretic peptide (Shionoiri and Kaneko, 1986), synthetic human atrial natriuretic peptide (Delabays *et al.*, 1989), alprenolol and metoprolol (Duchateau *et al.*, 1986 a), deamino-8-D-arginine vasopressin (Vilhardt and Lundin, 1986), gonadotrophin-releasing hormone (Rajifer *et al.*, 1986), 1-deamino-2-D-tyr(OEt)-4-thr-8-orn-vasotocin (Lundin *et al.*, 1986), insulin and glucagon (Pontiroli *et al.*, 1986 a), dihydroergotamine (Acllig and Rosenthaler, 1986), progesterone (Dalton *et al.*, 1987), cyanocobalamin (Colman *et al.*, 1988) and cocaine (Bromley and Hayward, 1988). There has been a brief review of the intranasal delivery of peptides and proteins (Su, 1986) and a review of recent advances in intranasal drug delivery systems (Su *et al.*, 1987). Despite all this activity, the only compounds which are commonly administered for their therapeutic systemic effects are lysopressin, desmopressin/DDAVP, vasopressin, oxytocin, gonadotrophin-releasing hormone and LHRH agonist.

The majority of papers in this voluminous literature only aim to demonstrate the utility of the nasal route for the particular compound involved. Little investigation of the factors involved in nasal absorption has been performed. An exception is the work on the use of agents employed to enhance or promote absorption. These promoters have been widely used with peptides, e.g. insulin (Salzman *et al.*, 1985; Gordon *et al.*, 1985; Flier *et al.*, 1985) or glucagon (Pontiroli *et al.*, 1985 b), and are generally surfactants (ionic, nonionic, bile salts). Some peptides are not absorbed by the intranasal route, or indeed by other routes, unless a promoter is present. This is presumed to be because peptides are hydrophilic and have to traverse lipophilic membranes to be absorbed (Kimura, 1984). Most reports have only quantified absorption by the physiological or pharmacological response to the applied compound and apparently the only two reported studies on the mechanism of nasal absorption in man are the electron microscopic studies by Crifo and Russo (1980) and Inagaki *et al.* (1985). Crifo and Russo (1980) demonstrated the absorption of IgA by pinocytosis while Inagaki *et al.* (1985) demonstrated the permeability of mucosal tight junctions by horseradish peroxidase. These latter workers concluded that goblet cell–goblet cell, and goblet cell–ciliated cell junctions were weaker than those of ciliated cell–ciliated cell.

The nasal cavity has a thin mucosa, is well supplied with blood, is covered with mucus, and has many cells with microvilli or cilia, which make it, theoretically, a powerful absorptive surface. Compared with the oral route, there is no delay due to factors such as disintegration of the dosage form or gastric emptying; any breakdown or metabolism in the lumen or wall of the gastrointestinal tract is avoided, and any first-pass effect of the liver is also circumvented. Some compounds with poor intrinsic oral absorption have been shown to be well absorbed from the nose, e.g. phenol red (Hirai *et al.*, 1981 a), clofilium tosylate (Su *et al.*, 1984), or sodium cromoglycate (Fisher *et al.*, 1985). Furthermore, the nasal route has, potentially, better patient acceptability compared with other routes used for long-term therapy, especially repeated injection (Hirai *et al.*, 1978; Pontiroli *et al.*, 1985 a).

The lack of systematic investigations on the absorption of compounds in man can be considered to be an inhibiting factor in the exploitation of the intranasal route for the systemic administration of drugs. The important parameters involved in absorption from the nose are not yet fully understood. Some of the deficiencies in the human data can probably be corrected by appropriate and relevant animal studies. This hopefully will allow the full benefits of intranasal application to be utilized.

Consequently this review will consider the types of compound applied to the nasal mucosa of animals with particular reference to the rat and the structure of the rat nasal cavity. The utility of animal species to predict effects in man, and the known mechanisms of nasal absorption, will also be covered.

2. Systemic absorption of compounds administered intranasally to animals

A large number of compounds has been administered intranasally to animals. Where an assessment can be made of systemic absorption, the compounds are shown in Table 1 (p. 92).

Some materials have been administered to the nose solely for their local or topical effect, for example to demonstrate efficacy or toxicity. Studies such as these, where only local responses are measured, have been excluded from Table 1. An illustration of a study on efficacy aspects is the comparison between the local effects of xylometazoline, natural prostaglandins E_1 and E_2, and synthetic prostaglandin E_2 (Jackson and Birnbaum, 1982). After nasal application of these compounds only nasal patency (resistance to airflow) was measured, although some material presumably must have crossed the nasal mucosa to stimulate vasoconstriction in the underlying blood vessels. In the case of toxicity, formaldehyde is well established as being toxic in the nasal cavity of rodents. Thus, nasal exposure to formaldehyde has been performed to investigate cellular toxicity (Chang *et al.*, 1983) or the effect on the mucociliary apparatus (Morgan *et al.*, 1983, 1986 a,b). Where the systemic absorption of a topical compound can be estimated (e.g. with an imidazoline decongestant [Munzel and Eichner, 1975]), this is included in Table 1.

Inorganic or particulate materials, sometimes one and the same, have been administered intranasally to animals to determine distribution and clearance patterns within the nasal cavity (Cuddihy *et al.*, 1973). Indeed there are several comprehensive reviews of disposition and clearance, although few concentrate on the nose and even less on animals (Heyder and Rudolf, 1975; Hounam and Morgan, 1977; Lippmann *et al.*, 1980; Andersen and Proctor, 1982; Schreider, 1986). Again, such nasal applications are excluded from Table 1. Some inorganics and particulates are included in the Table where systemic absorption was measured or a route across the mucosa was traced. The important use of the intranasal route for sensitization, vaccination or challenge (McCaskill *et al.*, 1984) has not been considered in this review.

The compounds listed in Table 1 have been divided into groups according to their chemical or physical form. Group 1.1, peptides and proteins, is quite large. Many of the compounds investigated are hormones or analogues thereof and the use of absorption promoters has been quite common. As new peptide and protein products are generated from genetic engineering techniques, and since the intranasal route avoids the degradation of these compounds by the gastrointestinal tract, it is likely that many more proteins and peptides will be applied intranasally. The steroids listed in Group 1.2 again reflects a large number of experiments. However, the number of compounds involved is limited. In addition to systemic experiments measuring steroid-derived material, the many and varied pharmacological and physiological effects of intranasally applied steroids have also been investigated. Gases and vapours (Group 1.3) have been passed into the nasal cavity mainly to examine physiological and toxicological effects. The absorption, or removal from the applied atmosphere, has been measured in some cases and those studies are listed. Groups 1.4, 1.5, 1.6 and 1.7 comprise inorganics, amino acids, carbohydrates and particulates respectively. Finally Group 1.8, other compounds, consists of a large number of miscellaneous and heterogeneous materials, most of which are pharmaceuticals.

Generally studies within groups are listed in chronological order. However, in addition, an attempt has been made to group together studies involving the same compound.

Experimental techniques

The animal species used have been, almost exclusively, common laboratory animals and in particular rat, dog and monkey.

An indication is made in Table 1 of the experimental procedure involved. This is because when an animal is anaesthetized, physiological functions can be affected, for example the deposition of aerosols in hamster lungs (Sweeney *et al.*, 1983), or reduction in the rate of mucociliary clearance, drainage or mechanical removal. While the inhibition of mucociliary clearance by anaesthesia has been demonstrated in rat trachea (Patrick and Stirling, 1977), the clearance of nasal mucus in the dog was not reduced by anaesthesia (Whaley *et al.*, 1987). Losses via drainage or mechanical removal will, to some extent, depend upon orientation of the animal.

The technique of choice is the *in vivo* one described by Hirai *et al.* (1981 a). Briefly, this consists of an anaesthetized rat, on its back, with a completely

Table 1. Systemic absorption of materials after intranasal administration to animals
1.1 *Peptides and proteins*

Compound	Species	Anaesthetized/ Conscious	In situ/ In vivo of Hirai	Method of administration	Parameter measured	Absorption	Authors
Egg albumin	Cat	Anaesthetized	—	Solution	Lymph egg albumin	Present	
	Dog	Anaesthetized	—	Solution	Lymph egg albumin	Present	
	Monkey	Anaesthetized	—	Solution	Lymph egg albumin	Present	Yoffey et al., 1938
Horse Serum	Cat	Anaesthetized	—	Solution	Lymph horse serum	Not detected	
	Monkey	Anaesthetized	—	Solution	Lymph horse serum	Not detected	
Horse serum–Evans blue complex	Cat	Anaesthetized	—	Solution	Lymph complex	Not detected	
Serum albumin	Cat	Anaesthetized	—	Solution	Lymph serum albumin	Not detected	
	Rabbit	Anaesthetized	—	Solution	Lymph serum albumin	Present	
Insulin	Dog	Anaesthetized	—	Spray altered pH plus surfactants	Plasma glucose and insulin	25–30% effective c.f. i.v.	Hirai et al., 1978
Insulin	Rat	Anaesthetized	In vivo	Solution	Blood glucose	Glucose down	Hirai et al., 1981 a
Insulin	Rat	Anaesthetized	In vivo	Solution	Plasma glucose	Glucose down 6% 30%	
Insulin	Rat	Anaesthetized	In vivo	Plus surfactants	Plasma glucose	Glucose down 0–64%	Hirai et al., 1981 b,c
Insulin	Sheep	Anaesthetized to dose	—	Solution plus surfactants	Serum insulin	16.4%	Longenecker, 1986; Longenecker et al., 1987
Insulin	Dog	Anaesthetized	—	Powder plus enhancers	Plasma glucose and insulin	Glucose down by up to 33%	Nagai et al., 1984
Insulin	Rat	Anaesthetized	In vivo	Solution	Plasma glucose	0.4–2.0% c.f. i.m.	Aungst et al., 1988
Insulin	Rat	Anaesthetized	In vivo	Plus promoter	Plasma glucose	47% c.f. i.m.	
Insulin	Rat	Anaesthetized	In vivo	Solution	Plasma glucose	0.4–2.0% c.f. i.m.	Aungst and Rogers, 1988
Insulin	Rat	Anaesthetized	In vivo	Plus promoters	Plasma glucose	3.5–28.7% c.f. i.m.	

Compound	Animal	State	Method	Formulation	Parameter	Result	Reference
Insulin	Rat	Anaesthetized	In vivo	Solution	Blood glucose and serum insulin	Not absorbed	Bjork and Edman, 1988
				Powder and microspheres	Plasma glucose and serum insulin	30%	
Insulin	Rabbit	Conscious	—	Solutions	Blood glucose, serum insulin	Low	Hermens et al., 1988
				Plus enhancers	Blood glucose, serum insulin	4%	
Insulin	Rat	Anaesthetized	In vivo	Solution	Plasma glucose and insulin	10% c.f. s.c.	Mishima et al., 1987
				Plus promoters	Plasma glucose and insulin	10–100% c.f. s.c.	
Insulin	Rat	Anaesthetized	In vivo	Solution, gel	Plasma glucose	Only gels reduced plasma glucose	Morimoto et al., 1985
[Asu^{1,7}]-eel calcitonin	Rat	Anaesthetized	In vivo	Solution, gel	Plasma calcium	Only gels reduced plasma calcium	
Salmon calcitonin	Rat	Anaesthetized	In vivo	Solution and enhancers	Serum calcium	Serum calcium falls, enhancers increase effect	Hanson et al., 1986
[Asu^{1,7}]-eel calcitonin	Rat	Anaesthetized	In vivo	Solutions at different pH	Plasma calcitonin	pH 3, 10% c.f. i.m.	Yamamoto et al., 1987
				Plus promoters	Plasma calcitonin	pH 6, 10% c.f. i.m.	
[1-Deamino-8-D-arginine]-vasopressin (DDAVP, desmopressin)	Rat	Conscious	—	Solution	Antidiuresis	Effective	Vavra et al., 1968
	Dog	Conscious	—	Solution	Antidiuresis	Effective	
Nafarelin acetate (LHRH agonist)	Monkey	Anaesthetized to dose and bleed	—	Sprayed solution	Plasma nafarelin	2%	Anik et al., 1984; Vickery et al., 1985
Des-Gly^{10}-[D-Leu^6]-LHRH-ethylamide (TAP-144, LHRH agonist)	Rat	Conscious	—	Solution	Serum TAP-144 Serum hormones	16%	Yamazaki, 1984

(continued).

Table 1. 1.1 *Peptides and Proteins (Continued)*

Compound	Species	Anaesthetized/ Conscious	In situ/ In vivo of Hirai	Method of administration	Parameter measured	Absorption	Authors
[N-Ac$_3$-D-p-Cl$_6$-Phe^{1,2} D-Trp^3,D-Arg^6, D-Ala^{10}]-LHRH (ORG 30276), LHRH antagonist	Monkey	Anaesthetized to bleed	—	Solution	Serum FSH and LH	16–26%	Asch et al., 1985
Leuprolide (LHRH analogue)	Rat	Conscious	—	Solution and enhancers	Induction of ovulation	0.1% solution 2–3% with enhancers	Okada et al., 1982
LHRH	Rat	Anaesthetized	—	Solution plus enhancer	Serum LH, Induction of ovulation	3 times increase over control, 2 times increase over control	Raehs et al., 1988 b
Buserelin (LHRH agonist)	Rat	Anaesthetized	—	Solution plus enhancer	Serum LH, Urinary Buserelin	2–9 times increase over control, 2 times increase over control	
Secretin	Rat	Anaesthetized	In vivo	Solution	Pancreatic juice secretion	11–25% of i.v.	Ohwaki et al., 1985
	Rat	Anaesthetized	In vivo	Altered pH	Pancreatic juice secretion	5–31% of i.v.	
	Rat	Anaesthetized	In vivo	Altered osmolarity	Pancreatic juice secretion	9–14% of i.v.	
Metkephamide (enkephalin)	Rat	Anaesthetized	In vivo	Solution	Serum metkephamide	65–100%	
	Rat	Anaesthetized	In vivo	Plus surfactant	Serum metkephamide	65–100%	Su et al., 1985; Su et al., 1986; Su et al., 1987;
[^{3}H]Tyr-D-Ala-Gly-L-Phe-D-Leu-OH([^{3}H])	Rat	Anaesthetized	In vivo	Solution	Blood DADLE	59%	
DADLE, enkephalin analogue	Rat	Anaesthetized	In vivo	Plus surfactant	Blood DADLE	94%	

Substance	Animal	State	In situ / In vivo	Formulation	Measurement	Result	Reference
Leucine enkephalin	Rat	Anaesthetized	In situ	Perfusion solution	Perfusate leucine enkephalin and its metabolite	< 10%	Hussain et al., 1985 b
Interferon β Interferon	Calf Rabbit	Conscious Conscious	— —	Solution Solution, powder and surfactants	Serum interferon Plasma interferon titre	Not detected None a one, 2.2% with surfactant	Gillespie et al., 1986 Maitani et al., 1986
Human interferon β	Rabbit	Conscious	—	Powder with enhancer plus excipients	Plasma human interferon β	3%	Igawa et al., 1988
[3H]Nor-muramyl dipeptide (nor-MDP)	Mouse	Anaesthetized	—	Solution	Tissue and blood radioactivity	Radioactivity present	
[3H]Muramyl tripeptide phosphatidylethanolamine (MTP-PE)	Mouse	Anaesthetized	—	Solution	Tissue and blood radioactivity	Radioactivity present	Fogler et al., 1985
Substance P	Rat	Anaesthetized	—	Solution	Plasma substance P	Plasma substance P rose	Karasek et al., 1986
Thyrotrophin-releasing hormone (TRH)	Rat	Anaesthetized	—	Gel	Plasma TRH	20%	
Alsactide (ACTH analogue)	Rat		—	Solution	Plasma cortisone. Adrenal ascorbic acid	12%	
LHRH agonists (D-Leu^6-ethylamide, D-Trp^6-ethylamide, D-Ser(But)^6-ethylamide [buserelin]	Rat	Anaesthetized to dose	—	—	Inhibition of ovulation	All equally effective (≈ 1% of i.v.)	Sandow and Petri 1985
IgG Caerulein	Rabbit Dog	— Anaesthetized	— —	Nebulizer Spray solution	Serum IgG Gall bladder stimulation	Absorbed Absorbed	Inagaki et al., 1984 Agosti and Bertaccini, 1969
[3H] SS6 (Somatostatin analogue)	Rat	Anaesthetized	In vivo	Solution	Plasma radioactivity and SS6	73%	McMartin and Peters; 1986;
Horseradish peroxidase (HRP)	Rat	Anaesthetized	In vivo	Solution	Blood HRP	0.6%	McMartin et al., 1987

(continued)

Table 1. 1.1 *Peptides and Proteins (Continued)*

Compound	Species	Anaesthetized/ Conscious	In situ/ In vivo of Hirai	Method of administration	Parameter measured	Absorption	Authors
Cholecystokinin octapeptide	Dog	Anaesthetized	—	Solution	Gall bladder contraction	As effective as i.v. at 80 times i.v. dose	Lonovics et al., 1980
Human epidermal growth factor	Rat	Anaesthetized	In vivo	Solution Plus promoters	Plasma hEGF / Plasma hEGF	Not detected / Up to 90%	Murakami et al., 1987
Recombinant human growth hormone	Rat	Anaesthetized	In vivo	Solution Plus surfactants	Plasma hGH / Plasma hGH	$<1\%$ / 11–80%	Daugherty et al., 1988
Growth hormone releasing hormone (GH-RH) analogues	Rat	Anaesthetized	—	Solution plus enhancer	Serum GH	4–10 times increase over control	Raehs et al., 1988 a
Synthetic rat atrial natriuretic factor	Rat	Anaesthetized	—	Solution	Diuresis and natriuresis	Increased diuresis and natriuresis	Shionori et al., 1987
SKF 101926 (vasopressin agonist)	Dog	Conscious	—	Solution	Antidiuretic response	3–21% c.f. i.v.	Liversidge et al., 1988
L-tyr-gly	Rat	Anaesthetized	In situ	In perfusate	Perfusate L-tyr-gly	Not absorbed	
L-tyr-L-arg (Kyotorphin)	Rat	Anaesthetized	In situ	In perfusate	Perfusate L-tyr-L-arg	Not absorbed	Tengamnuay and Mitra, 1988 b
L-tyr-D-arg	Rat	Anaesthetized	In situ	In perfusate Plus promoter	Perfusate L-tyr-D-arg / Perfusate L-tyr-D-arg	Not absorbed / Significant absorption	
[3H] [D-ala2] Met-enkephalinamide	Rabbit	Conscious	—	Solution via lacrymal sac/naso-lacrymal duct	Plasma radio-activity	17.6% c.f. i.v.	Stratford et al., 1988

Compound	Species	Anaesthetized/Conscious	In situ/In vivo of Hirai	Method of administration	Parameter measured	Absorption	Authors
Dermorphine and A-2 analogue	Rat	Conscious	—	Solution	Analgesic activity	Low dose strong and prolonged analgesia. Lost at high doses	Baturina et al., 1988
Glucagon	Rabbit	Conscious	—	—	Blood glucose	Rapid onset of action	Soerensen et al., 1988
[³H] Dalargin	Dog	Anaesthetized	—	—	Blood radioactivity	8%	Vinogradov et al., 1988

1.2 *Steroids*

Compound	Species	Anaesthetized/Conscious	In situ/In vivo of Hirai	Method of administration	Parameter measured	Absorption	Authors
[³H] Testosterone	Rat	Anaesthetized	In vivo	Solution	Blood testosterone	99 and 90%	Hussain et al., 1984 c Hussain et al., 1981; Bawarshi, 1981
[¹⁴C] Progesterone	Rat	Conscious	In vivo	Solution	Blood progesterone	100%	
[³H] Progesterone	Monkey	Conscious	—	Spray solvent	Serum and c.s.f. radioactivity	Radioactivity present	Sehgal et al., 1980
	Monkey	Conscious	—	Spray powder	Serum and c.s.f. radioactivity	Radioactivity present	
Progesterone	Monkey	Conscious	—	Nasal spray	Serum and c.s.f. progesterone	>100% in both c.f. i.v. over one hour.	David et al., 1981
Progesterone	Monkey	Conscious	—	Nasal drops	Serum and c.s.f. progesterone	43% serum, 14% c.s.f. c.f. i.v. over 1 hour.	
Progesterone	Monkey	Conscious	—	Nasal spray	Ovulation, serum progesterone, oestradiol and LH	Dose-related supression of ovulation Serum concentrations reduced	David et al., 1985
Progesterone	Monkey	Anaesthetized	—	Nasal spray	Serum and c.s.f. progesterone	100% from both fluids c.f. i.v. infusion	Anand Kumar et al., 1982

(continued)

Table 1.2 *Steroids (Continued)*

Compound	Species	Anaesthetized/Conscious	In situ/In vivo of Hirai	Method of administration	Parameter measured	Absorption	Authors
Progesterone	Monkey	Conscious	—	Nasal spray	Ovulation suppression from progesterone and oestradiol in serum.	Suppressed	Anand Kumar et al., 1977
Norethisterone	Monkey	Conscious	—	Nasal spray		Suppressed at higher doses	
Progesterone	Monkey	Conscious	—	Nasal spray	Serum testosterone, sperm count.	Decrease in sperm count	Moudgal et al., 1985
Norethisterone	Monkey	Conscious	—	Nasal spray	Serum testosterone, sperm count. Menstrual cycle length, circulating steroids and hormones	Decrease in all parameters	
[³H] Progesterone	Monkey	Conscious	—	Nasal spray	Plasma, c.s.f. and tissue radioactivity	Radioactivity present	Anand Kumar et al., 1974
[³H] 17β-Oestradiol	Monkey	Conscious	—	Nasal spray	Plasma, c.s.f. and tissue radioactivity	Radioactivity present	
Progesterone	Monkey	Conscious	—	Nasal spray	Serum and c.s.f. progesterone and inhibition of ovulation	Absorbed. Some suppression of ovulation	Anand Kumar et al., 1979
Norethisterone	Monkey	Conscious	—	Nasal spray	Serum and c.s.f. norethisterone and inhibition of ovulation	Absorbed. Some suppression of ovulation	

Compound	Animal				Parameters measured	Result	Reference
Progesterone	Monkey	Anaesthetized	—	Suspension	Plasma and c.s.f. progesterone	Absorbed. C.s.f. concentrations low	Öhman et al., 1978
Norethindrone	Monkey	Anaesthetized	—	Suspension	Plasma and c.s.f norethindrone	Absorbed. C.s.f. concentrations low	
Progesterone	Monkey	Conscious	—	Nasal spray	Testicular size, spermatogenesis, serum testosterone	All parameters reduced	Anand Kumar et al., 1980
Norethisterone	Monkey	Conscious	—	Nasal spray	Testicular size, spermatogenesis, serum testosterone	All parameters reduced	
17β-Oestradiol	Monkey	Conscious	—	Nasal spray	Testicular size, spermatogenesis, serum testosterone	All parameters reduced	
17β-Oestradiol	Monkey	Anaesthetized	—	Suspension	Plasma and c.s.f. oestradiol	Absorbed. C.s.f. concentrations low.	Öhman et al., 1980
	Monkey	Anaesthetized	—	Nasal spray			
17β-Oestradiol	Rat	Anaesthetized	In vivo	Solution	Blood oestrogens, oestradiol and oestrone	50–84% unchanged	Bawarshi, 1981
17α-Ethinyl oestradiol	Rat	Anaesthetized	In vivo	Solution	Blood 17α-ethinyl oestradiol	80–85%	
Norethisterone	Monkey	Conscious	—	Nasal spray	Ovulation, serum oestradiol, LH, progesterone	Some suppression of ovulation, serum concentrations down	Puri et al., 1986
5α-Androst-16-en-3-one	Pig	Conscious	—	Spray	Plasma oxytocin	Absorbed. Oxytocin released	Mattioli et al., 1986
[³H] Progesterone	Rat	Anaesthetized	In situ	In perfusate	Perfusate radioactivity	Absorbed	Gibson and Olanoff, 1987
[³H] Testosterone	Rat	Anaesthetized	In situ	In perfusate	Perfusate radioactivity	Absorbed	
[³H] Hydrocortisone	Rat	Anaesthetized	In situ	In perfusate	Perfusate radioactivity	Absorbed	

(continued)

Table 1. 1.2 *Steroids (Continued)*

Compound	Species	Anaesthetized/Conscious	In situ/In vivo of Hirai	Method of administration	Parameter measured	Absorption	Authors
Progesterone	Rabbit	Conscious	—	Solution from nasal device or spray	Plasma progesterone	72–82%	Corbo *et al.*, 1988
Progesterone and hydroxy derivatives	Rabbit	Conscious	—	Solution from spray or controlled release device	Plasma progesterone	61–97% or 78–88%	Corbo *et al.*, 1989
[14C] Progesterone	Rat	Anaesthetized	In vivo	Solution	Blood progesterone	100%	Bawarshi-Nassar *et al.*, 1989 a
17β-Oestradiol	Rat	Anaesthetized	In vivo	Solution	Blood oestradiol	50–84%	Bawarshi-Nassar *et al.*, 1989 b
17α-Ethinylol-oestradiol	Rat	—	—	Solutions	Blood 17α-ethinylol-oestradiol	80–85%	

1.3 *Gases and vapours*

Compound	Species	Anaesthetized/Conscious	In situ/In vivo of Hirai	Method of administration	Parameter measured	Absorption	Authors
Phosgene	Rabbit	Anaesthetized	—	Gas chamber	Chamber/nose phosgene	25%	
	Monkey	Anaesthetized	—	Gas chamber	Chamber/nose phosgene	33%	
Mustard gas	Rabbit	Anaesthetized	—	Gas chamber	Chamber/nose mustard gas	80%	Cameron *et al.*, 1946
	Monkey	Anaesthetized	—	Gas chamber	Chamber/nose mustard gas	80%	
Nitrogen mustard gas	Rabbit	Anaesthetized	—	Gas chamber	Chamber/nose nitrogen mustard	90%	

Substance	Animal	State		Method	Measurement	Absorption	Reference
Ozone	Dog	Anaesthetized	—	Face mask —nose only	Tracheal ozone	30–70%	Yokoyama and Frank, 1972
Ozone	Rabbit	Anaesthetized	—	Gas chamber	Tracheal/chamber ozone	50%	Miller et al., 1979
Ozone	Guinea pig	Anaesthetized	—	Gas chamber	Tracheal/chamber ozone	50%	
[35S] Sulphur dioxide	Dog	Anaesthetized	—	Face mask — nose only	Tracheal sulphur dioxide	100%	Frank et al., 1969; Brain, 1970
Acetaldehyde	Dog	Anaesthetized	—	Mask—nose only	Tracheal/mask acealdehyde	50–68%	Egle, 1972 a
Propionaldehyde	Dog	Anaesthetized	—	Mask—nose only	Mask/Tracheal propionaldehyde	60–80%	
Acrolein	Dog	Anaesthetized	—	Mask—nose only	Mask/tracheal acrolein	60–80%	Egle, 1972 b
Formaldehyde	Dog	Anaesthetized	—	Mask—nose only	Mask/tracheal formaldehyde	100%	
Hydrogen fluoride	Rat	Anaesthetized	—	Gas chamber	Tracheal/chamber/plasma hydrogen fluoride	100%	Morris and Smith, 1982
Carbon monoxide (in cigarette smoke)	Monkey	Anaesthetized	—	Face mask	Blood carbon monoxide	None	Schoenfisch et al., 1980
Polypropylene glycol monomethyl ether	Rat	Anaesthetized	—	Face mask	Tracheal concentration	96%	
Polypropylene glycol monomethyl ether acetate	Rat	Anaesthetized	—	Face mask	Tracheal concentration	94%	
Ethyl acrylate	Rat	Anaesthetized	—	Face mask	Tracheal concentration	66%	Stott et al., 1986
Nitroethane	Rat	Anaesthetized	—	Face mask	Tracheal concentration	65%	
Epichlorohydrin	Rat	Anaesthetized	—	Face mask	Tracheal concentration	61%	
Styrene	Rat	Anaesthetized	—	Face mask	Tracheal concentration	57%	
Ethylene dibromide	Rat	Anaesthetized	—	Face mask	Tracheal concentration	49%	
Methylene chloride	Rat	Anaesthetized	—	Face mask	Tracheal concentration	13%	

(continued)

1.4 *Inorganics*

Compound	Species	Anaesthetized/ Conscious	In situ/ In vivo of Hirai	Method of administration	Parameter measured	Absorption	Authors
Potassium ferrocyanide and iron ammonium citrate (Prussian blue particles on fixation)	Rabbit	Conscious	—	Solution	Blue particles	Observed in brain, lymph and blood vessels	le Gross Clark, 1929
Prussian blue	Cat	Conscious	—	Solution	Blue particles	Observed in lymphatic	Blumgart, 1924
Potassium iodide	Cat	Anaesthetized	—	Solution	Urinary KI	Present	
[137Cs] Caesium chloride	Hamster	Anaesthetized	—	Solution	Whole body counting	75%	
[85Sr] Strontium chloride	Hamster	Anaesthetized	—	Solution	Whole body counting	77%	Cuddihy and Ozog, 1973
[133Ba] Barium chloride	Hamster	Anaesthetized	—	Solution	Whole body counting	61%	
[144Ce] Cerium chloride	Hamster	Anaesthetized	—	Solution	Whole body counting	4%	
Zinc sulphate	Rat	Anaesthetized to dose	—	Solution	Weight loss	—	Thor and Flannelly, 1977
[75Se] Selenious acid	Dog	Conscious	—	Suspension	Whole body counting	80%	Weissman *et al.*, 1979
[75Se] Selenious acid	Rat	Anaesthetized	—	Suspension	Whole body counting	18%	
[75Se] Selenium	Rat	Anaesthetized	—	Suspension	Whole body counting	16%	Medinsky *et al.*, 1981

1.5 *Amino acids*

Compound	Species	Anaesthetized/ Conscious	In situ/ In vivo of Hirai	Method of administration	Parameter measured	Absorption	Authors
Glycine	Rabbit	—	—	—	Serum radioactivity	5% in 1 hour	Münzel and Eichner, 1975
Proline	Rabbit	—	—	—	Serum radioactivity	2% in 1 hour	
[14C] Glycine	Rabbit	Anaesthetized	—	Solution	Autoradiography	To lamina propria	Münzel, 1972
[14C] Serine	Rabbit	Anaesthetized	—	Solution	Autoradiography	To lamina propria	
[14C] Arginine	Rabbit	Anaesthetized	—	Solution	Autoradiography	To lamina propria	
[14C] Glutamic acid	Rabbit	Anaesthetized	—	Solution	Autoradiography	To lamina propria	
[14C] Proline	Rabbit	Anaesthetized	—	Solution	Autoradiography	To lamina propria	
L-Tyrosine	Rat	Anaesthetized	In situ	In perfusate	Perfusate L-tyrosine	None	Bawarshi, 1981
L-Tyrosine derivatives, O-Acyl, N-Acyl, carboxyl esters	Rat	Anaesthetized	In situ	In perfusate	Perfusate amino acid	All absorbed	Huang et al., 1985 b; Hussain et al., 1985 a
L-tyrosine	Rat	Anaesthetized	In situ	In perfusate	Perfusate L-tyr	26–74%	
D-tyrosine	Rat	Anaesthetized	In situ	In perfusate	Perfusate D-tyr	15–21%	Tengamnuay and Mitra, 1988 a
D-phenylalanine	Rat	Anaesthetized	In situ	In perfusate	Perfusate D-phe	5–27%	
L-phenylalanine	Rat	Anaesthetized	In situ	In perfusate Plus inhibitors	Perfusate L-phe	23–92% 26–48% of control	

(continued)

Progress in Drug Metabolism

1.6 *Carbohydrates*

Compound	Species	Anaesthetized/ Conscious	In situ/ In vivo of Hirai	Method of administration	Parameter measured	Absorption	Authors
D-Glucose	Rat	Anaesthetized	In situ	In perfusate	Perfusate glucose	None	Bawarshi, 1981
Inulin	Rat	Anaesthetized	Both	Solution/in perfusate	Cavity/perfusate inulin	None	
Fluorescein isothiocyanate (FITC) dextran	Rat	Anaesthetized	In situ	In perfusate	Perfusate FITC dextran	None	Kotani et al., 1983
[^{3}H] Inulin	Rat	Anaesthetized	Simplified	Solution	Plasma or urine radioactivity	15.5%	
[^{3}H] Dextran (Av. mol. wt 70 000)	Rat	Anaesthetized	Simplified	Solution	Plasma or bile and urine radioactivity	2.3%	Fisher et al., 1987
[^{3}H] Mannitol	Rat	Anaesthetized	In situ	In perfusate	Perfusate radioactivity	None	Gibson and Olanoff, 1987
[^{3}H] Inulin	Rabbit	Conscious	—	Solution via lacrymal sac/naso-lacrymal duct	Plasma radioactivity	6.5% c.f. i.v.	Stratford et al., 1988
FITC Dextrans	Rabbit	Conscious	—	Powder	Plasma FITC dextran	Not detected	
				Plus promoter	Plasma FITC dextran	Absorbed	Maitani et al., 1989
DEAE Dextrans	Rabbit	Conscious	—	Powder	Plasma DEAE dextran	Not detected	
				Plus promoter	Plasma DEAE dextran	Absorbed	

1.7 *Particulates*

Compound	Species	Anaesthetized/ Conscious	In situ/ In vivo of Hirai	Method of administration	Parameter measured	Absorption	Authors
Lead carbonate	Dog	Conscious	—	Atomizer	Lead in tissues	5%	Blumgart, 1923
	Cat	Conscious	—	Atomizer	Lead in tissues	10%	
Colloidal silver	Cat	Conscious	—	Suspension	Tissue silver	Present in lymph	Blumgart, 1924
Ivory black	Cat	Conscious	—	Suspension	Tissue black	Absent from lymph	
Fixed *Staphylococcus aureus*	Cat	Conscious	—	Suspension	Tissue organisms	Absent from lymph	
Graphite suspension	Cat	Anaesthetized	—	Suspension	Lymph graphite	None	Yoffey and Drinker, 1938
Vaccinia virus	Monkey	Anaesthetized to dose	—	Suspension	Lymphatic virus	Present (after 12 hours)	Yoffey and Sullivan, 1939
	Rabbit	Anaesthetized to dose	—	Suspension	Lymphatic virus	Present (after 12 hours)	
	Monkey	Anaesthetized	—	Suspension	Lymphatic virus	Absent (up to 12 hours)	
	Rabbit	Anaesthetized	—	Suspension	Lymphatic virus	Absent (up to 12 hours)	
	Cat	Anaesthetized	—	Suspension	Lymphatic virus	Absent (up to 12 hours)	
Mycobacterium leprae	Mouse	Anaesthetized to dose	—	Suspension	Histological examination	Penetration to subepithelium	Job et al., 1987
Cigarette smoke	Rabbit	Anaesthetized	—	Smoke stream	Removal of organics	32%	Dalhamn et al., 1971
Colloidal gold	Monkey	Conscious	—	Nasal spray	Electron microscopy of gold particles	Particles in olfactory neurones and blood vessels	Gopinath et al., 1978

(continued)

Table 1. 1.8 *Other compounds*

Compound	Species	Anaesthetized/Conscious	In situ/In vivo of Hirai	Method of administration	Parameter measured	Absorption	Authors
Phenol red	Cat	Anaesthetized	—	Solution	Urinary phenol red	Present	Blumgart, 1924
Trypan blue	Cat	Anaesthetized	—	Solution	Blood and lymph Trypan blue	Present	
	Dog	Anaesthetized	—	Solution	Blood and lymph Trypan blue	Present	
Evans blue	Cat	Anaesthetized	—	Solution	Blood and lymph Evans blue	Present	Yoffey and Drinker, 1938
	Dog	Anaesthetized	—	Solution	Blood and lymph Evans blue	Present	
	Rabbit	Anaesthetized	—	Solution	Blood and lymph Evans blue	Present	
	Monkey	Anaesthetized	—	Solution	Blood and lymph Evans blue	Present	
Propranolol	Rat	Anaesthetized	*In vivo*	Solution	Blood propranolol	100%	Hussain *et al.*, 1979
Propranolol	Rat	Anaesthetized	*In vivo*	Solution	Blood propranolol	100%	
Propranolol	Rat	Anaesthetized	*In vivo*	Sustained release formulations	Blood propranolol	94–100%	Hussain *et al.*, 1980 a; Bawarshi, 1981
	Dog	Anaesthetized	—	Solution	Blood propranolol	100%	
	Dog	Anaesthetized	—	Sustained release formulations	Blood propranolol	100%	
Indenolol	Rat	Anaesthetized	*In vivo*	Solution	Blood indenolol	Complete (99%)	Babhair and Tariq, 1988
[3H] Clonidine	Mice	—	—	—	Plasma	100%	Babhair *et al.*, 1988

Drug	Animal	State	Method	Formulation	Measurement	Result	Reference
Naloxone	Rat	Anaesthetized	In vivo	Solution	Plasma naloxone	100%	Hussain et al., 1984 a
Buprenorphine	Rat	Anaesthetized	In vivo	Solution	Plasma buprenorphine	95%	
Verapamil	Dog	Anaesthetized for dosing	—	Solution	Plasma verapamil	36%	Arnold et al., 1985
Meclizine	Rat	Anaesthetized	In vivo	Solution	Blood meclizine	51%	Chovan et al., 1985
	Dog	Anaesthetized initially	—	Solution	Blood meclizine	89%	
[111In] Diethylene triamine penta-acetic acid (DTPA)	Rat	Anaesthetized	—	Solution	Whole body counting	30%	Dudley et al., 1980 a
[111In] DTPA	Dog	Anaesthetized	—	Solution	Whole body counting	16%	Dudley et al., 1980 b
Ergotamine tartrate	Rat	Anaesthetized	In vivo	Solution	Plasma ergotamine	62%	Hussain et al., 1984 b
Nicardipine	Rat	Anaesthetized	—	Solution	Plasma nicardipine	73%	Visor et al., 1986
	Rat	Anaesthetized	—	Viscous solution	Plasma nicardipine	77%	
Gentamicin	Rabbit	Anaesthetized to dose	—	Viscous solution	Plasma gentamicin	None	Duchateau et al., 1986 b
	Rabbit	Anaesthetized to dose	—	Plus bile salts	Plasma gentamicin	11–41%	
Gentamicin	Rat	Anaesthetized	Simplified	Solution	Serum gentamicin	Low	Illum et al., 1988
				Plus promoter	Serum gentamicin	5 times solution AUC	
	Sheep	Conscious		Solution	Serum gentamicin	<1% c.f. i.v.	
				Plus promoter	Serum gentamicin	<1% c.f. ...v.	
				Microspheres	Serum gentamicin	10% c.f. ...v.	
				Plus promoter	Serum gentamicin	50% c.f. ...v.	
Aminodeoxy-kanamycin	Rabbit	—	—	Nebulizer	Serum aminodeoxykan-amycin	Absorbed	Inagaki et al., 1984
[14C] Xylometazoline	Rat	Anaesthetized	In vivo	Solution	Whole body autoradiography	Part	Kitagawa et al., 1974
[14C] Tramazolin	Rabbit	—	—	—	Serum radioactivity	1% in 1 hour	Munzel and Eichner, 1975

(continued)

Table 1. 1.8   *Other compounds (Continued)*

Compound	Species	Anaesthetized/ Conscious	In situ/ In vivo of Hirai	Method of administration	Parameter measured	Absorption	Authors
Polyethylene glycol (PEG) 4000 PEG 20000	Rat	Anaesthetized	In situ	In perfusate	Perfusate PEG 4000	40–50%	Kotani et al., 1983
	Rat	Anaesthetized	In situ	In perfusate	Perfusate PEG 20000	40–50%	
Polyethylene glycols 600–2000	Rat	—	—	Solutions Plus adjuvants	—	5–50% Variable	Donovan et al., 1988
Salicylic acid	Rat	Anaesthetized	In situ	In perfusate	Perfusate salicylic acid	75% in 1 hour	
	Rat	Anaesthetized	In vivo	Solution	Plasma salicylic acid	Well absorbed	
Aminopyrine	Rat	Anaesthetized	In situ	In perfusate	Perfusate aminopyrine	30% in 1 hour	Hirai et al., 1981 a
Phenol red	Rat	Anaesthetized	In situ	In perfusate	Perfusate phenol red	None	
Bucolome	Rat	Anaesthetized	In vivo	Solution	Urinary phenol red	>35%	
Sulbenicillin	Rat	Anaesthetized	In vivo	Solution	Plasma bucolome	Well absorbed	
	Rat	Anaesthetized	In vivo	Solution	Urinary sulbenicillin	>25%	
Cefazolin	Rat	Anaesthetized	In vivo	Solution	Urinary cefazolin	>40%	
Cephacetrile	Rat	Anaesthetized	In vivo	Solution	Urinary cephacetrile	>35%	
Benzoic acid	Rat	Anaesthetized	In situ	In perfusate different pH	Perfusate benzoic acid	13–44% depending on pH	
Sodium barbital	Rat	Anaesthetized	In situ	In perfusate	Perfusate barbiturate	5%	Bawarshi, 1981; Huang et al., 1985a; Hussain et al., 1985a
Sodium phenobarbital	Rat	Anaesthetized	In situ	In perfusate	Perfusate barbiturate	11%	
Sodium pentobarbital	Rat	Anaesthetized	In situ	In perfusate	Perfusate barbiturate	20%	
Sodium secobarbital	Rat	Anaesthetized	In situ	In perfusate	Perfusate barbiturate	24%	

Drug	Animal		In vivo/situ	Formulation	Measurement	Result	Reference
Hydralazine	Rat	Anaesthetized	In situ	In perfusate, different pH	Perfusate hydralazine	30–60% depending on pH	Kaneo, 1983
	Rat	Anaesthetized	In vivo	Solution, different vehicles	Plasma hydralazine	83–100%	
Antipyrene, D₂O, inulin and FITC dextran	Rat	Anaesthetized	In situ	In perfusate	Perfusate concentrations	Water influx and sieving co-efficient calculated	Hayashi *et al.*, 1985
[¹⁴C] Clofilium tosylate [4-(p-chloro-phenyl)butyl] diethyl-heptyl ammonium tosylate	Rat	Anaesthetized	In vivo	Solution	Blood and tissue radioactivity	29–70%, dose dependent	Su *et al.*, 1984; Su and Campanale, 1985; Su *et al.*, 1987
[¹⁴C] LY140091 (anti-asthma)	Rat	Anaesthetized	In vivo	Solution (of salt)	Blood radioactivity	100%	Su and Campanale, 1985
	Rat	Anaesthetized	In vivo	Suspension (of acid)	Blood radioactivity	35%	
Phenol red	Rabbit	Anaesthetized to dose	—	Viscous solution plus surfactants	Serum phenol red	21–98%	Duchateau *et al.*, 1987
Sodium guaiazulene-3-sulphonate (GAS)	Rat	Anaesthetized	In vivo / In situ	Solution	Plasma GAS	20–64% concentration dependent	Mukai *et al.*, 1985; Seki *et al.*, 1985
[¹⁴C] or [³H] sodium cromoglycate	Rabbit	Anaesthetized	—	Solution	Plasma GAS	25–47%	Fisher *et al.*, 1985
	Rat	Anaesthetized	In vivo & simplified	Solution	Plasma or bile radioactivity	69%	
[¹⁴C] nedocromil sodium	Rat	Anaesthetized	Simplified	Solution	Plasma radioactivity	76%	Brown *et al.*, 1986

(continued)

Table 1. 1.8 *Other compounds (Continued)*

Compound	Species	Anaesthetized/ Conscious	In situ/ In vivo of Hirai	Method of administration	Parameter measured	Absorption	Authors
[³H] 4-oxo-4H-1-benzopyran-2-carboxylic acid	Rat	Anaesthetized	Simplified	Solution	Plasma or bile and urine radioactivity	100%	Fisher *et al.*, 1987
[³H] Para-aminohippuric acid	Rat	Anaesthetized	Simplified	Solution	Plasma or bile and urine radioactivity	81%	
Dobutamine HCl	Rat	Anaesthetized	*In vivo*	Solution	Plasma dobutamine	Extensive. More complete from posterior of cavity	
	Dog	Anaesthetized		Solution	Plasma dobutamine, cardiac activity	Extensive	Su *et al.*, 1987
	Dog	Anaesthetized		Aerosol and solution plus sustained release agents	Cardiac activity	Prolonged activity from sustained release aerosol and some agents	

	Species				Detection	Result	Reference
[14C] Decanoic acid	Rat	Anaesthetized	In situ	In perfusate	Perfusate radioactivity	Absorbed	Gibson and Olanoff, 1987
[14C] Octanoic acid	Rat	Anaesthetized	In situ	In perfusate	Perfusate radioactivity	Absorbed	
[14C] Hexanoic acid	Rat	Anaesthetized	In situ	In perfusate	Perfusate radioactivity	Absorbed	
Hydromorphone	Rabbit	Anaesthetized	"In situ"	In perfusate	Plasma hydromorphone	Complete (103%)	Chang et al., 1988
Tetraethylammonia	Rat	—	—	—	—	80%	Kimura et al., 1987
[14C] Benzo[a]pyrene	Dog	Anaesthetized	—	Suspension in gelatine	Blood or urine radioactivity	Not detected	Petridou-Fischer et al., 1988
	Monkey	Anaesthetized	—	Suspension in gelatine	Blood or urine radioactivity	Not detected	
[3H] Dihydrosafrole	Dog	Anaesthetized	—	Suspension in saline	Blood or urine radioactivity	Absorbed	Petridou-Fischer et al., 1987
	Monkey	Anaesthetized	—	Suspension in saline	Blood or urine radioactivity	Absorbed	

isolated nasal cavity. After instillation of material into the nose, it is sealed, and blood or urine samples collected to determine the amount of material present. With the *in situ* recirculating technique of Hirai *et al.* (1981 a), the surgical preparation is similar but the nasal cavity is continually perfused with a solution containing the compound of interest. Concentrations of compound in the perfusate are periodically determined. The technique of Hirai *et al.* (1981 a) is indicated because using the *in vivo* preparation absorption should be maximal, while the results from the *in situ* technique are not always reliable. Indeed *in vivo* and *in situ* results with the same compound do not always agree as demonstrated by Hirai and colleagues themselves with phenol red (1981 a). Furthermore, Bawarshi (1981) concluded that L-tyrosine was not absorbed when using the *in situ* technique. However, later, the same laboratory, also using the *in situ* technique, demonstrated absorption of this compound (Huang *et al.*, 1985 b; Hussain *et al.*, 1985 a). A simplified version of the Hirai technique has been developed (Fisher *et al.*, 1985). This preparation also maximized absorption and is indicated for routine investigations.

The rat has been widely used in the studies listed in Table 1. There are several, conventional, reasons for using the rat. It is cheap to buy and maintain, it breeds readily, rapidly reaches maturity, and there are many well defined strains available. Most areas of the structure, anatomy and physiology have been well defined. Experimentally the rat is easy to handle and use, and relatively small amounts of dose material are required. The animal is easy to modify surgically, and, with regard to nasal studies, this yields a useful preparation.

Table 1 demonstrates that most compounds administered to the animal nasal cavity are absorbed. However, few of the studies listed examined or discussed the mechanisms of nasal absorption.

3. Structure of the rat nasal cavity

As discussed above, the rat is a commonly used and convenient laboratory species and it has been used by Hirai *et al.* (1981 a) and several others (Table 1) to study nasal absorption. Furthermore, it is a species widely used for inhalation toxicity studies as described in texts edited by Reznick and Stinson (1983) and Barrow (1986). The significance of the rat in inhalation studies is that because of the close apposition of the epiglottis and soft palate the animal is an obligatory nasal breather (Negus, 1958; Proctor and Chang, 1983).

The structure of the rat nose reflects its functions, which are conduction, olfaction, filtration, air conditioning, mucociliary transport, metabolism and resonance. To conduct air from the external atmosphere to the trachea and lungs requires a tube, or tubes, of suitable dimensions. The olfactory mucosa is logically located in the nose where it can continually monitor the environment. Negus throughout his comparative text (1958) considers the sense of smell to be the primary function of the nose. He maintains that the emphasis on the study of man, with his rather poor sense of smell, has distorted our view of the function of the nose in the rest of the animal kingdom. This idea has been borne out by subsequent publications and only recently has the importance of olfaction in animals been rediscovered (Schreider 1986).

The functions of filtration, air conditioning, mucociliary clearance and metabolism are all protective mechanisms for the animal in general, and for the lower respiratory tract in particular (Proctor, 1964; Brain *et al.*, 1977; Proctor and Andersen, 1982; Schreider, 1986). The ciliated, moist, mucous-lined and tortuous airways with enzymically active mucosa all play a part in protection. Filtration removes larger particles from the air which are then removed mechanically or trapped in the mucous coat and removed by muco-ciliary clearance. Material, particulate or soluble vapours, can be trapped directly in the mucous layer and then removed. Air conditioning warms and humidifies air on its way to the lungs and recovers moisture and heat from expired air. The nasal mucosa contains systems to metabolize both foreign and endogenous compounds (Brittebo *et al.*, 1986; Bond, 1986; Dahl, 1986), the production of less toxic material being an obvious protective mechanism. Lysozyme is also present to destroy bacteria. Some, or all, of these protective functions could also play a part in olfaction. Negus (1958) suggested that a moist environment is essential for olfaction, while Dahl (1986) suggests that by metabolism and production of less odiferous materials the acuity of the sense of smell is maintained.

The resonance of air in the nasal passages of man is very important in vocalization; it will, presumably, play a reduced role in other animal species.

The large amount of effort directed towards the study of the human nose, its structures and properties, in whole or in part, has produced many compre-hensive texts (Brain *et al.*, 1977, 1978; Proctor and Anderson, 1982). How-ever, the rat nasal cavity has, by comparison, been very poorly described. In 1946, Keleman and Sargent stated: 'Monographs on the anatomy of the rat are sketchy in regard to the nose, and illustrations of the nasal cavity are few; text books on comparative anatomy mention the conditions found in the nasal cavity of the rat in barest outline'. Nearly forty years later, Reznik (1983) stated that: 'Thorough descriptions of the nasal cavity of the rat are rare'. The following description is based upon Kelemen and Sargent (1946); Negus (1958); Rhodin (1974); Hebel and Stromberg (1976); Gross *et al.*, 1982; Proctor and Chang (1983); Reznik (1983); Menco (1983); Schreider (1986); Young (1986); Popp *et al.* (1986); and Morgan *et al.* (1986 a).

Gross anatomy

There are two, approximately symmetrical nasal cavities incompletely separ-ated by a cartilagenous nasal septum. The base of the cavity is separated from the buccal cavity by the palate and the posterior of the cavity is separated from the brain by the cribriform plate. This cribriform plate is perforated by olfactory nerve axons. At the anterior end of the cavity are the narrow

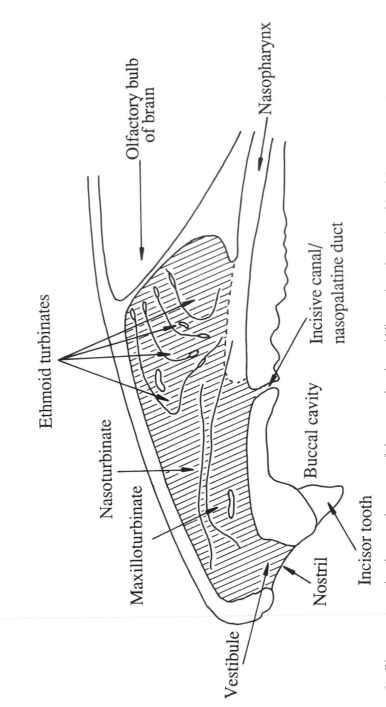
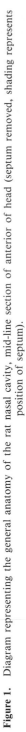

Figure 1. Diagram representing the general anatomy of the rat nasal cavity, mid-line section of anterior of head (septum removed, shading represents position of septum).

external openings, the nares, or nostrils; these lie on a narrow region of naked skin above the cloven upper lip, the rhinarium. The posterior exit from the cavity is into the nasopharynx. Surrounding the nasal cavities are the anterior bones of the skull. These bones are covered with cartilage, which projects and folds into the cavity forming turbinates. The entire surface of the nasal cavity, including the septum, is covered with a mucous epithelium.

Figure 1 represents a mid-line section of the nasal part of a rat head with the nasal septum removed. Immediately inside the nostrils is the vestibule region. Just inside and outside the vestibule are two folds of cartilage described as atrioturbinals. In the body of the nasal cavity projecting down from, and originating from, the nasal bone is the nasal turbinate, while projecting up from, and originating from, the maxillary bone is the maxillary turbinate. Both these turbinates have a folded structure described as a double scroll. There is a canal in the ventral floor of the cavity linking it to the buccal cavity; this is the incisive canal or nasopalatine duct. At the posterior of the cavity are the ethmoid turbinates which originate from the ethmoid bone. These turbinates are multiple and complexly folded structures. The number of them seems to be disputed, but generally there are considered to be five. They are not all illustrated in Figure 1 as those nearer the septum, the endoturbinates, overlie those nearer the lateral wall, the ectoturbinates.

The nasal septum is incomplete in rats and the two nasal cavities freely communicate in the posterior ventral region before they join to become the nasopharynx. Within the ventral surface of the septum is a paired tubular structure, the nasovomeral organ or organ of Jacobson, the function of which is unclear. Also in the ventral septum are swell bodies formed from vascular spaces. When collapsed, these swell bodies allow the free flow of air under the

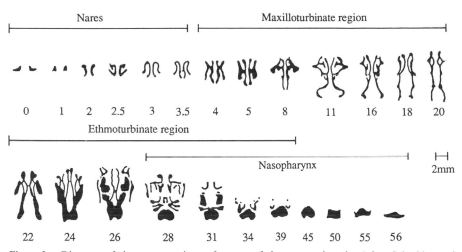

Figure 2. Diagram of the cross sections of a cast of the rat nasal cavity (after Schreider and Raabe, 1980, with permission). Numbers under each section correspond to the distance in mm from the tip of the nares.

maxilloturbinate, but when distended, air flows over the maxilloturbinate. Paranasal sinuses exist in the rat but the number and size of them is disputed. The maxillary sinus is described as high and narrow by Kelemen and Sargent (1946), small by Negus (1958), as a large recess by Hebel and Stromberg (1976) while Schreider (1986) just points out that they are present. Both Kelemen and Sargent (1946) and Negus (1958) state that the rat has no frontal sinus while Schreider (1986) states that it does. Only Negus (1958) mentions the sphenoid sinus, but only to dismiss it as small or absent. The complexity of the three-dimensional structure of the nasal cavity is difficult to visualize and describe. Thus, the problems with identifying the ethmoid turbinates or accessory sinuses are not surprising. However, Schreider and Raabe (1980, 1981) took casts of the entire respiratory tract of several species, and cut serial sections of the cast. Their cross sections of the rat nasal cavity are represented in Figure 2. This clearly demonstrates the complexity of the airway system.

Estimates have been made of the volume of the entire nasal cavity. These vary between 0.4 ml (Schreider and Raabe, 1980), 0.2–0.3 ml (Hirai *et al.*, 1981 a) and 0.257 ml (Gross *et al.*, 1982). The surface area has been estimated to be 13.4 cm^2 for a 290 g rat (Gross *et al.*, 1982) or 10.4 cm^2 for a 250 g rat (Schreider, 1986). A comparison will be made with man in a later section of this review.

Mucus

The surface of the nasal cavity is covered with a continuous sheet of mucus (Morgan *et al.*, 1986 a) which is secreted by various mucosal and submucosal glands. Mucus is composed of two phases, a gel-like epiphase which floats on a more watery hypophase. When viewed with an electron microscope there is a definite osmiophilic membrane on the luminal surface of the mucus. The mucous layer flows over both ciliated and non-ciliated regions, propelled by the beating action of cilia. The direction of mucous streaming was originally described by Lucas and Douglas (1933–34) and more recently, and in great detail, by Morgan *et al.* (1984). Briefly, there is a main ventral stream of mucus moving in a posterior direction along the floor of the nasal cavity to the nasopharynx. Mucus from the maxilliary sinus and ethmoid turbinates flows laterally into this main stream. There is a second major stream along the anterior half of the dorsal surface of the cavity. This flows in an anterior direction until it reaches the edge of the vestibule region when it transfers in a lateral direction to the ventral stream. Transfer of mucus laterally from dorsal to ventral streams takes place along the length of the cavity and down the septum. Morgan *et al.* (1984) give an informative and detailed description of the rat mucociliary apparatus. This group has extended their work to examine the effect of nasal irritants on the mucociliary apparatus (Morgan *et al.*, 1986 a,b).

The surface pH of the rat mucosa has been estimated to be 7.2 by Dietz (1944) and 7.39 by Hirai *et al.* (1981 a), i.e. it is neutral.

Nasal epithelia

There are three distinct types of epithelium in the rat nasal mucosa: squamous, respiratory and olfactory. The approximate distribution of these epithelia is indicated in Figure 3. Gross *et al.* (1982) estimated that in a 290 g rat the proportions of these epithelia were 3 per cent squamous, 47 per cent respiratory and 50 per cent olfactory.

Squamous epithelium lines the vestibule, the anterior part of the nasal turbinate, and the floor of the cavity up to the nasopalatine duct. It is a simple stratified squamous epithelium with some coarse hairs (vibrissae) present. The degree of keratinization is unclear; Proctor and Chang (1983) state that it is keratinized, Rhodin (1974) notes moderate keratinization, while Reznik (1983) states that it is not keratinized. It is likely that the amount of keratin decreases from the exterior surface to the interior of the cavity; thus, the degree of keratinization found will depend upon the position examined. The lamina propria beneath the epithelium consists of a simple collagenous stroma which contains few glands.

The respiratory epithelium is shown diagramatically in Figure 4. It is described as simple cuboidal or columnar pseudostratified and is similar to that found throughout the respiratory tract. There are generally four types of cell present, ciliated, non-ciliated, goblet and basal. A fifth type of cell, the brush cell, has been described by Popp and Martin (1984). The ciliated and non-ciliated cell surfaces are covered with microvilli, and the ciliated cells have numerous cilia. Within the nasal cavity there is a trend for increasing ciliary cell density and increasing ciliary length in an anterior to posterior

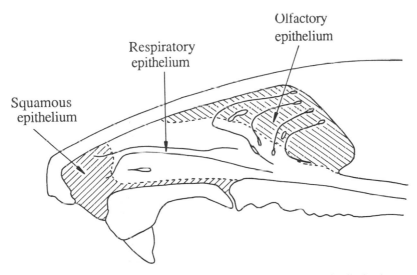

Figure 3. Diagram showing the approximate locations of different epithelia in the rat nasal cavity.

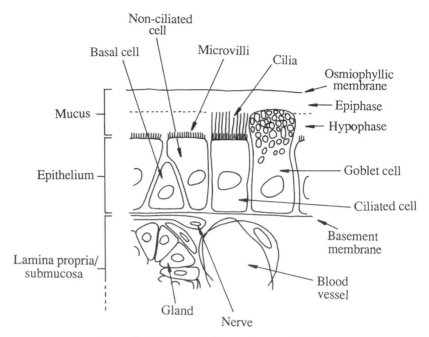

Figure 4. Diagram of the respiratory epithelium.

direction (Jiang *et al.*, 1983). There are many goblet cells in the epithelium that discharge on local stimulation. The epithelium sits on a thin basement membrane, below which is the lamina propria. This layer is collagenous and contains many glands, nerves and blood vessels. The glands are both serous and mucous types under the control of autonomic nerves. The blood supply is particularly rich: 0.5 per cent of cardiac output to upper respiratory tract in intact animals, 1 per cent with upper respiratory tract surgically isolated (Stott *et al.*, 1986); blood vessels are thin walled and subject to autonomic innervation, and there are many arteriovenous anastamoses (Hodde and de Blecourt, 1979; Nagai *et al.*, 1982, 1983). Yoffey and Courtice (1956) state that there are rich lymphatic plexes in the submucosa of the species studied, which did not include the rat. No other workers have commented on the lymphatic system of the rat nasal cavity; however, there is no reason to expect any differences from other species.

Figure 5 is a diagrammatic representation of the olfactory epithelium. It is a pseudostratified neuroepithelium with olfactory cells, sustentacular cells and basal cells. There are no ciliated or goblet cells present. The olfactory cells, or olfactory sensory neurones are unique in that they regenerate; their life span is estimated to be thirty to forty days (Doucette *et al.*, 1983) or thirty days (Schreider, 1986). These cells bear sensory cilia with knob-like endings which project into the mucous layer, and olfactory axons at the basal end which eventually combine to form the olfactory nerves. There are sustenta-

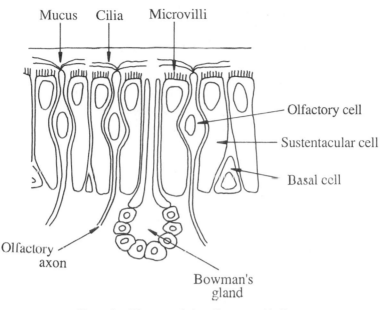

Figure 5. Diagram of the olfactory epithelium.

cular or support cells that have microvilli on their surface. These cells plus the basal cells, which may be the precursors for new neurons, all sit on a thin basal lamella. In the lamina propria is a rich blood supply, but not as rich as in the respiratory subepithelium, numerous nerve bundles of the olfactory nerve and numerous Bowman's glands, which are described as serous or mucoserous. There are no other submucosal glands present.

Enzymology

Except for the long established presence of lysozyme (e.g. Spector, 1956), one aspect of the nasal mucosa which has only become apparent in recent years, is that it has the ability to metabolize applied materials. Indeed, the cytochrome P450 content of the rat nasal mucosa, when expressed per gram of tissue, is second only to the liver (Dahl, 1986). Most of the published results on this topic come from either Brittebo, or Hadley and Dahl. Brittebo identified the rat nasal mucosa as a site of xenobiotic metabolism from the whole body autoradiographic distribution of systemically applied compounds. Investigations to date, which have not all been performed in the rat, include N-nitroso compounds (Brittebo and Tjalve, 1981; Brittebo *et al.*, 1981 a,b), aminopyrine (Brittebo, 1982 a), phenacetin (Brittebo, 1987), diethylnitrosamine (Longo *et al.*, 1986), progesterone (Brittebo, 1982 b), oestradiol (Brittebo, 1985), 3α- and 3β-hydroxysteroid dehydrogenases (Hancock and Gower, 1986), testosterone (Lupo *et al.*, 1986), cytochrome P450 studies (Hadley and Dahl, 1982, 1983; Dahl, 1982; Dahl *et al.*, 1982; Voigt *et al.*,

1985; Ding *et al.*, 1986; Reed *et al.*, 1986), including the potential for formaldehyde generation by thirty-two substrates (Dahl and Hadley, 1983), several reports of aminopeptidase activity (Stratford and Lee, 1986; Kashi and Lee, 1986), and carboxylesterase activity (Bogdanffy *et al.*, 1987). The work is briefly reviewed by Gram *et al.* (1986), while certain aspects are reviewed by Brittebo *et al.* (1986), Bond (1986) and Dahl (1986). With the increasing numbers of compounds applied to the nasal cavity, or the localization there of systemically administered materials, the metabolism, or lack of it, by the mucosa will become more important.

4. Validity of using the rat for intranasal studies

As described above, many compounds have been administered intranasally to man and animals. Furthermore, the structure of the nasal cavity is well understood in man and other species. However, the mechanisms of nasal absorption are not fully understood in any species. To justify the use of an animal model to predict nasal absorption in man the validity of using animals in general, and the rat in particular, must be considered.

A comparison of some features of rat and human nasal cavities is shown in Table 2. The values in this table are collected from a range of references previously cited in the section on the structure of the rat nasal cavity, which include some human data, and Spector (1956), Proctor (1964), Snyder *et al.* (1975) and Proctor and Andersen (1982).

Within the rat nasal cavity the structure is much more complex with a larger number of more folded turbinates. Man only has three simple turbinates in each half of the cavity and no ethmoid turbinates at all. However, in man paranasal sinuses are more numerous and larger in size. While sinuses are not located in the main nasal cavity itself, they are freely connected to it and lined with a simplified form of respiratory epithelium. The angle between the nasal cavity and the nasopharynx is only shallow in the rat but sharp in man, leading to an additional site for deposition by impaction.

As the rat is considerably smaller than man, the absolute dimensions of its nasal cavity are, obviously, much smaller. However, when nasal surface area is normalized for body weight, or body surface area, the rat has proportionally a much larger nasal surface area. This reflects the better developed sense of smell of the rat. If nasal cavity volume is similarly normalized, the results are equivocal. When normalized to body weight, nasal cavity volumes are similar, but when normalized for body surface area, the human nose has a proportionally larger volume. Any differences probably reflect the greater complexity of the rat nasal cavity.

The differences in structure and dimensions are related to the greater importance of the sense of smell to the rat. These factors will influence the deposition of aerosols, vapours and particles but not directly applied solutions. Extrapolations from rat to man, with regard to deposition, must be performed with caution.

Table 2. Comparison of rat and human nasal cavities.[1]

	Rat	Man
Weight (kg)	0.2–0.3	56–70
Body surface area (m^2)	0.03–0.05	1.7–1.8
Structure		
Turbinates		
Name, (total no.), form	Atrio-(4)	
	Naso-(2) double scroll	Superior (2) simple scroll
	Maxillo (2) double scroll	Middle (2) simple scroll
		Inferior (2) simple scroll
	Ethmoid-(10) complex	
Sinuses	Frontal—disputed	Frontal
	Sphenoid—unclear	Sphenoid
	Maxillary—size unclear	Maxillary
		Ethmoid
Septum	Incomplete	Complete
Organ of Jacobson	Present	Present but rudimentary
Lateral nasal gland	Present	Absent
Swell bodies	Present	Absent
Angle nasal cavity to nasopharynx	15°	90°
Dimensions		
Naris cross section (mm^2)	0.7	140
Greatest width (mm)	9.6	35–45
Length (cm)	2.3	7–14
Surface area (cm^2)		
Plus sinuses	10.4–13.4	—
without sinuses	—	120–181
Volume (cm^3)		
plus sinuses	0.2–0.4	53–80
without sinuses		15–20
sinus volume	—	37–60
Nasal surface area		
:body weight (cm^2.kg)	35–67	1.7–3.2
:body area (cm^2:m^2)	208–447	67–106
Nasal cavity volume with sinuses (without)		
:bodyweight (cm^3:kg)	0.7–2.0	0.8–1.4 (0.5–1.1)
:body area (cm^3:m^2)	4–13	29–47 (21–35)
Epithelia		
Structure	Very similar	Very similar perhaps more ciliated cells in respiratory epithelia
Area (%)		
Squamous	3	11–13 (includes all vestibule)
Respiratory	47	64–82
Olfactory	50	6–24
pH	Neutral	Slightly acid
Submucosa		
Structure	Very similar	Very similar
Physiology		
Nasal cycle	Present	Present
Breathing	Obligate nasal	Naso-oral
Temperature raised from ambient to body	Nostril to posterior nasal cavity	Nostril to lungs

[1] From several sources previously cited in the section on the structure of the rat nasal cavity, and Spector (1956), Proctor (1964), Snyder *et al.* (1975) and Proctor and Andersen (1982)

Table 3. Comparison of animal and human results following intranasal administration

Compound	Animal (from Table 1)		Human	
	Species	Result(s)	Result(s)	Reference(s)
Insulin	Rat	Variable, hypoglycaemia or no effect	Variable, hypoglycaemia and changes in insulin-related material or no effect	Chien and Chang, 1985; Flier et al., 1985
	Dog	Hypoglycaemia		
Insulin plus enhancer	Rat	30% of i.v. effect	10–20% of i.v. effect	Hirata et al., 1979; Flier et al., 1985
	Dog	25–30% of i.v. effect		
DDAVP	Rat	Effective antidiuresis	Prolonged and effective antidiuresis	Chien and Chang, 1985.
	Dog	Effective antidiuresis		
LHRH and analogues	Rat	0.1% (2–3% plus enhancer) or 16% absorbed	LH and FSH increased, 1% of i.v. effect	Chien and Chang, 1985.
Buserelin	Monkey	16–20% absorbed	1.25% absorbed	Bourguignon et al., 1974.
	Rat	Inhibition of ovulation 1% of i.v.	1–2.5% absorbed	Sandow and Petri, 1985.
Naferelin acetate	Monkey	2% absorbed	Inhibition of ovulation and ovarian levels reduced, 5% absorbed	Vickery et al., 1985
Alsactide	Rat	12% absorbed	Serum cortisone increased	Sandow and Petri, 1985.
TRH	Rat	20% absorbed	20% absorbed	Sandow and Petri, 1985.
Caerulein	Dog	Active gall bladder stimulation	Active gall bladder stimulation. Same degree of activity	Agosti and Bertaccini, 1969.
Salmon calcitonin	Rat	Fall in serum calcium Enhanced by promoters	Fall in serum calcium only with promoter	Hanson et al., 1986.

Substance	Animal		Reference
Salmon or eel calcitonin	Rat	Salmon as above. Eel only as gel reduced plasma calcium	Human calcitonin with surfactant. Large fall in serum calcium and rise in plasma calcitonin	Pontiroli *et al.*, 1986 b.
Cholecystokinin octapeptide	Dog	27–49% gall bladder contraction	20–45% gall bladder contraction	Lonovics *et al.*, 1980
17β-oestradiol	Rat	50–84% in blood	Absorption rapid and sustained, compound, LH and FSH measured	Chien and Chang, 1985.
	Monkey	Hormonal responses reduced, or radioactivity in body fluids		
Testosterone	Rat	90 or 99% absorbed	Rapid and significant rise in plasma testosterone	Danner and Frick, 1980.
Sulphur dioxide	Dog	100% absorbed	100% absorbed	Speizer and Frank, 1966; Proctor *et al.*, 1977
Ozone	Guinea pig	50% absorbed	40% absorbed	Andersen and Proctor, 1982.
	Rabbit	50% absorbed		
	Dog	30–70% absorbed		
Carbon monoxide	Monkey	None absorbed	None absorbed	Guyatt *et al.*, 1981.
Formaldehyde	Dog	100% absorbed	100% absorbed	Andersen and Proctor, 1982.
Propranolol	Rat	100% absorbed	100% absorbed	Hussair *et al.*, 1980 b; Chien and Chang, 1985.
Gentamicin	Rabbit	None absorbed	None absorbed	Chien and Chang, 1985.
Gentamicin plus enhancer	Rabbit	11–41% absorbed	Absorbed	

When the epithelia and submucosa of rat and man are compared they are found to be very similar. Rat has a larger proportion of olfactory epithelium, again reflecting its better developed sense of smell. Man, possibly, has more ciliated cells in his respiratory epithelium. However, the similarity between the membrane in the two species, and indeed most other mammals, must be stressed as it is highly significant. When soluble materials are applied directly onto the nasal mucosa of rat or man, the barriers to be crossed and the subsequent mechanisms for removal are thus very similar. Penetration of directly applied materials in solution should, therefore, be comparable between the species. A comparison of compounds which have been administered to both animals and man is shown in Table 3. The animal results are obtained from Table 1 and the human results are from the references cited. It can be seen that, for most compounds, there is a very good agreement between the animal and human results. This emphasizes the similarity between species in the membranes to be traversed by applied materials. Therefore, any of the species studied to date should be predictive for man.

Accordingly it can be concluded that the rat is a convenient and suitable species for the study of nasal absorption.

5. Mechanisms of nasal absorption

In 1972, Munzel stated that 'There is an inverted relation between the great number of substances applied and our knowledge about the chemical, physical and biological factors responsible for the resorption of these substances through the nasal mucosa into the organism'. Despite the wide and increasing use of the intranasal route, in both animals and man, since this

Table 4. Factors investigated that are involved in nasal absorption (references in text).

Factor investigated	Compound(s) used
Molecular size (water soluble compounds)	4-oxo-4H-1-benzopyran-2-carboxylic acid, para-amino hippuric acid, nedocromil sodium, sodium cromoglycate, inulin, dextran, FITC and DEAE dextrans
Lipid solubility	Barbiturates, steroids, progesterone and hydroxy derivatives
Ionization	Aminopyrine, benzoic acid, salicylic acid, hydralazine, alkanoic acids
Chemical modification	L-tyrosine
Carrier mediation	L-tyrosine, sodium guaiazulene-3-sulfonate, L-phenylalanine
Ion-pairing	Sodium guaiazulene-3-sulphonate
pH	Insulin, secretin
Blood flow	Desmopressin
Pinocytosis	IgA
Junctional permeability	Horse radish peroxidase
Charge	DEAE dextran

statement was made, much has still to be learned about the mechanisms of nasal absorption.

Possible mechanisms have only been previously examined in a limited number of animal studies, most of which have been performed over the last ten years. These studies have not been systematic and the results, at first examination, appear equivocal. A great range of compounds, with widely different physicochemical properties, are absorbed from the nose. Indeed, almost all compounds applied to the nose have been absorbed to some extent (see Table 1). However, if nasal absorption is simplified into two routes, one aqueous and one lipoidal, a pattern emerges. This hypothesis is supported by McMartin *et al.* (1987) who proposed two mechanisms of transport; a fast rate dependent upon lipophilicity and a slower, but significant, rate for low molecular weight polar compounds.

The factors that have been involved in nasal absorption, and the compounds used in those investigations, are summarized in Table 4.

Mechanism of absorption of water-soluble compounds

The absorption of compounds in our own studies (Fisher *et al.*, 1985; Brown *et al.*, 1986; Fisher *et al.*, 1987) depended upon several factors, including contact time with the nasal mucosa, rate of absorption of the compound through the nasal mucosa, binding to the nasal mucosa, breakdown and/or metabolism in the nasal cavity and damage to the nasal mucosa. Because of the nature of the compounds chosen, the last three factors (binding, breakdown and/or metabolism and damage) were not important. Contact time was maintained for the duration of the experiments, which was as long as practical (generally six hours). This meant that for the smallest compounds (4-oxo-4H-1-benzopyran-2-carboxylic acid and para-aminohippuric acid), contact time was sufficiently long for nasal absorption to be complete. This leaves the rate of absorption of the compound through the nasal mucosa as the most important factor in the nasal absorption process. The water-soluble hydrophilic compounds used in these studies were assumed to cross the mucosal membrane by the passive process of diffusion through aqueous channels or pores.

Theoretical considerations and results

The process of diffusion depends upon the physical properties of the system. A diffusion coefficient can be defined by using the Einstein–Stokes equation (Stein, 1962):

$$D = \frac{kT}{6\pi r\eta}$$

where D is the diffusion coefficient, k is the Boltzmann constant, T is the absolute temperature, r is the radius of the molecule used and η is the viscosity. Thus the diffusion coefficient (D), a measure of the rate of diffusion, is related to molecular size (*r*). This relationship was originally derived for large spherical molecules. It can be rewritten in a more general form for all solutes with the introduction of a molecular weight term (Stein, 1962):

$$D = \frac{kT}{fM^{1/n}\eta}$$

where *M* is molecular weight and *f* and *n* are modifying factors to allow for the shape and size respectively. The equation defines the direct relationship between diffusion and molecular weight.

The proportions of the dose absorbed (per cent) for each individual compound studied, calculated from both the plasma and the bile and urine data, are collated in Table 5. There is an apparent inverse relationship between molecular weight and the proportion of the intranasal dose absorbed. This relationship is more clearly seen when the log of the proportion absorbed is

Table 5. Proportion of the intranasal dose absorbed for all compounds investigated (after Fisher *et al.*, 1985; Brown *et al.*, 1986; Fisher *et al.*, 1987).

Compound	Molecular weight	Proportion absorbed (%)
4-Oxo-4H-1-benzopyran -2-carboxylic acid	190	100
Para-aminohippuric acid	194	84
FPL 59002 (Nedocromil sodium)	371	76
Sodium cromoglycate	512	69
Inulin	5 200	15.5
Dextran	70 000	2.3

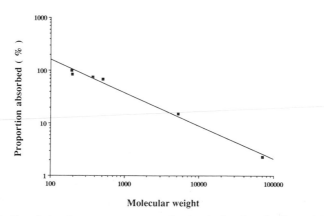

Figure 6. Correlation between percent nasally absorbed and molecular weight.

plotted against the log of the molecular weight (Figure 6). The line drawn is that of best fit calculated by linear least squares regression analysis and the correlation coefficient is -0.994 and the slope is -0.629. Consequently there is an excellent correlation between the log of the proportion of the dose absorbed and the log of the molecular weight. Thus, for water-soluble hydrophilic compounds there is an inverse relationship between the proportion of the dose absorbed and the molecular weight. By extrapolation from the regression line it can be predicted that all water-soluble hydrophilic compounds with a molecular weight below 200 will freely diffuse across the nasal mucosa.

There is further qualitative support for this proportion absorbed/molecular weight relationship from both the sodium cromoglycate results after administration of different dose concentrations (Fisons, data on file), and the results from other compounds (Brown *et al.*, 1986; Fisher *et al.*, 1987). Sodium cromoglycate has the property of forming larger aggregates in solution as the solution strength increases (Cox *et al.*, 1971; Smith, 1983). As the strength of intranasally administered sodium cromoglycate dose solution increases from 1 to 10 to 100 mM, the time taken to reach peak plasma concentrations is delayed from 8 to 20 to 69 min.

The shape of the peak in plasma concentrations becomes broader with increasing strength of dose solution. The rate of drug excretion in bile also shows a broadening peak in value as the concentration of dose solution increases. Therefore, the rate of absorption of sodium cromoglycate is reduced as the concentration of dose solution is increased, as a consequence of the increasing size of aggregates in that solution. With other compounds, the time to achieve peak plasma concentrations is delayed from 19 to 43 to 79 min for 4-oxo-4H-1-benzopyran-2-carboxylic acid, para-aminohippuric acid and inulin respectively, while dextran plasma concentrations continue to rise over 6 hours. As the molecular weight increases, the shape of the plasma concentration curve changes from a peak with 4-oxo-4H-1-benzopyran-2-carboxylic acid and para-aminohippuric acid to a plateau with inulin. Again, the biliary and urinary excretion results reflect the plasma results. Thus, with increasing aggregate size, sodium cromoglycate, or increasing molecular weight, all compounds, peak concentrations occur later and last longer. This indicates a slower rate of absorption with increasing molecular size. Therefore, it is likely that molecular size affects mainly the rate of absorption.

There are many factors that are involved in the absorption of compounds across biological membranes. However, for non-volatile, water-soluble, hydrophilic compounds, such as those used in our own studies, one of the main factors is molecular size. This has been demonstrated for a wide range of other biological membranes, both of plant and animal origin. Mammalian systems investigated include the lungs, where much work has been performed by Schanker (reviewed by himself in 1978 and with Hemberger, 1983), gastrointestinal tract (Loehry *et al.*, 1970, 1973; Chadwick *et al.*, 1977 a,b), placenta (Thornburg and Faber, 1977; Stulc and Stulcova, 1986), gall bladder

(Smulders and Wright, 1971) and capillary wall (Renkin, 1977; Rippe and Haraldsson, 1986). The molecular size/absorption relationship for hydrophilic water-soluble compounds is so well established that it is incorporated in most standard texts (Schanker, 1971; Schou, 1971; Scheler and Blank, 1977; Cohn, 1979 and Gennaro, 1985). These studies (Fisher *et al.*, 1987; Fisons, data on file) were the first experimental evidence for a correlation between molecular size and the nasal absorption of non-volatile, water-soluble, hydrophilic compounds. The study of McMartin *et al.* (1987) also supports an inverse relationship between molecular size and nasal absorption. These workers looked for correlations between published values for the nasal absorption of compounds, and the physicochemical properties of those compounds. The best correlation was between molecular size and nasal absorption, consistent with non-specific diffusion through aqueous channels, as demonstrated in Figure 7. Maitani *et al.* (1989) examined the influence of molecular weight on nasal absorption in rabbits using a range of fluorescein isothiocyanate (FITC) dextrans as neutral macromolecules and a range of diethylaminoethyl (DEAE)

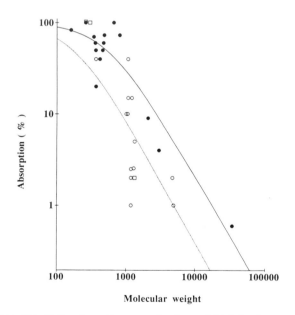

Figure 7.   Log-log plot of the absorption vs molecular weight following nasal administration (after McMartin *et al.*, 1987, with permission).

Key: Rat   ●
        Human   ○
        Other species □
The curves are the results of least-squares fitting of the function:

$$\% \text{ Absorption} = 100/[1 + a \, (\text{mol.wt.})^b]$$

where rat $a = 0.0003$, $b = 1.3$ ———
and human $a = 0.001$, $b = 1.35$ ·········

dextrans as charged macromolecules. As the molecular size of the dextran increased, the plasma concentrations detected decreased, and so this work is further evidence for the inverse relationship between molecular size and nasal absorption. However, these workers were unable to show any dextran absorption without coadministration of sodium glycocholate as a promoter. Although it was shown that the plasma concentrations of similarly sized FITC and DEAE dextrans were different, the effect of different charges could not be explained.

Nature of aqueous channels

Although the absorption of water-soluble, hydrophilic compounds is assumed to take place through channels or pores in the membrane, the question of the number, size and location of these pores is unresolved. There may be a transcellular route where hydrophilic regions in the membrane form aqueous channels (Kotyk, 1973). Such channels are possible considering the molecular components of membranes, but have never been visualized. The alternative route of transport (paracellular transport; Fromter and Diamond, 1972) has some electron microscopic support. Bundgaard (1984), with serial sectioning, has mapped clefts between the strands that join adjacent capilliary cells. Rippe and Haraldsson (1986) have combined both routes of transport in the capilliary wall with the notion of two pore sizes, transcellular transport being equivalent to small pores, and paracellular transport being equivalent to large pores. Similarly, both routes may operate in the eye (Lee *et al.*, 1986). Here it was stated that inulin did not penetrate via a carrier mechanism or by endocytosis, but it did penetrate via a paracellular route. When concentrations of inulin increased, penetration also occurred via a transcellular route. Various distributions of pore sizes have been suggested including three sizes of pore in the lungs (Schanker, 1978), two pore sizes in the capilliary (Rippe and Haraldsson, 1986) or a continual range of pore sizes in the stomach or intestine (Altamirano and Martinoya, 1966; Loehry *et al.*, 1970). The presence of pores in the nasal mucosa has been suggested by Hirai *et al.*, (1981 a) and Kaneo, (1983) and Hayashi *et al.*, (1985) Gibson and Olanoff (1987) suggested that aqueous pores do not exist as they could not demonstrate mannitol penetration using the *in situ* technique. In 1985, Hayashi *et al.* studied water influx and the sieving coefficient in rat jejunal, rectal and nasal membranes. Unfortunately these authors used inulin as a non-absorbable marker, and the present study has shown that this is significantly absorbed. Compared to jejunum the nasal membrane has a greater water flux because it has four times the number of water channels with a smaller, 4–8Å, pore size. Pores of this size cannot explain the transnasal passage of the larger compounds used in the present study. The Stokes (molecular) radius of sodium cromoglycate can be estimated, from its density, using:

$$r = 3 \sqrt{\frac{\text{Gram molecular weight} \times 3}{\text{Density} \times \text{Avagadro's Number} \times 4\pi}}$$

to be approximately 5Å, inulin has an established Stokes radius of 14–15Å (Egan, 1980) and dextran with a molecular weight of 76000 has a Stokes radius of approximately 60Å (Granath and Kvist, 1967). Thus, the pore size must be large enough to allow the passage of these molecules and must be considerably larger than that calculated by Hayashi *et al.* (1985). However, the issue is not as clear as this. Dextran, and to a certain degree inulin, are both flexible linear molecules with very little branching. Dextran molecules form loose and randomly coiled hydrated spheres in free solution (Ogston and Woods, 1953; Rennke *et al.*, 1979) which does not conflict with the essentially rod-like structure described in gel solutions (Laurent and Killander, 1964). Inulin may assume a more compact shape in solution because of the fructose 1 → 2 linkages and branching (Granath and Kvist, 1967; Ogston and Woods, 1953). When considering a straight chain polysaccharide, Laurent and Killander (1964) used a radius of 2–3Å, but with flexible and branched molecule dextran, a radius of 7Å was used. The linear nature and flexibility of both dextran and, to a lesser degree inulin, would allow them to pass end-on through smaller pores than predicted from Stokes radii. This is supported by work with microporous artificial membranes (Munch *et al.*, 1979) where the passage of a flexible polyelectrolyte (hydrolysed polacrylamide) was compared with a rigid spherical polyelectrolyte (bovine serum albumin). The flexible molecule passed through pores that had less than half the hydrodynamic radius of the molecule. Munch stresses that the behaviour of flexible linear molecules cannot be predicted from a rigid spherical model. The process of end-on transport is also supported by the work of Rennke *et al.* (1979). These latter authors studied the passage of horseradish peroxidase, a rigid globular protein, and dextran, with similar hydrodynamic radii, across the glomerular capilliary wall. The passage of horseradish peroxidase was restricted relative to the dextran. It was concluded that this was *in vivo* evidence of end-on movement of dextran through the membrane which results in a smaller effective molecular radius. The flexibility of the dextran molecule helps the negotiation of any obstruction. More work is required to elucidate the size of the pore, or pores, in the nasal mucosa. Also the process by which linear molecules cross membranes, and the critical dimensions of such molecules needs to be clarified.

Relationship between molecular size and nasal absorption of peptides

Previously, the relationship between molecular size and nasal absorption has only been considered, briefly, for peptides. These correlations have been based on data generated for other purposes, not from specific experiments designed to investigate the relationships between size and absorption. The conclusions are contradictory. Sandow and Petri (1985) and Harris (1986) claimed a relationship between size and bioavailability whereas Hussain *et al.* (1985 a) and Su (1986) stated that there was no relationship between size and absorption. However, peptides are complicated by being variously charged, variously shaped, molecules and their size measured, unreliably, in terms of amino acid units. It is possible to select peptide results to illustrate, or confound, any correlation!

Long-established studies of nasal absorption mechanisms

Although many studies which have investigated the factors involved in nasal absorption have been performed recently (i.e. over the last ten years), reports of substances administered to the nose have been made since 1922 (Blumgart), if not earlier. The early results of intranasal administration were correlated by Yoffey and Courtice (1956) when they were considering lymph and the lymphatics. They drew conclusions with respect to the nasal penetration of groups of compounds they called 'water, crystalloids and other small molecules, colloids, inanimate particles, viruses and bacteria'. The 'crystalloids', including saline, prussian blue, phenol-sulphonphthalein, potassium iodide, pituitrin, lead carbonate and mecholyl, plus water, all crossed the nasal mucosa, and it was assumed to be via diffusion. Additionally, with prussian blue, histological examination of cat, rabbit and mouse nasal mucosa showed blue grains in and between olfactory cells, in loose connective tissue of the submucosa and in the lumen of some lymphatics and blood vessels. Thus, it was concluded that 'small crystalloids' entered the body mainly by diffusion through the olfactory region. The 'colloids' considered were trypan blue, Evans blue, egg albumin, serum albumin, horse serum and horse serum—Evans blue complex. Trypan blue, Evans blue and egg albumin all passed through the nasal mucosa into the lymph; serum albumin was detected in the lymph of cat but not rabbit; horse serum and the horse serum—Evans blue complex were not detected in the lymph. It was concluded that molecules up to the size of egg albumin normally penetrated the nasal mucosa, but larger molecules did not. The conclusions reached from the two groups of compounds considered so far, which both include compounds with some degree of water solubility, are well supported by more recent investigations, including our own. Penetration specifically through the olfactory epithelium has not been studied in recent years with the notable exception of Anand Kumar and co-workers (e.g. Gopinath *et al.*, 1978; Anand Kumar, 1982). The 'inanimate particles' considered by Yoffey and Courtice were lead carbonate, ivory black and carbon black. The lead carbonate penetrated into lymph, but it was considered that such particles were solubolized after phagocytosis. Neither of the other compounds was detected in lymph. Thus 'inert particles', unless soluble, did not penetrate the nasal mucosa. The viruses considered were vaccinia, measles, chicken-pox, small-pox, common cold and poliomyelitis. Penetration of the nasal mucosa could not be predicted from size; and it appeared that only viruses that multiplied in the mucosa could enter lymph in significant amounts. The last group considered by Yoffey and Courtice were bacteria, which included fixed staphylococcus and live meningococcus, *Haemophilus influenzae*, pneumococci and *Salmonella enteriditis*. There was penetration of the mucosa by most live bacteria using a variety of routes. For bacteria which multiplied in or on the mucosa then spread to other parts of the body, the mucosa could be damaged leading to penetration or there could be penetration of the olfactory mucosa between the olfactory cells.

Recent investigations into mechanisms of nasal absorption

Lipid solubility alone is of some importance in intranasal absorption as shown by Bawarshi (1981) and Gibson and Olanoff (1987). Both groups of workers used the *in situ* technique. Bawarshi (1981) demonstrated that with a range of barbiturates, as the partition coefficient increased so did the extent of absorption. Similarly, Gibson and Olanoff (1987), with a range of steroids, showed that the absorption rate constant increased as the partition coefficient increased, and this was pH independent. Good correlations like these would be expected from a series of chemically similar compounds (Schanker, 1962) such as the barbiturates or steroids used above.

The bioavailibility of progesterone and its hydroxy derivatives in rabbits could not be correlated with octanol/water partition coefficients (Corbo *et al.*, 1989). However, these authors defined and determined a 'nasal mucosal partition coefficient' which was the degree of partitioning of a compound into an isolated sample of nasal mucosal tissue. They showed a hyperbolic correlation between bioavailability and 'nasal mucosal partition coefficient'.

When lipid soluble compounds also contain ionizable groups, absorption is conventionally described by the pH-partition hypothesis (e.g. Shore *et al.*, 1957; Schanker, 1962; Cohn, 1979; Gennaro, 1985). For a lipid-soluble compound to diffuse through a lipoidal membrane it must be in its unionized form. Thus, absorption is maximal when the compound is applied at a pH at which it is largely unionized. To date, published reports do not clearly support the pH-partition hypothesis alone as an important factor in nasal absorption. The absorption of the weakly ionized compound aminopyrine, is strongly dependent upon pH. It is passively absorbed in its unionized form and absorption is constant whatever the concentration (Hirai *et al.*, 1981 a). Benzoic acid (Bawarshi, 1981; Huang, 1985 a; Hussain *et al.*, 1985 a) salicylic acid (Bawarshi, 1981; Hirai *et al.*, 1981 a) and hydralazine (Kaneo, 1983) are all absorbed to a greater extent in their unionized forms, but there is significant absorption of the ionized species. Therefore, these compounds do not follow classical pH-partition theory. However, if these compounds are considered to be absorbed by both a lipoidal and an aqueous route, the results can be explained. The unionized form will cross membranes via the lipoidal route while the ionized form will cross via the aqueous route. There is some support for this idea as benzoic and salicylic acids also demonstrate deviation from the classical pH-partition hypothesis in the small intestine (Huang *et al.*, 1985 a). Furthermore, hydralazine reaches a maximum absorption when the pH is much less than the pKa, and Kaneo (1983) suggests that this indicates an aqueous channel mechanism. It is interesting to note that Hirai *et al.* (1981 a) demonstrated that salicylic acid absorption decreased as the concentration increased. It was suggested that either there was an increased binding of the compound to the nasal mucosa or mucosal damage was occurring. Gibson and Olanoff (1987) demonstrated that for a series of alkanoic acids (decanoic, octanoic and hexanoic), the maximum absorption rate constant was obtained when the pH was approximately equal to the pKa. The absorption rate constant decreased at both higher and lower pH values. Moreover, the maximum absorption rate constant of each compound had a similar value despite differences in partition coefficients. These compounds do not follow classical pH-partition theory and penetration via aqueous and lipoidal routes could explain the results. The authors, however, suggest that an aqueous boundary layer may be present which, under certain conditions, will affect the nasal absorption of charged compounds. Gibson and Olanoff (1987) considered these results together with their steroid and mannitol results; they concluded that the nasal mucosal membrane was essentially a modified lipophilic transport barrier.

Structural modifications of L-tyrosine have been prepared to study if they have any effect on nasal absorption, as monitored using the *in situ* technique (Huang *et al.*, 1985 b; Hussain *et al.*, 1985 a). Several O-acyl esters were produced which were more lipophilic than L-tyrosine but the absorption rate was similar for all compounds. The N-acetyl derivative, with a similar partition coefficient to the parent compound, was absorbed at a similar rate. However, esters of the carboxylic acid produced a series of compounds whose absorption rate constants increased as partition coefficient increased. Thus, the effect of lipophilicity alone was ambiguous. However, the authors concluded that L-tyrosine and its O-acyl esters were absorbed in zwitterionic form, hence they were absorbed at similar rates despite differences in lipophilicity. When the negative charge is masked by esterification of the carboxylic acid, increased absorption occurs for this group of compounds. The absorption of L-tyrosine was pH independent but concentration dependent. This led to the conclusion that L-tyrosine was absorbed by a pH-independent carrier mechanism. Thus, it appears that L-tyrosine and its analogues are intrinsically absorbed through the nasal mucosa. This is apparently regardless of charge and only in some circumstances dependent upon lipophilicity. Again, the results can be explained if these compounds cross the nasal mucosa by both aqueous and lipophilic routes; the proportion crossing by either route is determined by the physicochemical properties of the compound.

Tengamnuay and Mitra (1988 a) also used the *in situ* technique for tyrosine and phenylalanine. They similarly concluded that both L-amino acids were absorbed by a stereo-specific, saturable, active transport system, which required sodium and metabolic energy. When both L-amino acids were perfused together there was competitive inhibition, indicating at least one common carrier. To explain some discrepancies in their results with D-amino acids these workers suggested that active and passive transport processes were occurring together. It has been suggested that sodium guaiazulene-3-sulphonate is absorbed via two kinds of transport system (Seki *et al.*, 1985). The first mechanism is observed with low concentrations of compound and is an ouabain-sensitive carrier-mediated system. At higher concentrations of compound the mechanism proposed was a hydrophobic interaction with a mucosal constituent increased by ion-pair formation with a cation.

The peptides insulin (Hirai *et al.*, 1978) and secretin (Ohwaki *et al.*, 1985) were both absorbed to a greater extent from the nasal cavity as the pH was lowered. Hirai *et al.* (1978) suggested that for insulin this was due to changes in the physicochemical properties (aggregation) of the compound. At increased pH, insulin was either becoming insoluble or forming polymers. It is possible that the same may be happening with secretin. However, both pH and osmolarity also affect the structure of the nasal mucosa (Ohwaki *et al.*, 1987).

The rest of the published literature contains only a limited number of reports that indicate factors which may be important in nasal absorption. As the nasal mucosa contains secretory glands, water transport and consequently solvent drag may be important. Kotani *et al.* (1983) point out that there are more secretory glands in the nose compared to the intestine, hence solvent drag could be increased. Later Hayashi *et al.* (1985) stated that water influx in the nose was much higher than in the jejunum and rectum. It has been observed, but not always explained, that compounds with high water solubility and low lipophilicity, hence poor intrinsic oral absorption, such as phenol red, sulbenicillin, cefazolin, cephacetryl, insulin (Hirai *et al.*, 1981 a) clofilium tosylate (Su *et al.*, 1984) and sodium cromoglycate (Fisher *et al.*, 1985), are all well absorbed nasally. Such compounds must penetrate the nasal mucosa through an aqueous route. Moreover, the aqueous route must be more important in the nose than the gastrointestinal tract, which agrees with the study of Hayashi *et al.* (1985) outlined above.

It is possible that modifying nasal blood flow could affect the absorption of intranasally applied materials. This has been investigated in man with desmopressin (Olanoff *et al.*, 1987). It was shown that intranasal histamine increased local blood flow. When desmopressin was administered intranasally, following histamine pretreatment, the antidiuretic effect was enhanced compared to desmopressin alone. It was suggested that the systemic activity of intranasal desmopressin was enhanced because the increased nasal blood flow was leading to a greater absorption of the compound. Macromolecules may be absorbed by pinocytosis and this has been demonstrated in the human nose with IgA (Crifo and Russo, 1980). Inagaki *et al.* (1985) have studied the permeation of the nasal mucosa tight junctions by horseradish peroxidase. They stated that goblet cell–goblet cell, and goblet cell–ciliated cell junctions were weaker than ciliated cell–ciliated cell junctions.

Variables in the *in situ* technique of Hirai

In addition to being widely used to study nasal absorption, the variables in the *in situ* technique itself have also been reported (Huang *et al.*, 1985 a; Hussain *et al.*, 1985 a). The rate of perfusion does not affect the absorption of phenobarbitone. If the volume of perfusing fluid is reduced absorption increases. Some compounds, however, are not shown to be absorbed using the *in situ* technique, but are shown to be absorbed using the *in vivo* technique, e.g. phenol red (Hirai *et al.*, 1981 a) and inulin (Kotani *et al.*, 1983; Fisher *et al.*, 1987).

In vitro studies

There are two recent reports where tissue chambers (Ussing chambers) have been used to investigate the *in vitro* permeability of pieces of nasal mucosa. Hersey and Jackson (1987) used rabbit or dog mucosae and investigated the transport of radiolabelled water, sucrose, polyethylene glycol 5000 and cholecystokinin octapeptide. They suggested that, for water-soluble compounds, transport was not just by simple diffusion as the nasal mucosa was acting as a selective permeability barrier. Accordingly agents that alter the barrier should alter permeability. This idea was supported when 0.5 per cent deoxycholate was added to the chamber leading to increased transport. Subsequent histological examination of the tissue revealed cell damage; thus, the barrier had been permanently altered. The authors suggest that care should be taken when using bile salts in the nose. Wheatley *et al.* (1988) using sheep nasal mucosa, also looked at a series of model compounds, inulin, mannitol and propranolol, in the presence and absence of deoxycholate. Transport in both directions was at equivalent rates consistent with a passive transport mechanism. Inulin was transported at 3 per cent of the mannitol rate and, as both compounds would be expected to cross via passive diffusion through paracellular spaces, this indicated that molecular weight had an effect. The molecular weight of propranolol is about equal to that of mannitol, but the more lipid-soluble compound was transported at five times the mannitol rate, thus indicating a transcellular route for propranolol. This was more evidence for the idea of aqueous and lipoidal routes. At 0.1 per cent, deoxycholate increased the transport of mannitol and inulin ten to twenty times without causing tissue necrosis. Deoxycholate at 1.0 per cent did cause tissue necrosis. Thus, these two *in vitro* studies correlate well with the *in vivo* work.

Use of absorption promoters

Other approaches have included the use of promoters to increase the nasal absorption of such compounds as β-interferon (Maitani *et al.*, 1986), leuprolide (Okada *et al.*, 1982), insulin (Morimoto *et al.*, 1985; Hirai *et al.*, 1978, 1981 b,c; Flier *et al.*, 1985; Gordon *et al.*, 1985; Longenecker *et al.*, 1987), calcitonin (Morimoto *et al.*, 1985), hydralazine (Kaneo, 1983) and gentamicin (Duchateau *et al.*, 1986 b; Illum *et el.*, 1987 a). Indeed, it is stated that β-interferon (Maitani *et al.*, 1986), calcitonin (Morimoto *et al.*, 1985) and gentamicin (Duchateau *et al.*, 1986 b; Illum *et al.*, 1987 a) are not absorbed without promoters. Sustained release preparations of propranolol were tested by Hussain *et al.* (1980 a) and the use of bioadhesive microspheres has been investigated in man (Illum, 1986; Illum *et al.*, 1987 b) and animals (Illum *et al.*, 1988; Bjork and Edman, 1988). However, these studies have not considered the basic mechanisms by which compounds cross the nasal mucosa.

6. Conclusions

It can be concluded that although some work has been performed to study the mechanisms of nasal absorption, it is fragmentary and has not been performed in a systematic way. The information that is available can be rationalized by considering that there are basically two mechanisms for crossing the nasal mucosa, an aqueous route and a lipoidal route. There is established an aqueous route for highly water-soluble hydrophilic compounds. However, such a route is probably available to all compounds exhibiting some water solubility. The absorption of water-soluble compounds by the nose is very effective, indeed more effective than the gastrointestinal tract. A lipoidal route for nasal absorption also exists. However, more detailed systematic work is required to define this mechanism. Thus, we have made some progress since 1972, when Munzel pointed out our lack of knowledge with respect to the factors responsible for nasal absorption, but more work is still required.

To exploit the advantages of the intranasal route for systemic administration, or to optimize the use of topically acting compounds, it is essential to establish the absorption mechanisms involved. More comprehensive, basic information is required about the physicochemical properties which are involved in nasal absorption including molecular size and shape, lipophilicity, pH and pKa. These parameters should be examined in an established well controlled animal model, similar to those described by Hirai *et al.* (1981) and Fisher *et al.* (1985). Then, various other aspects can be considered including the effects of anaesthesia, method of administration of the dose, site of deposition of the dose and its significance, mucocilliary clearance, drainage, blood flow, disease, stability of the compound and its metabolism in the nasal cavity. When considerably more of these variables have been studied and understood extrapolation to man can be made with greater confidence. At this stage intranasal administration of compounds to man, the ultimate objective, could be studied on a more scientific basis than, apparently, exists at the present time.

Acknowledgements

I would like to thank Professor S. S. Davis and Dr D. A. Smith for their helpful discussions and useful comments, and Mrs P. Spavold for typing the manuscript.

References

Aellig, W. H. and Rosenthaler, J. (1986), *Europ. J. Clin. Pharmacol.*, **30**, 581.

Agosti, A. and Bertaccini, G. (1969), *Lancet*, **1**, 580.

Altamirano, M. and Martinoya, C. (1966), *J. Physiol.*, **184**, 771.

Anand Kumar, T. C., David, G. F. X., Umberkoman, B. and Saini, K. D. (1974), *Curr. Sci.*, **43**, 435.

Anand Kumar, T. C., David, G. F. X. and Puri, V. (1977), *Nature*, **270**, 532.

Anand Kumar, T. C., David, G. F. X. and Puri, V. (1979), in *Recent Advances in Reproduction and Regulation of Fertility* (G. P. Talwar, ed), p. 49, Elsevier, Amsterdam.

Anand Kumar, T. C., Sehgal, A., David, G. F. X., Bajaj, J. S. and Prasad, M. R. N. (1980), *Biol. Reprod.*, **22**, 935.

Anand Kumar, T. C., David, G. F. X., Sankaranarayanan, A., Puri, V. and Sundram, K. R. (1982), *Proc. Nat. Acad. Sci.* (USA), **79**, 4185.

Andersen, I. and Proctor, D. F. (1982), in *The Nose: Upper Airway Physiology and the Atmospheric Environment* (D. F. Proctor and I. Andersen, eds), p. 423, Elsevier, Amsterdam.

Anik, S. T., McRae, G., Nerenberg, C., Worden, A., Forman, J., Hwang, J-Y., Kushinsky, S., Jones, R. E. and Vickery, B. (1984), *J. Pharmaceut. Sci.*, **73**, 684.

Arnold, T. H., Tackett, R. L. and Vallner, J. J. (1985), *Biopharmaceut. Drug Dispos.*, **6**, 447.

Asch, R. H., Balmacedra, J. P., Neves de Castro, M. and Schally, A. V. (1985), *Adv. Contracept.*, **1**, 109.

Aungst, B. J. and Rogers, N. J. (1988), *Pharmaceut. Res.*, **5**, 305.

Aungst, B. J., Rogers, N. J. and Shefter, E. (1988), *J. Pharmacol. Exp. Therap.*, **244**, 23.

Babhair, S. A. and Tariq, M. (1988), *Res. Commun. Chem. Pathol. Pharmacol.*, **59**, 137.

Babhair, S. A., Tariq, M. and Abdullah, M. E. (1988), *Pharmaceut. Res.*, **5**(Suppl.), S97.

Barrow, C. S. (ed) (1986), *Toxicology of the Nasal Passages*, Hemisphere, Washington.

Baturina, E. Y., Sarycheva, N. Y., Deigin, Y. I., Yarova, E. P., Kamenskii, A. A. and Asharin, I. P. (1988), *Bull. Exp. Biol. Med.*, **105**, 202.

Bawarshi, R. N. (1981), *A Study of the Utility of the Nasal Route for Drug Administration*, PhD Thesis, University of Kentucky.

Bawarshi-Nassar, R. N., Hussain, A. A. and Crooks, P. A. (1989 a), *Drug Metab. Dispos.*, **17**, 248.

Bawarshi-Nassar, R. N., Hussain, A. and Crooks, P. A. (1989 b), *J. Pharmacy Pharmacol.*, **41**, 214.

Bjork, E. and Edman, P. (1988), *Int. J. Pharmaceut.*, **47**, 233.

Blumgart, H. L. (1922), *Arch. Intern. Med.*, **29**, 508.

Blumgart, H. L. (1923), *J. Indust. Hyg.*, **5**, 153.

Blumgart, H. L. (1924), *Arch. Intern. Med.*, **33**, 415.

Bogdanffy, M. S., Randall, H. W. and Morgan, K. T. (1987), *Toxicol. Appl. Pharmacol.*, **88**, 183.

Bond, J. A. (1986), in *Toxicology of the Nasal Passages* (C. S. Barrow, ed), p. 249, Hemisphere, Washington.

Bourguignon, J. P., Burger, H. G. and Franchimont, P. (1974), *Clin. Endocrinol.*, **3**, 437.

Brain, J. D. (1970), *Annals Otol. Rhinol. Laryngol.*, **79**, 529.

Brain, J. D., Proctor, D. F. and Reid, L. M. (eds) (1977), *Respiratory Defense Mechanisms Part I*, Marcel Dekker, New York.

Brain, J. D., Proctor, D. F. and Reid, L. M. (eds) (1978), *Respiratory Defense Mechanisms Part II*, Marcel Dekker, New York.

Brittebo, E. B. (1982 a), *Acta Pharmacol. Toxicol.*, **51**, 227.

Brittebo, E. B. (1982 b), *Acta Pharmacol. Toxicol.*, **51**, 441.

Brittebo, E. B. (1985), *Acta Pharmacol. Toxicol.*, **57**, 285.

Brittebo, E. B. (1987), *Cancer Res.*, **47**, 1449.

Brittebo, E. B. and Tjalve, H. (1981), *Carcinogenisis*, **2**, 959.

Brittebo, E., Lofberg, B. and Tjalve, H. (1981 a), *Xenobiotica*, **11**, 619.

Brittebo, E. B., Lofberg, B. and Tjalve, H. (1981 b), *Chemico-Bio. Interact.*, **34**, 209.

Brittebo, E. B., Castonguay, A., Rafter, J. J., Kowalski, B., Ahlman, M. and Brandt, I. (1986), in *Toxicology of the Nasal Passages* (C. S. Barrow, ed), p. 211, Hemisphere, Washington.

Bromley, L. and Hayward, A. (1988), *Anaesthesia*, **43**, 356.

Brown, K., Chauhan, P. B., Collington, J. W., Fisher, A. N., Foulds, R. A., Hewitt, S., Lockley, W. J. S., Mead, B., Neale, M. G., Parkin, S. C., Plumb, A. P., Smith, D. A. and Wilkinson, D. J. (1986), Poster at: *Inflammation: its Clinical Relevance in Airway Diseases*, Amsterdam, 16–17 March.

Bundgaard, M. (1984), *J. Ultrastruct. Res.*, **88**, 1.

Cameron, G. R., Gaddum, J. H. and Short, R. H. D. (1946), *J. Pathol. Bacteriol.*, **58**, 449.

Chadwick, V. S., Phillips, S. F. and Hofmann, A. F. (1977 a), *Gastroenterology*, **73**, 241.

Chadwick, V. S., Phillips, S. F. and Hofmann, A. F. (1977 b), *Gastroenterology*, **73**, 247.

Chang, J. C. F., Gross, E. A., Swenberg, J. A. and Barrow, C. S. (1983), *Toxicol. Appl. Pharmacol.*, **68**, 161.

Chang, S-F., Moore, L. and Chien, Y. W. (1988), *Pharmaceut. Res.*, **5**, 718.

Chien, Y. W. and Chang, S. F. (1985), in *Transnasal Systemic Medications* (Y. W. Chien, ed), p. 1, Elsevier, Amsterdam.

Chien, Y. W. and Chang, S. F. (1987), *CRC Crit. Rev. Therapeut. Drug Carrier Systems*, **4**, 67.

Chovan, J. P., Klett, R. P. and Rakieten, N. (1985), *J. Pharmaceut. Sci.*, **74**, 1111.

Cohen, M. B., Ecker, E. E., Breitbart, J. R. and Rudolph, J. A. (1930), *J. Immunol.*, **18**, 419.

Cohn, V. H. (1979), in *Fundamentals of Drug Metabolism and Drug Disposition* (B. N. LaDu, G. H. Mandel and E. E. Way, eds), p. 3, Robert E. Krieger, Huntingdon, New York.

Colman, N., DeMartino, L. and McAleer, E. (1988), *Fed. Am. Soc. Exp. Biol. J.*, **2**, A1086.

Corbo, D. C., Huang, Y. C. and Chien, Y. W. (1988), *Int. J. Pharmaceut.*, **46**, 133.

Corbo, D. C., Huang, Y. C. and Chien, Y. W. (1989), *Int. J. Pharmaceut.*, **50**, 253.

Cox, J. S. G., Woodward, G. D. and McCrone, W. C. (1971), *J. Pharmaceut. Sci.*, **60**, 1458.

Crifo, S. and Russo, M. (1980), *Acta Oto-Laryngol.*, **89**, 214.

Cuddihy, R. G. and Ozog, J. A. (1973), *Health Physics*, **25**, 219.

Cuddihy, R. G., Brownstein, D. G., Raabe, O. G. and Kanapilly, G. M. (1973), *Aerosol Sci.*, **4**, 35.

D'Agostino, H. R., Barnett, C. A., Zielinski, X. J. and Gordan, G. S. (1988), *Clin. Orthopaed. Related Res.*, **230**, 223.

Dahl, A. R. (1982), *Drug Metab. Dispos.*, **10**, 553.

Dahl, A. R. (1986), in *Toxicology of the Nasal Passages* (G. S. Barrow, ed), p. 263, Hemisphere, Washington.

Dahl, A. R. and Hadley, W. M. (1983), *Toxicol. Appl. Pharmacol.*, **67**, 200.

Dahl, A. R., Hadley, W. M., Hahn, F. F., Benson, J. M. and McClellan, R. O. (1982), *Science.*, **216**, 57.

Dalhamn, T., Rosengren, A. and Rylander, R. (1971), *Arch. Env. Health*, **22**, 554.

Dalton, M. E., Bromham, D. R., Ambrose, L. L., Osborne, J. and Dalton, K. D. (1987), *Br. J. Obstet. Gynaec.*, **94**, 84.

Danner, Ch. and Frick, J. (1980), *Int. J. Androl.*, **3**, 429.

Daugherty, A. L., Liggitt, H. D., McCabe, J. G., Moore, J. A. and Patton, J. S. (1988), *Int. J. Pharmaceut.*, **45**, 197.

David, G. F. X., Puri, C. P. and Anand Kumar, T. C. (1981), *Experimentia*, **37**, 533.

David, G. F. X., Puri, V., Dubey, A. K., Puri, C. P. and Anand Kumar, T. C. (1985), *Acta Endocrinol.*, **110**, 461.

Delabays, A., Porchet, M., Waeber, B., Nussberger, J. and Brunner, H. R. (1989), *J. Cardiovasc. Pharmacol.*, **13**, 173.

Dietz, A. A. (1944), *Proc. Soc. Exp. Biol. Med.*, **57**, 339.

Ding, X., Koop, D. R., Crump, B. L. and Coon, M. J. (1986), *Molec. Pharmacol.*, **30**, 370.

Donovan, M. D., Amidon, G. L. and Flynn, G. L. (1988), *Pharmaceut. Res.*, **5**(Suppl.), S97.

Doucette, J. R., Kiernan, J. A. and Flumerfelt, B. A. (1983), *J. Anat.*, **136**, 673.

Duchateau, G. S. M. J. E., Zuidema, J., Albers, W. M. and Merkus, F. W. H. M. (1986 a), *Int. J. Pharmaceut.*, **34**, 131.

Duchateau, G. S. M. J. E., Zuidema, J. and Merkus, F. W. H. M. (1986 b), *Int. J. Pharmaceut.*, **31**, 193.

Duchateau, G. S. M. J. E., Zuidema, J. and Basseleur, S. W. J. (1987), *Int. J. Pharmaceut.*, **39**, 87.

Dudley, R. E., Muggenburg, B. A., Cuddihy, R. G. and McClellan, R. O. (1980 a), *Health Phys.*, **38**, 763.

Dudley, R. E., Muggenburg, B. A., Cuddihy, R. G. and McClellan, R. O. (1980 b), *Am. Indust. Hyg. Assoc. J.*, **41**, 5.

Edsbacker, S., Andersson, K-E. and Ryrfeldt, A. (1985), *Europ. J. Clin. Pharmacol.*, **29**, 177.

Egan, E. A. (1980), *J. Appl. Physiol.*, **49**, 1032.

Egle, J. L. (1972 a), *Arch. Env. Health*, **24**, 354.

Egle, J. L. (1972 b), *Arch. Env. Health*, **25**, 119.

Fisher, A. N., Brown, K., Davis, S. S., Parr, G. D. and Smith, D. A. (1985), *J. Pharmacy Pharmacol.*, **37**, 38.

Fisher, A. N., Brown, K., Davis, S. S., Parr, G. D. and Smith, D. A. (1987), *J. Pharmacy Pharmacol.*, **39**, 357.

Flier, J. S., Moses, A. C., Carey, M. C., Gordon, G. S. and Silver, R. S. (1985), in *Transnasal Systemic Medications* (Y. W. Chien, ed), p. 217, Elsevier, Amsterdam.

Fogler, W. E., Wade, R., Brundish, D. E. and Fidler, I. J. (1985), *J. Immunol.*, **135**, 1372.

Frank, R. N., Yoder, R. E., Brain, J. D. and Yokoyama, E. (1969), *Arch. Env. Health*, **18**, 315.

Fromter, E. and Diamond, J. (1972), *Nature (NB)*, **235**, 9.

Gennaro, A. R. (ed) (1985), *Remington's Pharmaceutical Sciences*, 17th edn, p. 713, p. 820, Mack Publishing, Easton, Penn.

Gibson, R. E. and Olanoff, L. S. (1987), *J. Controlled Release*, **6**, 361.

Gillespie, J. H., Scott, F. W., Geissinger, C. M., Czarniecki, C. W. and Scialli, V. T. (1986), *J. Clin. Microbiol.*, **24**, 240.

Gopinath, P. G., Gopinath, G. and Anand Kumar, T. C. (1978), *Curr. Therap. Res.*, **23**, 596.

Gordon, G. S., Moses, A. C., Silver, R. D., Flier, J. S. and Carey, M. C. (1985), *Proc. Nat. Acad. Sci. (USA)*, **82**, 7419.

Gram, T. E., Okine, L. K. and Gram, R. A. (1986), *Ann. Rev. Pharmacol.*, **26**, 259.

Granath, K. A. and Kvist, B. E. (1967), *J. Chromatog.*, **28**, 69.

Gross, E. A., Swenberg, J. A., Fields, S. and Popp, J. A. (1982), *J. Anat.*, **135**, 83.

Guyatt, A. R., Holmes, M. A. and Cumming, G. (1981), *Europ. J. Respir. Dis.*, **62**, 383.

Hadley, W. M. and Dahl, A. R. (1982), *Toxicol. Lett.*, **10**, 417.

Hadley, W. M. and Dahl, A. R. (1983), *Drug Metab. Dispos.*, **11**, 275.

Hancock, M. R. and Gower, D. B. (1986), *Biochem. Soc. Trans.*, **14**, 1033.

Hanson, M., Gazdick, G., Cahill, J. and Augustine, M. (1986), in *Delivery Systems for Peptide Drugs* (S. S. Davis, L. Illum and E. Tomlinson, eds), p. 233, Plenum Press, New York and London.

Harris, A. S. (1986), in *Delivery Systems for Peptide Drugs* (S. S. Davis, L. Illum and E. Tomlinson, eds), p. 191, Plenum Press, New York and London.

Harris, A. S., Nilsson, I. M., Wagner, Z. G. and Alkner, U. (1986), *J. Pharmaceut. Sci.*, **75**, 1085.

Harris, A. S., Hender, P. and Vilhardt, H. (1987), *J. Pharmacy Pharmacol.*, **39**, 932.

Harris, A. S., Ohlin, M., Lethagen, S. and Nilsson, I. M. (1988), *J. Pharmaceut. Sci.*, **77**, 337.

Hayashi, M., Hirasawa, T., Muraoka, T., Shiga, M. and Awazu, S. (1985), *Chem. Pharmaceut. Bull.*, **33**, 2149.

Hebel, R. and Stromberg, M. W. (1976), *Anatomy of the Laboratory Rat*, p. 55, Williams and Wilkins, Baltimore.

Hermens, W. A. J. J., Romeijn, S. G. and Merkus, F. W. H. M. (1988), *Pharmaceut. Weekbl. Sci. Ed.*, **10**, 54.

Hersey, S. J. and Jackson, R. T. (1987), *J. Pharmaceut. Sci.*, **76**, 876.

Heyder, J. and Rudolf, G. (1975), *Inhaled Particles*, **4**, 107.

Heykants, J., Van Peer, A., Woestenborghs, R., Geuens, I., Rombaut, N. and Van den Bussche, G. (1985), *Arch. Int. Pharmacodyn. Therap.*, **274**, 329.

Hirai, S., Ikenaga, T. and Matsuzawa, T. (1978), *Diabetes*, **27**, 296.

Hirai, S., Yashiki, T., Matsuzawa, T. and Mima, H. (1981 a), *Int. J. Pharmac.*, **7**, 317.

Hirai, S., Yashiki, T. and Mima, H. (1981 b), *Int. J. Pharmaceut.*, **9**, 165.

Hirai, S., Yashiki, T. and Mima, H. (1981 c), *Int. J. Pharmaceut.*, **9**, 173.

Hirata, Y., Yokosuka, T., Kasahara, T., Kikuchi, M. and Ooi, K. (1979), in *Proceedings of a Symposium on Proinsulin, Insulin and C-peptide* (S. Baba, T. Kaneko and N. Yanihara, eds), p. 319, Tokushima, July 1978, Excerpta Medica, Amsterdam.

Hodde, K. C. and de Blecourt, C. V. (1979), *J. Anat.*, **129**, 206.

Hounam, R. F. and Morgan, A. (1977), in *Respiratory Defense Mechanisms part 1* (J. D. Brain, D. F. Proctor and L. M. Reid, eds), p. 125, Marcel Dekker, New York.

Huang, C. H., Kimura, R., Bawarshi-Nassar, R. and Hussain, A. (1985 a), *J. Pharmaceut. Sci.*, **74**, 608.

Huang, C. H., Kimura, R., Bawarshi-Nassar, R. and Hussain, A. (1985 b), *J. Pharmaceut. Sci.*, **74**, 1298.

Hussain, A. A., Hirai, S. and Bawarshi, R. (1979), *J. Pharmaceut. Sci.*, **68**, 1196.

Hussain, A., Hirai, S. and Bawarshi, R. (1980 a), *J. Pharmaceut. Sci.*, **69**, 1411.

Hussain, A., Foster, T., Hirai, S., Kashihara, T., Batenhorst, R. and Jones, M. (1980 b), *J. Pharmaceut. Sci.*, **69**, 1240.

Hussain, A. A., Hirai, S. and Bawarshi, R. (1981), *J. Pharmaceut. Sci.*, **70**, 466.

Hussain, A., Kimura, R., Huang, C-H. and Kashihara, T. (1984 a), *Int. J. Pharmaceut.*, **21**, 233.

Hussain, A., Kimura, R., Huang, C-H. and Mustafa, R. (1984 b), *Int. J. Pharmaceut.*, **21**, 289.

Hussain, A. A., Kimura, R. and Huang, H. H. (1984 c), *J. Pharmaceut. Sci.*, **73**, 1300.

Hussain, A. A., Bawarshi-Nassar, R. and Huang, C. H. (1985 a), in *Transnasal Systemic Medications* (Y. W. Chien, ed), p. 121, Elsevier, Amsterdam.

Hussain, A., Faraj, J., Aramaki, Y. and Truelove, J. E. (1985 b), *Biochem. Biophys. Res. Commun.*, **133**, 923.

Igawa, T., Maitani, Y., Machida, Y. and Nagai, T. (1988), *Chem. Pharmaceut. Bull.*, **36**, 3055.

Illum, L. (1986), in *Delivery Systems for Peptide Drugs* (S. S. Davis, L. Illum and E. Tomlinson, eds), p. 205, Plenum Press, New York and London.

Illum, L., Davis, S. S. and Farraj, N. (1987 a), *J. Pharmaceut. Sci.*, **76**, S74.

Illum, L., Jorgensen, H., Bisgaard, H., Krogsgaard, O. and Rossing, N. (1987 b), *Int. J. Pharmaceut.*, **39**, 189.

Illum, L., Farraj, N., Critchley, H. and Davis, S. S. (1988), *Int. J. Pharmaceut.*, **46**, 261.

Inagaki, M., Sakakura, Y., Majima, Y. and Miyoshi, Y. (1984), *Nippon Jibinkoka Gakki Kaiho*, **87**, 213.

Inagaki, M., Sakakura, Y., Itoh, J., Ukai, K. and Miyoshi, Y. (1985), *Rhinology*, **23**, 213.

Jackson, R. T. and Birnbaum, J. E. (1982), *Otolaryngol.—Head and Neck Surg.*, **90**, 594.

Jiang, X. Z., Buckley, L. A. and Morgan, K. T. (1983), *Toxicol. Appl. Pharmacol.*, **71**, 225.

Job, C. K., Chehl, S., McCormick, G. T. and Hastings, R. C. (1987), *Indian J. Leprosy.*, **59**, 356.

Kaneo, Y. (1983), *Acta Pharmaceut. Suecica*, **20**, 379.

Karesek, E., Rathsack, R., Fechner, K. and Grafenberg, M. (1986), *Pharmazie*, **41**, 289.

Kashi, S. D. and Lee, V. H. L. (1986), *Life Sci.*, **38**, 2019.

Kelemen, G. and Sargent, F. (1946), *Arch. Otolaryngol.*, **44**, 24.

Kimmerle, R. and Rolla, A. R. (1985), *Am. J. Med.*, **79**, 535.

Kimuira, T. (1984), *Pharmacy Int.*, **5**, 75.

Kimura, K., Miwa, M. and Kato, Y. (1987), *J. Pharmaceut. Sci.*, **76**, S77.

Kitagawa, H., Yokoshima, T., Nanpo, M. T. and Takemoto, M. (1974), *Oyo Yakuri*, **8**, 391.

Kotani, A., Hayashi, M. and Awazu, S. (1983), *Chem. Pharmaceut. Bull.*, **31**, 1097.

Kotyk, A. (1973), *Biochem. Biophys. Acta*, **300**, 183.

Laurent, T. C. and Killander, J. (1964), *J. Chromatog.*, **14**, 317.

Le Gros Clark, W. E. (1929), *Report on Public Health and Medical Subjects, No. 54*, HMSO, Ministry of Health, London.

Lee, V. H. L., Carson, W. and Takemoto, K. A. (1986), *Int. J. Pharmaceut.*, **29**, 43.

Lippmann, M., Yeates, D. B. and Albert, R. E. (1980), *Br. J. Indust. Med.*, **37**, 337.

Liversidge, G. C., Wilson, C. G., Sternson, L. and Kinter, L. B. (1988), *J. Appl. Physiol.*, **64**, 377.

Loehry, C. A., Axon, A. T. R., Hilton, P. J., Hider, R. C. and Creamer, B. (1970), *Gut*, **11**, 466.

Loehry, C. A., Kingham, J. and Baker, J. (1973), *Gut*, **14**, 683.

Longenecker, J. P. (1986), in *Delivery Systems for Peptide Drugs* (S. S. Davis, L. Illum and E. Tomlinson, eds), p. 211, Plenum Press, New York and London.

Longenecker, J. P., Moses, A. C., Flier, J. S., Silver, R. D., Carey, M. C. and Dubovi, E. J. (1987), *J. Pharmaceut. Sci.*, **76**, 351.

Longo, V., Citti, L. and Gervasi, P. G. (1986), *Carcinogenesis*, **7**, 1323.

Lonovics, J., Nari, G. and Varro, V. (1980), *Materia Medica Polona*, **4**, 229.

Lucas, A. M. and Douglas, L. C. (1933–34), *Proc. Soc. Exp. Biol. Med.*, **31**, 320.

Lundin, S., Akerlund, M., Fagerstrom, P-O., Hauksson, A. and Melin, P. (1986), *Acta Endocrinol.*, **112**, 465.

Lupo, C., Lodi, L., Canonaco, M., Valenti, A. and Dessi-Fulgheri, F. (1986), *Neurosci. Lett.*, **69**, 259.

Maitani, Y., Igawa, T., Machida, Y. and Nagai, T. (1986), *Drug Design Delivery*, **1**, 65.

Maitani, Y., Machida, Y. and Nagai, T. (1989), *Int. J. Pharmaceut.*, **49**, 23.

Mattioli, M., Galaeti, G., Conte, F. and Seren, E. (1986), *Theriogenology*, **25**, 399.

McCaskill, A. C., Hosking, C. S. and Hill, D. J. (1984), *Immunology*, **51**, 669.

McKendry, J. B. R., Schwarz, H. and Hall, M. (1954), *Can. Med. Ass. J.*, **70**, 244.

McMartin, C. and Peters, G. (1986), in *Delivery Systems for Peptide Drugs* (S. S. Davis, L. Illum and E. Tomlinson, eds), p. 255, Plenum Press, New York and London.

McMartin, C., Hutchinson, L. E. F., Hyde, R. and Peters, G. E. (1987), *J. Pharmaceut. Sci.*, **76**, 535.

Medinsky, M. A., Cuddihy, R. G. and McClellan, R. O. (1981), *J. Toxicol. Env. Health*, **8**, 917.

Menco. B. Ph. M. (1983), in *Nasal Tumours in Animals and Man* (G. Reznick and S. F. Stinson, eds), p. 45, CRC Press, Boca Raton, Florida.

Michels, M. I., Smith, R. E. and Heimlich, E. M. (1967), *Annals Allergy*, **25**, 569.

Miller, F. J., McNeal, C. A., Kirtz, J. M., Gardner, D. E., Coffin, D. L. and Menzel, D. B. (1979), *Toxicology*, **14**, 273.

Mishima, M., Wakita, Y. and Nakano, M. (1987), *J. Pharmacobiodynamics*, **10**, 624.

Morgan, K. T., Patterson, D. L. and Gross, E. A. (1983), in *Formaldehyde— Toxicology, Epidemiology, Mechanisms* (J. J. Clary, J. E. Gibson and R. S. Waritz, eds), p. 193, Marcel Dekker, New York.

Morgan, K. T., Jiang, X-Z, Patterson, D. L. and Gross, E. A. (1984), *Am. Rev. Resp. Dis.*, **130**, 275.

Morgan, K. T., Patterson, D. L. and Gross, E. A. (1986 a), in *Toxicology of the Nasal Passages* (C. S. Barrow, ed), p. 123, Hemisphere, Washington.

Morgan, K. T., Patterson, D. L. and Gross, E. A. (1986 b), *Toxicol. Appl. Pharmacol.*, **82**, 1.

Morimoto, K. Morisaka, K. and Kamada, A. (1985), *J. Pharmacy Pharmacol.*, **37**, 134.

Morris, J. B. and Smith, F. A. (1982), *Toxicol. Appl. Pharmacol.*, **62**, 81.

Moudgal, R. N., Rao, A. J., Murthy, G. S. R. C., Neelakanta, R., Banavar, S. R., Kotagi, S. G. and Anand Kumar, T. C. (1985), *Fert. Steril.*, **44**, 120.

Mukai, H., Sugihara, K. and Sugiyama, M. (1985), *J. Pharmacobiodynamics*, **8**, 329.

Munch, W. D., Zestar, L. P. and Anderson, J. L. (1979), *J. Membrane Sci.*, **5**, 77.

Munzel, M. (1972), *Rhinology*, **10**, 114.

Munzel, M. and Eichner, H. (1975), *Laryngol., Rhinol., Otol.*, **54**, 875.

Murakami, T., Kishimoto, M., Kawakita, H., Higashi, Y., Yata, N., Amagase, H., Nojima, N. and Fuwa, T. (1987), *J. Pharmaceut. Sci.*, **76**, S85.

Nagai, M., Nagai, T. and Morimitsu, T. (1982), *Arch. Oto-Rhino-Laryngol.*, **237**, 67.

Nagai, M., Nagai, T. and Tono, T. (1983), *Arch. Oto-Rhino-Laryngol.*, **238**, 115.

Nagai, T., Nishimoto, Y., Nambu, N., Suzuki, Y. and Sekine, K. (1984), *J. Controlled Release*, **1**, 15.

Negus, Sir V. (1958), *The Comparative Anatomy and Physiology of the Nose and Paranasal Sinuses*, Livingstone, Edinburgh.

Ogston, A. G. and Woods, E. F. (1953), *Nature*, **171**, 221.

Öhman, L., Hahnenberger, R. and Johansson, E. D. B. (1978), *Contraception*, **18**, 171.

Öhman, L., Hahnenberger, R. and Johansson, E. D. B. (1980), *Contraception.*, **22**, 349.

Ohwaki, T., Ando, H., Watanabe, S. and Miyake, Y. (1985), *J. Pharmaceut. Sci.*, **74**, 550.

Ohwaki, T., Ando, H., Kakimoto, F., Uesugi, K., Watanabe, S., Miyake, Y. and Kayano, M. (1987), *J. Pharmaceut. Sci.*, **76**, 695.

Okada, H., Yamazaki, I., Ogawa, Y., Hirai, S., Yashiki, T. and Mima, H. (1982), *J. Pharmaceut. Sci.*, **71**, 1367.

Olanoff, L. S., Titus, C. R., Shea, M. S., Gibson, R. E. and Brooks, C. D. (1987), *J. Clin. Invest.*, **80**, 890.

Patrick, G. and Stirling, C. (1977), *J. Appl. Physiol.*, **42**, 451.

Petridou-Fischer, J., Whaley, S. L. and Dahl, A. R. (1987), *Chemico-Biol. Interact.*, **64**, 1.

Petridou-Fischer, J., Whaley, S. L. and Dahl, A. R. (1988), *Toxicology*, **48**, 31.

Pontiroli, A. E., Alberetto, M. and Pozza, G. (1985 a), *Br. Med. J.*, **290**, 1390.

Pontiroli, A. E., Alberetto, M. and Pozza, G. (1985 b), *Acta Diabetol. Latina*, **22**, 103.

Pontiroli, A. E., Alberetto, M., Calderara, A., Pajetta, F. and Pozza, G. (1986 a), in *Delivery Systems for Peptide Drugs* (S. S. Davis, L. Illum and E. Tomlinson, eds), p. 243, Plenum, New York and London.

Pontiroli, A. E., Alberetto, M., Calderara, A., Pajetta, E., Manganelli, V., Tessari, L. and Pozza, G. (1986 b), in *Delivery Systems for Peptide Drugs* (S. S. Davis, L. Illum and E. Tomlinson, eds), p. 249, Plenum, New York and London.

Popp, J. A. and Martin, J. T. (1984), *Am. J. Anat.*, **169**, 425.

Popp, J. A., Monteiro-Riviere, N. A. and Martin, J. T. (1986), in *Toxicology of the Nasal Passages* (C. S. Barrow, ed), p. 37, Hemisphere, Washington.

Proctor, D. F. (1964), in *Handbook of Physiology, Section 3, Respiration, Volume I* (W. O. Fenn and H. Rahn, eds), p. 309, American Physiological Society, Washington.

Proctor, D. F. and Andersen, I. (eds) (1982), *The Nose–Upper Airway Physiology and the Atmospheric Environment*, Elsevier, Amsterdam.

Proctor, D. F. and Chang, C. F. (1983), in *Nasal Tumours in Animals and Man, Volume 1* (G. Reznick and S. Stinson, eds), p. 1, CRC Press, Boca Raton, Florida.

Proctor, D. F., Andersen, I. and Lundqvist, G. (1977), in *Respiratory Defense Mechanisms, Part 1* (J. D. Brain, D. F. Proctor and L. M. Reid, eds), p. 427, Marcel Dekker, New York

Puri, V., David, G. F. X., Dubey, A. K., Puri, C. P. and Anand Kumar, T. C. (1986), *J. Reprod. Fert.*, **76**, 215.

Raehs, S. C., Sandow, J. and Merkle, H. P. (1988 a), in *Proc. Int. Symp. Controlled Release of Bioactive Materials* (*15*), p. 72, Controlled Release Society, Inc., Lincolnshire, Illinois.

Raehs, S. C., Sandow, J., Wirth, K. and Merkle, H. P. (1988 b), *Pharmaceut. Res.*, **5**, 689.

Rajifer, J., Handelsman, D. J., Swerdolff, R. S., Farrer, J. II. and Sikka, S. C. (1986), *Fert. Steril.*, **45**, 794.

Reed, C. J., Lock, E. A. and De Matteis, F. (1986), *Biochem. J.*, **240**, 585.

Renkin, E. M. (1977), *Circulation Res.*, **41**, 735.

Rennke, H. G., Venkatachalam, M. A. and Patel, Y. (1979), *J. Clin. Invest.*, **63**, 713.

Reznik, G. (1983), in *Nasal Tumours in Animals and Man, Volume 1* (G. Reznik and S. F. Stinson, eds), p. 35, CRC Press, Boca Raton, Florida.

Reznik, G. and Stinson, S. F. (eds) (1983), *Nasal Tumours in Animals and Man* (3 vols), CRC Press, Boca Raton, Florida.

Rhodin, J. A. G. (1974), *Histology—a Text and Atlas*, p. 607, Oxford University Press, New York.

Rippe, B. and Haraldsson, B. (1986), *Acta Physiol. Scand.*, **127**, 289.

Salzman, R., Manson, J. E., Griffing, G. T., Kimmerle, R., Ruderman, N., McCall, A., Staltz, E. I., Mullin, C., Small, D., Armstrong, J. and Melby, J. C. (1985), *New Engl. J. Med.*, **312**, 1078.

Sandow, J. and Petri, W. (1985), in *Transnasal Systemic Medications* (Y. W. Chien, ed), p. 183, Elsevier, Amsterdam.

Schanker, L. S. (1962), *Pharmacol. Rev.*, **14**, 501.

Schanker, L. S. (1971), in *Concepts in Biochemical Pharmacology, Part 1* (B. B. Brodie and J. R. Gillette, eds), p. 9, Springer-Verlag, Berlin.

Schanker, L. S. (1978), *Biochem. Pharmacol.*, **27**, 381.

Schanker, L. S. and Hemberger, J. A. (1983), *Biochem. Pharmacol.*, **32**, 2599.

Scheler, W. and Blanck, J. (1977), in *Kinetics of Drug Action* (J. M. van Rossum, ed), p. 3, Springer-Verlag, Berlin.

Schoenfisch, W. H., Hoop, K. A. and Struelens, B. S. (1980), *Arch. Env. Health.*, **35**, 152.

Schou, J. (1971), in *Concepts in Biochemical Pharmacology, Part 1* (B. B. Brodie and J. R. Gillette, eds), p. 47, Springer-Verlag, Berlin.

Schreider, J. P. (1986), in *Toxicology of the Nasal Passages* (C. S. Barrow, ed), p. 1, Hemisphere, Washington.

Schreider, J. P. and Raabe, O. G. (1980), *J. Env. Pathol. Toxicol.*, **4**, 427.

Schreider, J. P. and Raabe, O. G. (1981), *Anat. Rec.*, **200**, 195.

Sehgal, A., David, G. F. X., Dubey, S. K. and Anand Kumar, T. C. (1980), *Indian J. Exp. Biol.*, **18**, 707.

Seki, J., Mukai, H. and Sugiyama, M. (1985), *J. Pharmacobiodynamics*, **8**, 337.

Shionoiri, H. and Kaneko, Y. (1986), *Life Sci.*, **38**, 773.

Shionoiri, J., Oda, H., Yasuda, G., Takasaki, I., Kato, Y. and Gotoh, E. (1987), *Curr. Ther. Res.*, **42**, 1189.

Shore, P. A., Brodie, B. B. and Hogben, C. A. M. (1957), *J. Pharmacol. Exp. Ther.*, **119**, 361.

Smith, D. A. (1983), Personal communication.

Smulders, A. P. and Wright, E. M. (1971), *J. Membrane Biol.*, **5**, 297.

Snyder, W. S. (chair), Cook, M. J., Nasset, E. S., Karhausen, L. R., Parry Howells, G. and Tipton, I. H. (1975), *Int. Commission Radiological Protection, Publication No. 23, Report of the Task Group on Reference Man*, Pergamon, Oxford.

Soderman, P., Sahlberg, D. and Wiholm, B-E. (1984), *Lancet*, **1**, 573.

Soerensen, A. R., Drejer, K., Engesgaad, A., Guldhammer, B., Hansen, P., Hjortkaer, R. K. and Mygind, N. (1988), *Diabet. Res. Clin. Prac.*, **5**(Suppl. 1), S165.

Spector, W. S. (ed) (1956), *Handbook of Biological Data*, p. 29, Saunders, Philadelphia.

Speizer, F. E. and Frank, N. R. (1966), *Arch. Env. Health*, **12**, 725.

Stein, W. D. (1962), in *Comprehensive Biochemistry, Vol. 2, Organic and Physical Chemistry*, p. 283, Elsevier, Amsterdam.

Stott, W. T., Ramsey, J. C. and McKenna, M. J. (1986), in *Toxicology of the Nasal Passages* (C. S. Barrow, ed), p. 191, Hemisphere, Washington.

Stratford, R. E. and Lee, V. H. L. (1986), *Int. J. Pharmaceut.*, **30**, 73.

Stratford, R. E., Carson, L. W., Dodda-Kashi, S. and Lee, V. H. L. (1988), *J. Pharmaceut. Sci.*, **77**, 838.

Stulc, J. and Stulcova, B. (1986), *J. Physiol.*, **371**, 1.

Su, K. S. E. (1986), *Pharmacy Int.*, **7**, 8.

Su, K. S. E. and Campanale, K. M. (1985), in *Transnasal Systemic Medications* (Y. W. Chien, ed), p. 139, Elsevier, Amsterdam.

Su, K. S. E., Campanale, K. M. and Gries, C. L. (1984), *J. Pharmaceut. Sci.*, **73**, 1251.

Su, K. S. E., Campanale, K. M., Mendelsohn, L. G., Kerchner, G. A. and Gries, C. L. (1985), *J. Pharmaceut. Sci.*, **74**, 394.

Su, K. S. E., Campanale, K. M., Mendelsohn, L. G., Kerchner, G. A. and Gries, C. L. (1986), in *Delivery Systems for Peptide Drugs* (S. S. Davis, L. Illum and E. Tomlinson, eds), p. 221, Plenum, New York and London.

Su, K. S. E., Wilson, H. C. and Campanale, K. M. (1987), in *Drug Delivery Systems: Fundamentals and Techniques* (P. Johnson and J. G. Lloyd-Jones, eds), p. 224, Verlagsgesellschaft, Weinheim, FRG.

Sweeney, T. D., Brain, J. D. and le Mott, S. (1983), *J. Appl. Physiol.*, **54**, 37.

Tarquini, B., Cavallini, V., Cariddi, A., Checchi, M., Sorice, V. and Cecchettin, M. (1988), *Chronobiol. Int.*, **5**, 149.

Tengamnuay, P. and Mitra, A. K. (1988 a), *Life Sci.*, **43**, 585.

Tengamnuay, P. and Mitra, A. K. (1988 b), *Pharmaceut. Res.*, **5**(Suppl.), S96.

Thor, D. H. and Flannelly, K. J. (1977), *Physiol. Psychol.*, **5**, 261.

Thornburg, K. L. and Faber, J. J. (1977), *Am. J. Physiol.*, **233**, C111.

Van Dellen, T. R., Bruger, M. and Wright, I. S. (1937), *J. Pharmacol. Exp. Ther.*, **59**, 413.

Vavra, I., Machova, A., Holecek, V., Cort, J. H., Zaoral, M. and Sorm, F. (1968), *Lancet*, **1**, 948.

Vicente, V., Alberca, I., Gonzalez, R. and Alegre, A. (1985), *Annals Intern. Med.*, **103**, 807.

Vickery, B. H., Anik, S., Chaplin, M. and Henzkl, M. (1985), in *Transnasal Systemic Medications* (Y. W. Chien, ed), p. 201, Elsevier, Amsterdam.

Vilhardt, H. and Lundin, S. (1986), *Gen. Pharmacol.*, **17**, 481.

Vinogradov, V. A., Kalenikova, E. I. and Sokolov, A. S. (1988), *Biulleten Eksperimentalnoi Biologii I Meditsiny*, **105**, 48.

Visor, G. C., Bajka, E. and Benjamin, E. (1986), *J. Pharmaceut. Sci.*, **75**, 44.

Voigt, J. M., Guengerich, F. P. and Baron, J. (1985), *Cancer Lett.*, **27**, 241.

Weissman, S. H., Cuddihy, R. G. and Burkstaller, M. A. (1979), Conf. *Trace Substances in Environmental Health 13*, p. 477, Columbia, Missouri, June 4–7.

Whaley, S. L., Wolff, R. K. and Muggenburg, B. A. (1987), *Am. J. Vet. Res.*, **48**, 204.

Wheatley, M. A., Dent, J., Wheeldon, E. B. and Smith, P. L. (1988), *J. Controlled Release*, **8**, 167.

Yamamoto, N., Sakakibara, II., Mizuno, K. and Murase, J. (1987), *J. Pharmaceut. Sci.*, **76**, S307.

Yamazaki, I. (1984), *J. Reprod. Fert.*, **72**, 129.

Yoffey, J. M. and Courtice, F. C. (1956), *Lymphatics, Lymph and Lymphoid Tissue*, p. 152, Edward Arnold, London.

Yoffey, J. M. and Drinker, C. K. (1938), *J. Exp. Med.*, **68**, 629.

Yoffey, J. M. and Sullivan, E. R. (1939), *J. Exp. Med.*, **69**, 133.

Yoffey, J. M., Sullivan, E. R. and Drinker, C. K. (1938), *J. Exp. Med.*, **68**, 941.

Yokoyama, E. and Frank, R. (1972), *Arch. Env. Health*, **25**, 132.

Young, J. T. (1986), in *Toxicology of the Nasal Passages* (C. S. Barrow, ed), p. 27, Hemisphere, Washington.

CHAPTER 4

Use of NMR spectroscopy in drug metabolism studies: recent advances

Nicholas E. Preece and John A. Timbrell*

Department of Physics, Royal College of Surgeons,
35–43 Lincoln Inn's Fields, London WC2A 3PN

*Toxicology Unit, School of Pharmacy, University of London,
29/39 Brunswick Square, London WC1N 1AX, England, UK

1. Introduction

It is assumed that the reader will have at least some familiarity with modern nuclear magnetic resonance (NMR) spectroscopy as it is beyond the scope of this review to describe the theory and practice of the technique fully, and several excellent texts on NMR are now available (Sanders and Hunter, 1987). We shall therefore only discuss theoretical considerations when they are relevant to the methodology. Indeed the theory and application of NMR with particular reference to drug metabolism have also been reviewed (Case, 1973; Calder, 1979). However improvements in the resolution, analytical power and sensitivity of NMR spectroscopy have changed the way the technique is used in drug metabolism studies. In addition, NMR spectroscopy is increasingly being directed to specific sites *in vivo* and when allied with magnetic resonance imaging, information about the location of drug metabolism may be generated. (Bell *et al.*, 1990).

Originally, NMR spectroscopy was used by chemists who generally studied samples with few components which were of defined purity. Subsequently the emphasis was on NMR as a means of structural elucidation in association with other analytical techniques with purification of drug metabolites before analysis. However, drugs and their metabolites and endogenous compounds in body fluids such as urine, plasma and bile are typically complex mixtures of several low and high molecular weight components, some of which are amenable to NMR observation without purification. Indeed proton, ^{31}P and ^{13}C NMR spectroscopy, and to some extent ^{14}N NMR spectroscopy are capable of analysing the endogenous components of biofluids simultaneously in addition to the drug and its metabolites. Preselection of conditions is not necessary and so unexpected metabolites and incorporation products may be detected. In contrast to this, most other assay techniques must be devised based on assumptions of the likely chemical structure of unknown metabolites.

Awareness of the advantages of NMR (Table 1) led those in the life sciences to begin using it for the study of components of complex biofluids and ultimately metabolism, *in vivo*. In this review, we shall show how metabolites can often be directly identified *in vivo*. Such metabolites may be too short-lived to be excreted or too unstable to be purified. Major developments in the NMR field are only slowly being utilized for drug metabolism studies. It is hoped that the examples chosen will exemplify the usefulness of the technique in studying the metabolism of foreign compounds, both quantitatively and qualitatively and in discovering novel and unexpected metabolites. Furthermore, the examples will illustrate that other information regarding biochemical changes in the drug-treated organism can be obtained simultaneously. The examples chosen will emphasize the wealth of additional information NMR can provide about pharmacokinetics, toxicity, drug–biomolecule interactions and biochemical changes associated with drug administration. Other articles recently published which also review the advances made in the field of NMR spectroscopy in drug metabolism are those by Nicholson and Wilson (1987) and Malet-Martino and Martino (1989).

Table 1. Unique features of NMR making it ideally suited to drug metabolism studies.

1. Unlike many other analytical techniques NMR does not require preselection of conditions based on a knowledge of the substance to be analysed.
2. There is no destruction of the sample and so it is available for analysis by a subsequent alternative technique.
3. There is often no sample pretreatment necessary.
4. An analytical technique does not have to be designed for each new application.
5. It can be a rapid technique and only requires a small volume of sample depending on the observed nuclei.
6. There is no destruction or perturbation of unstable metabolites.
7. The technique gives both qualitative/structural and can give quantitative information.
8. It can be used *in vivo*.

2. Sensitivity

NMR spectroscopy is intrinsically an insensitive technique, the reason for this lying in the very small population difference in excitable low energy spins upon which the NMR radiofrequency absorption phenomena depend. However, a number of developments, such as pulsed Fourier transform (FT)-NMR techniques, mathematical processing of digitized data to improve signal-to-noise ratios, improved probe design and increasing magnetic field strengths (2–14 tesla) in use (Table 2) have considerably improved the sensitivity achievable with NMR in recent years. The inherent sensitivity is proportional to the cube of the magnetogyric ratio, γ, of the observed nuclide. Relative sensitivity (rs) for an equal number of nuclei is expressed in this review as a percentage relative to 1H-NMR for easy comparison. The observed sensitivity is also related to the natural abundance (na) of the nuclei. Such data are readily available from an NMR periodic table (see also Table 2). Sensitivity problems associated with low natural abundance may be overcome by using enriched materials and such a strategy may be advantageous for spectral interpretation if background signals interfere with the signals of interest from the labelled drug and its metabolites. Finally, it is not always recognized that sensitivity is proportional to the concentration of the observed (equivalent) nuclei in the sample. It is foolish to use expensive labelled materials if the metabolites of interest cannot be concentrated in the sample above micromolar concentrations. Sensitivity problems cannot usually be overcome by simply increasing the accumulation time even when instrument time is abundant, which it generally is not. This is because although the signal will increase in proportion to n, the number of accumulated scans, transients or free induction decays (FID), the noise will also increase in proportion to the square root of n. There-

Table 2. Important characteristics of NMR observable nuclei.

	Resonance frequency[a]	Relative sensitivity[b] (rs) (%)	Natural abundance (na) (%)	Spin
Tritium	533.3	121	0	½
Proton	500.0	100	99.98	½
Fluorine-19	470.4	83.3	100	½
Phosphorus-31	202.4	6.6	100	½
Carbon-13	125.7	1.6	1.1	½
Deuterium	76.8	1	0.02	1
Nitrogen-15	50.7	0.1	0.37	½
Nitrogen-14	36.1	0.1	99.63	1

[a] at 11.75 tesla in MHz
[b] for an equal number of nuclei compared to 1H-NMR
Spectrometers are often referred to by the resonance frequency of the proton in Megahertz, e.g. 60–600 MHz. However, other nuclei resonate at frequencies dependent on the field strength measured in tesla (1 tesla = 10 kilogauss) and their specific magnetogyric ratios.

fore improvements seen with time take progressively longer to manifest themselves in the resultant spectrum. Consequently, the pulse width or flip angle and the associated relaxation delay should be chosen to maximize the resultant accumulated signal by use of the Ernst angle. The chemical composition of the sample or the magnetic homogeneity essential for high resolution work may fluctuate with time. *In vivo* experiments may also be limited by other time constraints.

Sensitivity may be improved by observing the combined signal resulting from nuclei in identical magnetic environments. Thus methyl protons often give intense singlets (when uncoupled) in ^{1}H-spectra and for similar reasons the trifluoromethyl group has proved a particular favourite in ^{19}F-NMR studies when sensitivity is a problem. Signals of interest likely to be split are best observed while decoupling the coupled nucleus. The intensity of the resultant singlet is increased by multiplet collapse and in low molecular weight compounds by the nuclear Overhauser effect (nOe). The population difference between the spins α^- and β^-, of hetero-nuclei may be altered by various polarization-transfer techniques (e.g. INEPT, DEPT*) so increasing the inherent sensitivity. Apart from these specialized experiments the sensitivity of two-dimensional (2D) NMR is usually less than the single pulse experiment. Overall, however, it is now possible to study a drug metabolite successfully in the 0.1−1 mmolar range with NMR spectroscopy of the high magnetogyric nuclides. A well designed NMR experiment can push this detection limit an order of magnitude lower.

3. Proton-NMR

Solvent suppression

Proton-NMR (^{1}H-NMR; rs = 100 per cent) is the most widely used in drug metabolism studies because of its high sensitivity and the large number of observable protons in most drugs and their metabolites (na = 99.98 per cent). Unfortunately, because the drug and its metabolites are initially obtained in an aqueous sample, the intense water signal present must be either eliminated, suppressed or edited out of the spectrum. The water, or for that matter any other protonated solvent used, will be greater than four orders of magnitude higher in concentration than the dissolved metabolites. Consequently, its signal will simply overload the receiver amplifier of the spectrometer when it is set to the attenuation required for observation of the metabolites. In addition, the water signal will be digitized in preference to the weaker signals of interest by the analog-to-digital converter (ADC), to an extent which will depend on the ADC's word length. Very recently, however, some instrument manufacturers have introduced spectrometers of greatly improved dynamic

---

* See Appendix

range which will simplify the problem (1988–89). Freeze-drying the sample and reconstitution in a deuterated solvent such as deuterium oxide (^2H_2O; D_2O) or extraction into a non-miscible solvent such as deuterochloroform is a simple solution and also offers an opportunity to concentrate the sample and add a deuterium lock signal. However, care must be taken not to lose volatile components or modify metabolites in the process. The deuteration of any slowly exchangeable protons present in the solutes of interest may eliminate useful signals but an appreciation of this effect can often help with structural elucidation. The substitution of deuterium oxide for water during *in vivo* studies poses a more fundamental problem, namely the modification of drug metabolism because of kinetic isotope effects (Nicholson *et al.*, 1985 a). However, this may also be of advantage in drug metabolism studies as investigations using deuterium-labelled drugs have demonstrated.

Analysis can be performed in protonated solvents such as H_2O by suppressing the signal. The simplest method is *selective saturation* and involves secondary irradiation at the solvent frequency. Although the technique can efficiently decrease the signal intensity of the solvent a thousand fold, the homonuclear decoupling power required for further reduction is considerable. The spectrum is often distorted and suppressed around the solvent peak in proportion to the decoupler power. Further, the decoupler coil used is no longer available for manipulation of any metabolite spin systems as an aid to structural elucidation. Slowly exchangeable protons will be simultaneously suppressed by saturation transfer. The efficiency of suppression tends to vary with the spectrometer used. Selective saturation is probably best used with freeze-dried biofluid samples which have been reconstituted in D_2O to eliminate the signal from residual H_2O.

Briefly *selective relaxation* involves first inverting the magnetization vector of the solvent with a (180°) pulse. A delay is then chosen during which the solvent only half recovers and is subsequently nulled. Relatively high molecular weight compounds which usually includes the drug and its metabolites tend to relax longitudinally (T1) more rapidly and as a result have passed their null points during the delay. Consequently, only those components of interest elicit signals when a 90° observation pulse is subsequently applied. This technique is most successful when the T1 relaxation times of the compounds of interest are known to be much shorter than the solvents, otherwise these are also partially suppressed.

An alternative approach to solvent suppression is to supplement the sample with an agent capable of greatly shortening the spin-spin or transverse (T2) relaxation of the solvent. In the case of H_2O, molar quantities of simple amino compounds which rapidly exchange protons with water at specific pH values such as ammonium, guanidine, hydroxylamine (Rabenstein and Fan, 1986), urea (Connor *et al.*, 1987 a) or hydrazine may be used. Alternatively, millimolar quantities of paramagnetic ions such as Mn^{2+} or Gd^{3+} (Brindle *et al.*, 1979; Eads *et al.*, 1986) which can efficiently relax rapidly exchanging liganded solvent molecules, are added to the sample. During the multiple inversions in a cumulative spin echo experiment or Carr-Purcell-Meiboom-Gill (CPMG) sequence, the magnetization of the solvent rapidly undergoes T2-relaxation to zero while significant signals from the low molecular weight components of interest remain. These methods are best applied in association with the suppression of interfering broad signals resulting from biological macromolecules such as protein and lipid seen in some biofluid samples (Rabenstein and Nakishima, 1979; Nicholson *et al.*, 1983). Unfortunately, these relaxation agents may broaden and suppress other important signals and the metal ions are apt to bind inaccessibly to proteins (Connor *et al.*, 1987 b). Signals with shifts identical to the solvent can be seen by these methods. A useful property of Hahn spin-echo experiments is to phase modulate the signals such that singlets and triplets remain upright while doublets and quartets are inverted. This may facilitate the identification of such multiplets.

Selective excitation or 'jump and return' involves applying a 90° pulse to the sample and waiting for the magnetization vector of the solvent to precess exactly 180°. A second 90° pulse applied with the opposite phase leaves the solvent with no net magnetization. Other components of the sample which precess at different rates can still be observed, however. Their signals are more intense the further they resonate from the chemical shift of the solvent. With D_2O (^2H_2O) as solvent the method proves most useful for examining signals at the periphery of the spectrum. The original 1–1 hard pulse (Clore *et al.*, 1983) has been improved by adding successive half pulses at the ends of the pulse sequence in the manner of a binomial expansion. The 1–3–3–1 pulse is considered by many to be the most successful (Hore, 1983). Another useful method of solvent suppression is data shift accumulation (Roth *et al.*, 1980).

Paracetamol

As the metabolism of paracetamol (acetaminophen) is well documented it has proved a useful model to study by ^1H-NMR, particularly as metabolite standards are available. NMR has been used to study the metabolism of paracetamol both in humans *in vivo* and in isolated rat hepatocytes *in vitro*.

In Vivo Studies. Human volunteers were given a single 1 g dose of paracetamol (APAP) and urine was collected hourly for the first 6 hours and then a final collection was made after 24 hours. Direct analysis of these urine samples by proton-NMR (9.4–11.8 tesla) revealed that a number of novel resonances could be detected in comparison with control urine samples (Bales *et al.*, 1984). By reference to NMR spectra of metabolite standards it was possible to assign these resonances. The CH_3 group of the N-acetyl moiety of paracetamol and its metabolites (Figure 1) gave resonances in the region of 2.13–2.19 ppm which were well resolved following apodization of the accumulated transients before Fourier transformation. The acetyl resonances

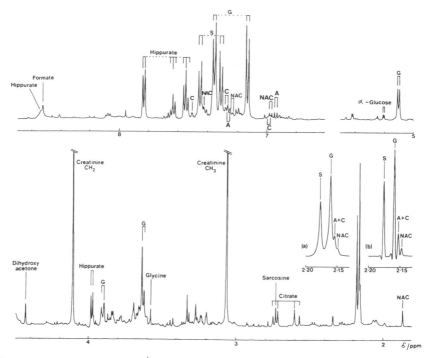

Figure 1. 500 MHz (11.8 tesla) ¹H-NMR spectrum of a urine sample collected 6 hours after acetaminophen ingestion showing the aromatic (upper) and aliphatic (lower) regions. A = acetaminophen; G = glucuronide conjugate; S = sulphate conjugate; C = L-cysteinyl conjugate; NAC = N-acetyl-L-cysteinyl conjugate. From Bales *et al.*, 1984. Copyright American Association for Clinical Chemistry.

detected were derived from: paracetamol, paracetamol glucuronide, paracetamol sulphate, paracetamol cysteine conjugate and paracetamol N-acetylcysteine conjugate. The acetyl resonances from paracetamol itself and the cysteine conjugate were not well resolved (see below under 2D-NMR). Peak identity was confirmed by the addition of authentic standards to the urine.

Paracetamol and its metabolites also give observable resonances due to the aromatic protons and those on the conjugating moiety. The protons on the glucuronic acid moiety (such as the β-anomeric proton doublet at 5.11 ppm) and the cysteine and N-acetylcysteine residues (N-acetyl resonance 1.84 ppm) will also contribute resonances to the spectrum. One particular advantage of ¹H-NMR is that there are often several resonances from one molecule which allow greater confidence in metabolite assignment.

The importance of this study was in showing that high resolution ¹H-NMR was able to detect and readily discriminate between the metabolites of paracetamol after a therapeutic dose to human volunteers. Quantitation of metabolites and calculation of amounts excreted agreed with previous studies using HPLC and other methods. As well as metabolism in humans after therapeutic doses, NMR has been applied to the study of the urinary metabolic profile following paracetamol overdose by Bales *et al.* (1988). These studies revealed that the proportion of glucuronide and sulphate conjugates of paracetamol were very different after an overdose. Thus the ratio (glucuronide : sulphate) was found to be 1.4, 6 hours after the 1 g dose whereas in overdosed patients this ranged from between 4.2 and 5.7, 24 hours after overdose and between 10.2 and 77.6, two to three days afterwards. Also noted was a large apparent increase in the N-acetylcysteine conjugate.

IN VITRO METABOLISM. The disposition of paracetamol in isolated rat hepatocytes was also studied by proton-NMR (Nicholson *et al.*, 1985 a). When whole hepatocytes were examined by NMR there were no resonances detectable from paracetamol or its metabolites. However, spin-echo spectra of cell extracts showed resonances for paracetamol, and its glucuronic acid and sulphate conjugates. When the metabolites were added to the hepatocyte suspension, resonances were readily detectable. This indicates that the metabolites formed inside the hepatocyte are not NMR visible probably because of binding to proteins or chemical exchange. GSH cannot be detected in hepatocytes by NMR but it is readily visible in erythrocytes (Brown *et al.*, 1977). This may be because of binding to specific proteins within the hepatocyte. An isotope effect was detected when the hepatocytes were incubated with paracetamol in ^2H_2O buffer. The glucuronidation of paracetamol was significantly slower in this latter buffer. There was selective deuteration at the C_2 of glucose which was also detectable in the C_2 of the glucuronide conjugate from the splitting pattern (spin-spin coupling) at the β-anomeric carbon. This finding suggested to the authors that futile cycling through part of the glycolytic pathway had occurred.

The original studies with paracetamol revealed that ^1H-NMR could be applied to the study of drug metabolism where standards were available and the metabolism was known. To be particularly useful, however, the technique needs to be applicable to the study of new compounds with unknown metabolic profiles.

p-aminophenol

Gartland *et al.* (1989 a) studied the metabolism and toxicity of the model nephrotoxin *p*-aminophenol, in the rat. The major metabolite, paracetamol sulphate, which results from N-acetylation and sulphate conjugation, was observed by ^1H-NMR in the urine of treated animals. Dose-related increases of lactate, acetate and glucose excretion and a decrease in citrate excretion indicative of renal failure was observed by NMR and confirmed by conventional methods. The change in urinary components were found to be associated with histologically observed proximal tubular necrosis. Further investigation (Gartland *et al.*, 1990) identified paracetamol sulphate and paracetamol glucuronide and tentatively identified *p*-aminophenol sulphate and *p*-aminophenol glucuronide as the biliary metabolites of *p*-aminophenol using spin-echo NMR.

Following on from these studies and earlier studies on mercury (Nicholson *et al.*, 1985 b), these workers have studied several nephrotoxins by ^{1}H-NMR urinalysis in an attempt to identify metabolite profiles indicative of regio-specific damage to the kidney (Gartland *et al.*, 1989 c). Foxall *et al.* (1989) have also used NMR to monitor a patient following a massive acute exposure to phenol and dichloromethane.

SPEC-NMR

Wilson and Ismail (1986) and Wilson and Nicholson (1987) successfully used medium-field strength instruments (4.7–5.9 tesla) in further ^{1}H-NMR studies of drug metabolism. They were able to simplify spectra of human urine samples by rapid and simple solid-phase extraction chromatography (SPEC-NMR) using disposable C-18 columns. Variable deuteromethanol/deuterium oxide (CD_3OD/D_2O) mixtures were used to selectively elute drug metabolites, and endogenous components which interfered in spectra of the original urine samples. These authors (Nicholson and Wilson, 1987) have argued that only limited purification of biofluids containing drug metabolites is necessary to effect component identification. Their approach contrasts with the more complicated HPLC-NMR technique exemplified by the studies of Laude and Wilkins (1987) which tend to be less adaptable and more time-consuming.

Using this SPEC-NMR technique Wilson and Ismail (1986) identified the glucuronides of *naproxen* (Figure 2) and its O-desmethyl metabolite in the urine of a patient being treated for osteoarthritis. They also showed that with this technique lower field strength NMR spectrometers were quite adequate.

Similarly, Wilson and Nicholson (1987) were able to identify the glucuronide conjugates of *ibuprofen* (Figure 3) and a metabolite formed by hydroxylation of the isobutyl side-chain in the urine of a human volunteer following a therapeutic dose. In addition, the metabolite produced by further oxidation of the side-chain was detected. The SPEC-NMR technique was able in this case to concentrate and semi-purify enough of the metabolites for fast atom bombardment-mass spectrometry (FAB-MS) and even ^{13}C-NMR characterization (see below).

Hydrazine

The hepatotoxin *hydrazine* is a small molecule, the metabolism (Figure 4) of which cannot be studied easily by conventional means as it is not possible to incorporate a radioactive isotope with a usable half-life which will not exchange in aqueous solution. Two approaches have been used to study the metabolism using single pulse NMR; either using proton-NMR to study metabolites in which NMR visible protons have been added metabolically or using

¹⁵N-NMR and ¹⁵N-labelled hydrazine (see below). Hydrazine itself may be detected by proton-NMR if the pH of the medium is sufficiently low.

In urine from rats dosed with hydrazine a number of novel resonances were detected by proton-NMR (Sanins *et al.*, 1988). Two singlets (1.95 ppm and 2.06 ppm) were identified as being due to the methyl groups of monoacetyl and diacetylhydrazine (Figure 5) by the use of authentic standards. Two triplets were detected at 2.55 ppm and 2.85 ppm. These were identified as being

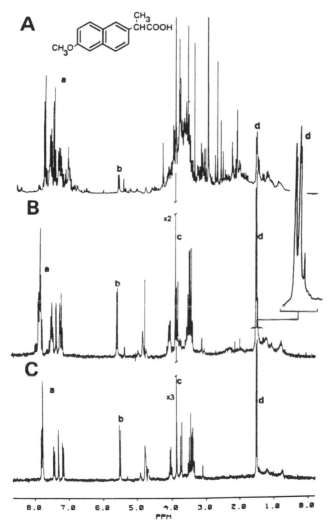

Figure 2. Proton NMR spectrum of (A) human urine sample after treatment with naproxen; (B) urine after elution from a Bond Elut column with acidified D₂0/CD₃0D (60 : 40); expansion shows region between 1 and 2 ppm with signals from α-methyl group of drug and O-demethyl metabolite; (C) urine after elution from a Bond Elut column with D₂0/CD₃0D (40 : 60) showing naproxen glucuronide a = aromatic protons; b = anomeric proton of D-glucuronide conjugate; c = O-methyl group; d = α-methyl group. From Wilson and Ismail, 1986, with permission.

due to tetrahydro-3-oxo-pyridazine 6-carboxylic acid (THOPC), the cyclized hydrazone formed between hydrazine and 2-oxoglutarate. Other possible metabolites were also detected but not identified. As well as metabolites of the hydrazine, changes in endogenous metabolites could also be detected. Thus excretion of lactate, methylamine and the amino acid taurine were elevated

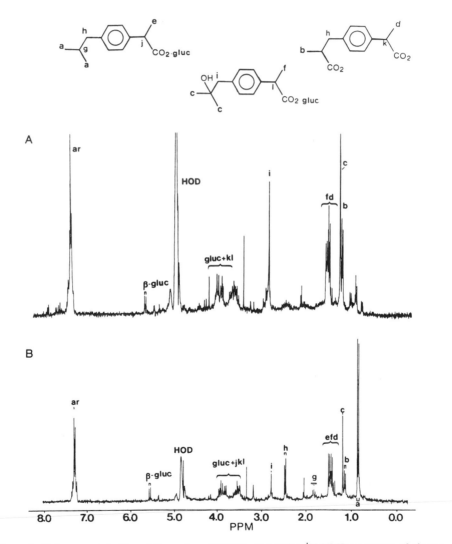

Figure 3. Urinary metabolites of ibuprofen. 400 MHz (9.4 tesla) ^{1}H-NMR spectrum of eluates from a C18 SPE column; (A) Eluates obtained with 40 : 60 methanol : water and (B) eluates obtained with 60 : 40 methanol : water. Urine collected 2–4 hours after an oral dose of ibuprofen (400 mg) to a human subject and 2 ml placed on the column. Letters refer to protons on structures shown. Fraction shown in A is mainly 2-[4(1-hydroxy-2-methyl-propyl)-phenyl] propionic acid glucuronide and 2-[4-(1-carboxy-2-methylpropyl)-phenyl] propionic acid. Fraction shown in B is mainly ibuprofen glucuronide and some of material eluting in 40 : 60 fraction. From Nicholson and Wilson, 1987, with permission.

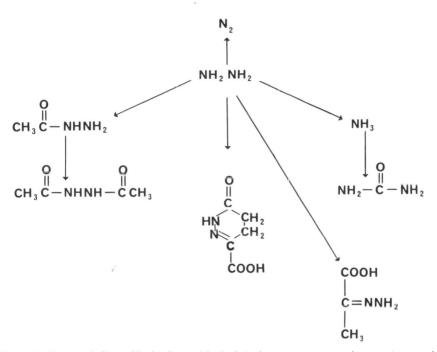

Figure 4. The metabolism of hydrazine to (clockwise) nitrogen gas, ammonia, urea (presumably via ammonia), pyruvate hydrazone, THOPC (the cyclized hydrazone of 2-oxoglutarate) and diacetylhydrazine via monoacetylhydrazine.

whereas other endogenous substances such as 2-oxoglutarate were notably absent.

Proton-NMR has also been used to study the disposition of hydrazine in liver extracts after dosing animals with hydrazine. Again the metabolites acetylhydrazine, diacetylhydrazine and THOPC could be detected in these extracts. Also changes in endogenous compounds such as increases in β-alanine, alanine and lactate were observed. Single pulse proton spectra of isolated hepatocytes are usually dominated by endogenous protein and lipid resonances in the aliphatic region (Figure 6). The cells can be removed easily by centrifugation and the medium examined for metabolites or spin-echo techniques can be used (Nicholson *et al.*, 1985 a). A study of the disposition of hydrazine in isolated rat hepatocytes by proton-NMR analysis of hepatocyte medium (Preece *et al.*, 1989) also revealed that metabolism to acetylhydrazine was taking place and THOPC was forming during incubation of metabolically competent cells with hydrazine (Figure 7). The appearance of acetylhydrazine was quantitated by NMR. Increases in lactate and alanine and a decrease in 3-hydroxybutyrate were also observed and quantitated.

N-methylformamide

Another small molecule recently studied by NMR is *N-methylformamide* (NMF). This potential anticancer drug is hepatotoxic and consequently its metabolism is of particular interest. The urinary metabolites of NMF in rats and mice dosed with the compound were investigated by proton-NMR as well as by conventional techniques (Tulip *et al.*, 1986). A number of clearly resolved resonances were detected in the spectra of urine from rats after dosing with NMF (Figure 8). The methyl group in NMF gave rise to the major peak (2.77 ppm; *anti*-isomer) which was a doublet at the low pH used to inhibit N–H or N–D exchange, due to splitting from the proton on the

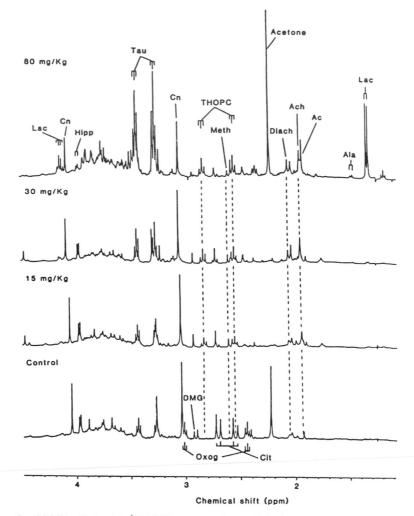

Figure 5. 400 MHz (9.4 tesla) ¹H-NMR spectra of the aliphatic region of urine collected 0–6 hours after treating rats with hydrazine. Ach = acetylhydrazine; Diach = diacetylhydrazine; THOPC = cyclized hydrazone with 2-oxoglutarate; Meth = methylamine. Endogenous components: Lac = lactate; Cn = creatinine; Hipp = hippurate; Tau = taurine; Ac = acetate; Ala = alanine. From Sanins *et al.*, 1988, with permission.

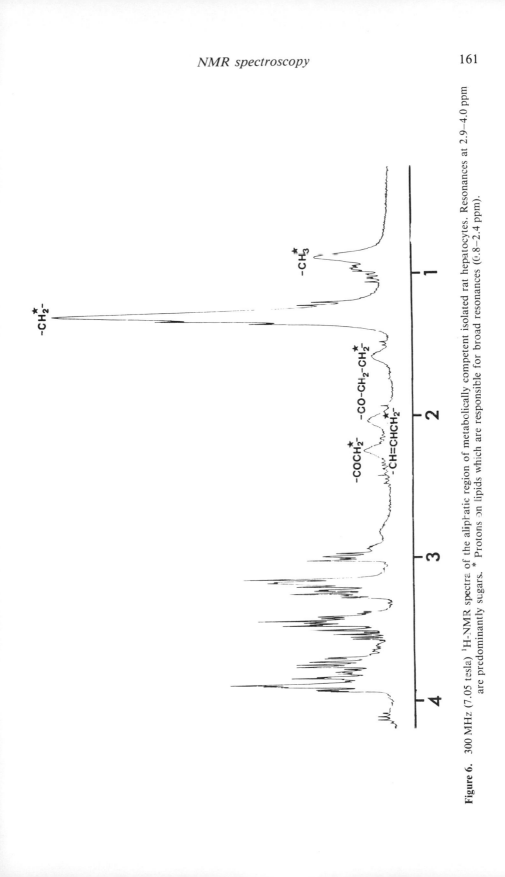

Figure 6. 300 MHz (7.05 tesla) ^{1}H-NMR spectra of the aliphatic region of metabolically competent isolated rat hepatocytes. Resonances at 2.9–4.0 ppm are predominantly sugars. * Protons on lipids which are responsible for broad resonances (0.8–2.4 ppm).

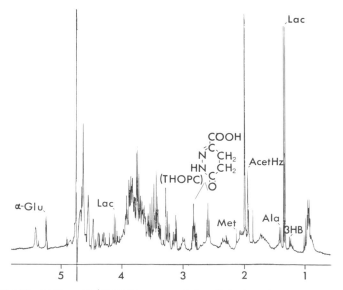

Figure 7. 300 MHz (7.05 tesla) ^{1}H-NMR spectra of the aliphatic region of hepatocyte isolation medium of cells removed after 2 hours incubation with hydrazine. AcetHz = acetylhydrazine; Ala = alanine; α-Glu = α-D-glucose; 3HB = 3-hydroxybutyrate: Lac = lactate; Met = methionine; THOPC = cyclized hydrazone with 2-oxoglutarate. From Preece and Timbrell, 1989.

nitrogen atom. A second signal of less intensity at 2.91 ppm was due to the *syn*-isomer of NMF (the compound exists in *syn* and *anti* forms in the ratio 1 : 9). As well as these resonances from the unchanged compound, there was a number of other, novel resonances. A singlet at 2.61 ppm was identified as due to methylamine. Although this is an endogenous metabolite the amounts in control urine were very small compared to those in urine from NMF treated mice or rats. Methylamine had not previously been described as a metabolite. Its presence was confirmed by GC-MS and quantitated by HPLC methods. Another singlet detected in the NMR spectrum at 8.46 ppm was identified as formate. The proposed metabolite N-hydroxymethyl formamide (NMF-OH) could not be detected as the CH_2 resonance was obscured by residual H_2O.

A number of other novel resonances was also detected in the urine from both rats and mice but especially in those urine samples collected between 24 and 48 hours after dosing (Figure 9). These resonances were assumed to be as follows: a doublet from a N-methyl group which was 0.02 ppm downfield from the N-methyl signal of NMF (2.79 ppm), a singlet from an acetyl CH_3 group (2.03 ppm), a multiplet from two methylene protons (3.4 ppm) and a

Figure 8. 400 MHz (9.4 tesla) ^{1}H-NMR spectra (aliphatic region) of urine from control and N-methylformamide (NMF)-treated rat. NMF_1 and NMF_2 refer to the *anti-* and *syn*-isomers of NMF; a, b, c, and d refer to the N-acetyl-L-cysteinyl derivative shown in Figure 9; A_1 and A_2 refer to resonances thought to be due to acetyl groups from uncharacterized metabolites. From Tulip *et al.*, 1986, with permission.

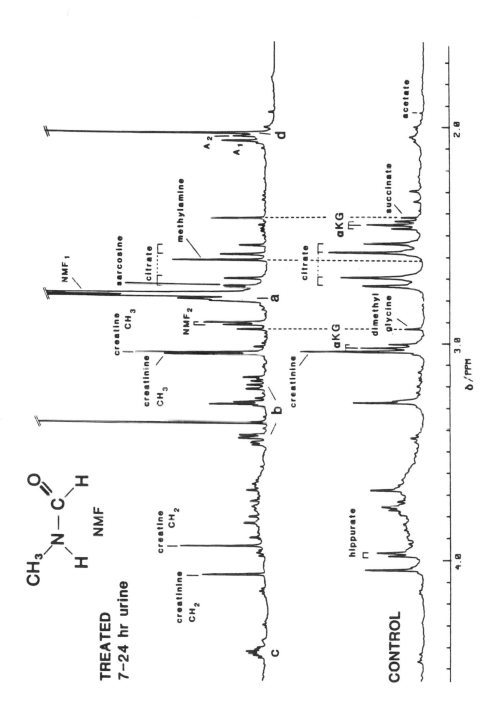

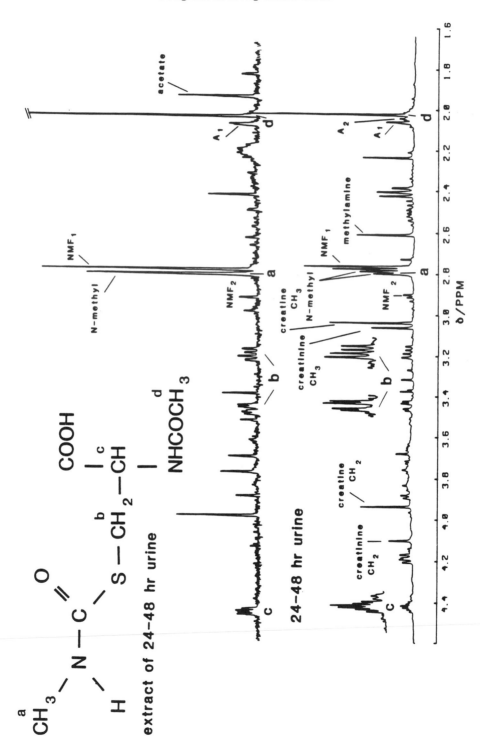

multiplet from an α-CH proton (4.42 ppm). There were good intensity correlations between these resonances. Extraction of urine samples with ethyl acetate under acidic conditions yielded an extract which on redissolving in ^2H_2O gave a much clearer spectrum. This spectrum of the extract allowed a tentative identification of the metabolite as an N'-acetylcysteine conjugate: N'-acetyl-S-(N-methyl-carbamoyl-)-L-cysteine (Figure 9). 2D-NMR also helped in elucidation of the structure by confirming that the α-proton and β-methylene protons were spin-spin coupled (see below and Figure 39). Synthesis of this compound confirmed the assignments and thin-layer chromatography confirmed its presence as a urinary metabolite. This N-acetylcysteine conjugate was therefore both detected and identified as a consequence of using the NMR approach.

N,N-dimethylformamide

A similar approach has been adopted to study the metabolism of N,N-dimethylformamide (DMF) the industrial solvent (Tulip *et al.*, 1989; Kestell *et al.*, 1986). High resolution NMR has revealed a number of novel metabolites. The major metabolite of DMF is hydroxymethyl N-methylformamide and unlike NMF-OH, the CH_2 protons can be readily seen in the spectra (Figure 10). Two singlet resonances from the N-methyl of DMF itself (*syn*- and *anti*-isomers) can be easily recognized as can a singlet resonance from dimethylamine. Downfield of these resonances, those of the formyl proton of DMF and N-hydroxymethyl-N-methylformamide are well resolved (Figure 10). In the urine collected 48–72 hours after dosing and extracted with ethyl acetate under acidic conditions, resonances from NMF were also detected. The complex pattern characteristic of the N-acetylcysteine conjugate, previously shown to be excreted as a metabolite of NMF (Figure 9) was also observed (Tulip *et al.*, 1989). DMF metabolism has also been studied using the ^{15}N labelled compound (see below).

Metronidazole

Allars *et al.* (1986) studied the metabolism of metronidazole (I; Figure 11) the antimicrobial drug and radio sensitizing agent, in the isolated perfused rat liver. The drug was introduced into the perfusate which was monitored at intervals by removing samples which, after lyophilization, were redissolved in

---

Figure 9. 400 (9.4 tesla) MHz ^1H-NMR spectra of urine from an NMF-treated rat (24–48 hours) before and after extraction with ethyl acetate. a, b, c and d refer to the resonances from the N-acetyl-L-cysteinyl conjugate, the structure of which is shown. The spectra were plotted after Gaussian resolution enhancement. As the extract was dissolved in ^2H_2O the N-methyl resonances collapsed to singlets due to loss of adjacent NH protons. From Tulip *et al.*, 1986, with permission.

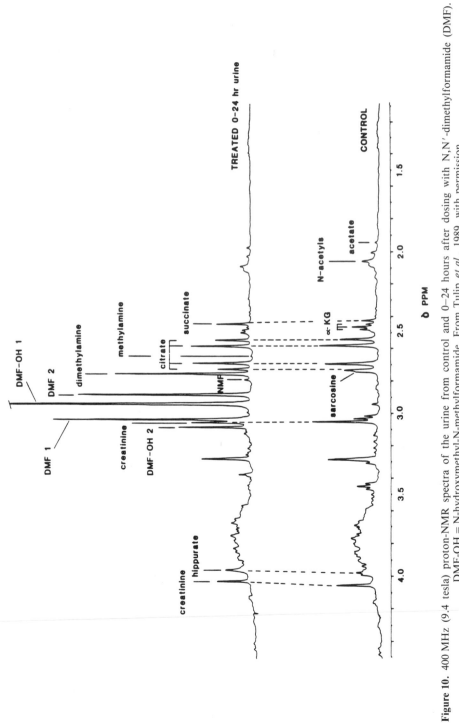

Figure 10. 400 MHz (9.4 tesla) proton-NMR spectra of the urine from control and 0–24 hours after dosing with N,N′-dimethylformamide (DMF). DMF-OH = N-hydroxymethyl-N-methylformamide. From Tulip *et al.*, 1989, with permission.

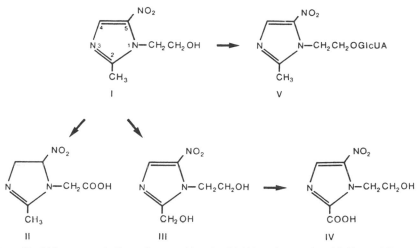

Figure 11. Urinary metabolites of metronidazole. GlcUA = glucuronic acid. From Allars *et al.*,
1986, with permission.

^2H_2O and analysed in the spectrometer. The acidic metabolite II and the glucuronide conjugate, metabolite V, were detected in the perfusate by ^1H-NMR
(7.05 tesla), along with the parent compound following metronidazole exposure. The major metabolite, the glucuronide conjugate, (V) was identified
from the resonances at 2.53 ppm (C-2 methyl group), 8.04 ppm (C-4 proton)
and the doublet at 4.38 ppm coupled to one at 3.20 ppm from the C-1′ and
C-2′ protons of the glucuronyl moiety. This assignment was confirmed by the
modulation of the signals following treatment with β-glucuronidase. The
singlet from the CH_3 group (2.53 ppm) was found to be the most satisfactory
for quantitating the disappearance of the parent compound and appearance
of the glucuronide (V). Metabolism was enhanced by using the livers from
phenobarbitone-pretreated rats. The lack of specific signals from the C-4
protons (approx. 8 ppm) of the other metabolites (III) and (IV) indicated they
were absent from the perfusate.

In subsequent studies, Coleman and Norton (1986) were able to detect and
quantitate all the major metabolites of metronidazole in human urine after an
oral dose of 400 mg by ^1H-NMR. In addition, a variety of endogenous metabolites were detectable. The major metabolites detected were (I), (II), (III) and
(V). For their procedure, urine samples were repeatedly lyophilized and
redissolved in ^2H_2O. This was necessary to allow the methylene resonance of
II, which is close to the resonance due to HO^2H, to be observed. Otherwise
this procedure would not have been necessary and the urine could have been
examined directly using secondary irradiation to reduce the intensity of
the water resonance. The authors found good agreement between values for
metabolite concentrations determined by HPLC methods and by ^1H-NMR.

Oxpentifylline

Wilson *et al.* (1987) studied the metabolism of oxpentifylline, an anti-hypertensive drug, in human volunteers and compared the results between ^{1}H-NMR and HPLC methods. Interestingly they also compared data generated from spectrometers with medium (5.9 tesla) and high (9.4 tesla) field strengths. Predictably, ^{1}H-NMR of the human urine gave poorer quality spectra at the lower field strength because of insufficient signal dispersion. Oxpentifylline is metabolized extensively to the metabolite CPDX (Figure 12) which has a number of NMR visible protons. The N-CH$_3$ proton signals were particularly strong, as was the C-8 proton in reconstituted urine samples. Comparison of the quantitation of the C-8 proton peak by NMR and of CPDX by HPLC showed that there was good correlation, using spectrometers of either field strength. However, when the N-3 methyl peak was used for

Structure of 1-(3′-carboxypropyl)-3,7-dimethylxanthine (CPDX).

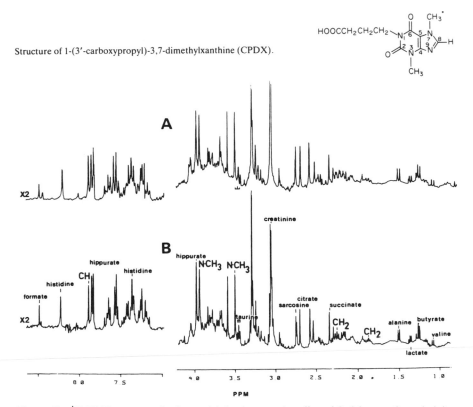

Figure 12. ^{1}H-NMR spectra of a freeze-dried urine sample collected 0–2 hours after administration of oxpentifylline (600 mg) to a human subject. The sample was redissolved in ^{2}H$_2$O at five times original concentration. Spectra A, 250 MHz (5.9 tesla); spectra B, 400 MHz (9.4 tesla). The resonances labelled on the spectra are from the protons shown in the structure of CPDX, the major metabolite. From Wilson *et al.*, 1987, with permission.

quantitation there was only good correlation with the HPLC data when using the 9.4-tesla spectrometer, despite that fact that this resonance was more intense than that from the C-8 proton. At 5.9 tesla this signal was not completely resolved from the endogenous taurine triplet. The C-8 proton peak fortunately resonated in an area of the spectra the authors termed a 'chemical window' which was devoid of other signals or 'chemical noise', as distinct from 'physical noise' which is a product of the spectrometer.

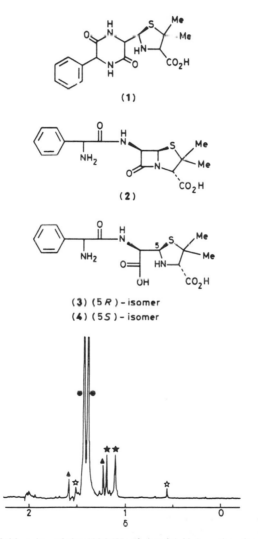

Figure 13. The high-field region of the 400 MHz (9.4 tesla) Hahn spin-echo ^{1}H-NMR spectrum of rat urine 0–2 hours after dosing with ampicillin (700 mg/kg). (1) diketopiperazine metabolite; (2) ampicillin; (3) 5R isomer of penicilloic acid; (4) 5S isomer of penicilloic acid. From Everett *et al.*, 1984, with permission.

Penicillins

Everett *et al*. (1984) studied the metabolism of ampicillin (Figure 13; structure 2) in the rat using spin-echo ¹H-NMR spectroscopy. Penicillins and their metabolites are readily detectable by a pair of characteristic sharp singlets due to the *gem*-dimethyl groups. Ampicillin and stereoisomers of the known metabolite penicilloic acid (Figure 13; 3 and 4), which form as a result of epimerization at C-5 of the thiazolidine ring, are detectable by their methyl resonances. In addition a new metabolite, diketopiperazine (Figure 13; 1), which is formed by an intramolecular cyclic rearrangement, was also detected by the two singlets from the *gem*-dimethyl groups. These resonances are particularly useful as they occur in a 'window' (1–1.6 ppm) in the spectra of urine from ampicillin-treated rats. The identification of the new metabolite was confirmed by HPLC methodology. Connor *et al*, (1987 a) found that elimination of the water peak by exchange broadening (specifically by addition of 1.2 M urea at pH 3.4, and utilization of a CPMG sequence) facilitated the observation of the C-6 proton of penillic acid in the urine of benzylpenicillin treated rats (Figure 14; see also flucloxacillin below).

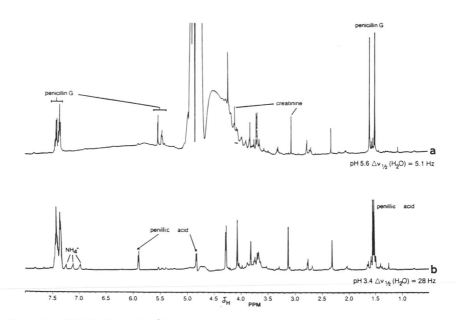

Figure 14. 400 MHz (9.4 tesla) ¹H-NMR spectra of the urine from a human following an oral dose of benzylpenicillin. (a) normal spectrum using homogated irradiation to effect partial solvent suppression; (b) CPMG spin-echo ¹H-NMR spectrum of the same urine following addition of urea to 1.2 M and adjustment of pH to 3.4. The sample has degraded to penillic acid, the C6 proton of which can be seen despite being coincident with the water resonance. From Connor *et al*., 1987 a, with permission

4. Tritium-NMR

The ^{3}H nucleus has the highest magnetogyric ratio and therefore tritium-NMR (^{3}H-NMR) is theoretically the most sensitive available (rs = 121 per cent) and might appear ideal for drug metabolism studies. This is because initial radiolabelling studies on the disposition of drugs labelled with tritium (na = 0 per cent) could be rapidly followed with ^{3}H-NMR studies of tissue extracts. Unfortunately, despite its high sensitivity the tritium concentrations required for rapid NMR studies are still several orders of magnitude greater than those required for safe radiolabelling studies. In addition most instruments are not allowed to be used or are not even equipped for tritium-NMR. Consequently, to our knowledge ^{3}H-NMR has been used only to confirm the site of tritiation prior to radiolabelling studies.

Deuterium-NMR. See page 194.

5. ^{19}F-NMR

^{19}F-NMR has also received considerable attention in drug metabolism studies because of its relatively high sensitivity (rs = 83 per cent), the large chemical shift range and the increasing use of fluorinated compounds as pharmaceuticals (Walsh, 1983).

Compounds studied

Flucloxacillin

In further NMR studies of the metabolism of penicillin analogues, Everett *et al.* (1985) were able to distinguish four metabolites of flucloxacillin in rat urine by ^{19}F-NMR, even though the structural differences between them were 6–8 bonds from the single fluorine atom present (Figure 15). Sensitivity was greatly increased by proton-decoupling due to multiplet collapse and the nOe. Following opening of the β-lactam ring, ^{19}F-NMR like ^{1}H-NMR, was able to distinguish the R and S forms of the penicilloic acid. These isomers had previously been indistinguishable by the published HPLC method. These workers have also applied two-dimensional techniques to further study flucloxacillin (see below).

Profluralin

Jacobson and Gerig (1988) have used ^{19}F-NMR and other techniques to study the complex metabolism of profluralin, a trifluoromethylated dinitroaniline herbicide in the rat. A hydroxylamine derivative following reduction of a nitro-group was the first urinary metabolite observed and among several other metabolites, benzimidazole structures have been identified following intramolecular cyclisations. The metabolism has also been investigated *in vivo*. These workers have also used ^{19}F-NMR to study the metabolism of *flumecinol*, an inducer of cytochrome P450b.

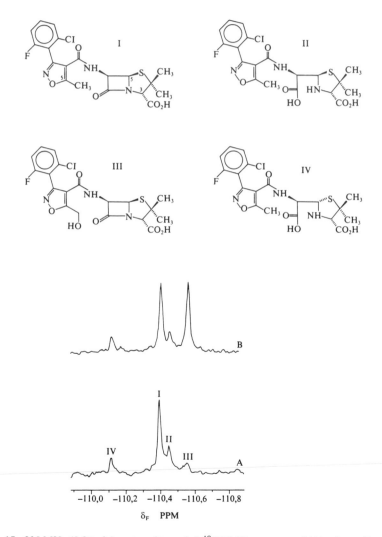

Figure 15. 235 MHz (5.9 tesla) proton decoupled ^{19}F-NMR spectrum of (A) urine collected from a rat 2–4 hours after dosing with sodium flucloxacillin (200 mg/kg i.v.) showing fluorine resonances from the parent compound (I) and major metabolites, penicilloic acid (II), the 5′-hydroxymethyl derivative (III) and the (5S)-flucloxacillin penicilloic acid (IV); (B) as above but with an extra spike of (III). Each spectrum required a 14.5-min accumulation time and was referenced to external $CFCl_3$. From Nicholson and Wilson, 1987, with permission. Original spectra courtesy of Dr J Everett.

Trifluoromethylaniline

Wade *et al.* (1988) have studied the metabolism of 4-trifluoromethylaniline (TFMA) in rats (Figure 16). Following ring hydroxylation, the glucuronide conjugate of the hydroxy-TFMA product is responsible for one of the four peaks detected in urine (Figure 17). Also present is an oxanilic acid derivative suggesting the trifluoromethyl group can facilitate the ω-hydroxylation of N-acetyl TFMA once formed. These workers have also used ^{19}F-NMR to study the metabolism of the NSAID *flurbiprofen* and *fluoroacetanilide*.

2-Fluoro-2-deoxyglucose

Nakada *et al.* (1986) studied the metabolism of 2-fluoro-2-deoxyglucose (FDG) in rat brain *in vivo*. Following administration of FDG, signals were observed from FDG and/or its 6-phosphate, and also 2-fluoro-2-deoxy-phosphogluconolactone and/or its gluconate produced via the pentose phosphate pathway. In addition, a third major signal was identified as 2-fluoro-2-deoxyglycerol and its intensity was found to be modulated by co-administration of sorbinil, an aldose reductase inhibitor (Nakada and Kwee, 1987).

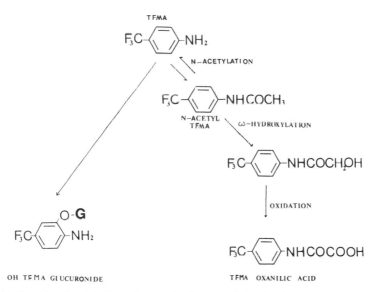

Figure 16. Postulated metabolic pathways of trifluoromethylaniline in the rat. From Wade *et al.*, 1988, with permission.

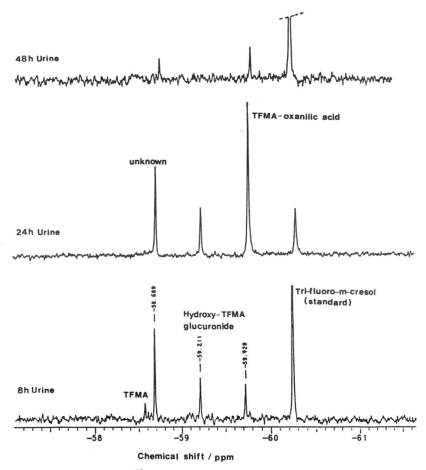

Figure 17. 376 MHz (9.4 telsa) ^{19}F-NMR spectra of urine from a rat given trifluoromethylaniline (TFMA; 19 mg/kg). From Wade *et al.*, 1988, with permission.

Difluorobenzoates

In their studies of aromatic hydrocarbon metabolism by microorganisms, Cass *et al.* (1987) utilized ^{19}F-NMR to study the metabolism of difluoroben-zoates in a mutant strain of *Pseudomonas putida*. Following incubation of 3,5-difluorobenzoate (3,5-DFB) with the mutant, its single peak gradually disappeared over 160 min while the two signals due to the 1,2-dihydrodiol of 3,5-DFB increased in intensity. This metabolite accumulated as the mutant was unable to catalyse the re-aromatization of the difluorocarboxydihydrodiol to the equivalent catechol, which leads to ring opening and further metab-olism (Figure 18). A small amount of fluoride was also observed indicating that this further metabolism was not completely inhibited. However, when

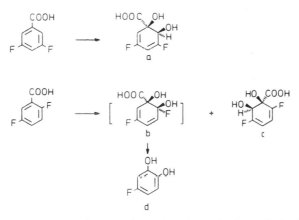

Figure 18. Proposed dioxygenation reactions for the oxidation of 3,5-difluorobenzoate; 2,5-difluorobenzoate by *P. putida* JT103. From Cass *et al.*, 1987, with permission.

2,5-difluorobenzoate was studied, F was the major metabolite. The authors concluded that dioxygenation at the carboxyl-substituted carbon and the adjacent flourine-substituted carbon would produce a difluorocarboxydihydrodiol which could then decarboxylate and spontaneously eliminate F⁻ to give the 4-fluorocatechol.

Fluorinated anaesthetics

Several studies have now been performed on the disposition and more recently the metabolism, of fluorinated anaesthetics using ¹⁹F-NMR. Many of these studies have been performed *in vivo*. There is an obvious advantage to studying the disposition of an anaesthetic as it also immobilizes the animal which is necessary while accumulating the spectra. Additional anaesthesia with either ketamine/xylazine or a short action, long duration barbiturate has often been necessary for time-course studies however. Burt *et al.* (1982) investigated *methoxyflurane* disposition (Figure 19) in dog blood by circulation through a narrow bore NMR spectrometer via indwelling cannulas. These workers concluded that the broad irregular spectrum observed indicated that methoxyflurane occupied multiple population sites in blood. Wyrwicz *et al.* (1983) observed methoxyflurane, *halothane* and *isoflurane* in rabbit brain. In one experiment, a ¹⁹F signal was still apparent 98 hours after a 30-min exposure to 1 per cent halothane. Evers *et al.* (1987) identified two distinct sites for halothane in rat brain. The short T2 relaxation time and kinetics of occupancy of the site related to the anaesthetic effect, was characteristic of a specific interaction of limited rotational freedom with a high molecular weight cellular component. Similarly Wyrwicz *et al.* (1987 a) described two sites for halothane and two sites for isoflurane (Wyrwicz *et al.*, 1987 b) in rabbit brain

$$HCCl_2CF_2\text{-}O\text{-}CH_3$$

Methoxyflurane

$$CF_3CHClBr$$

Halothane

$$CF_3CHCl\text{-}O\text{-}CHF_2$$

Isoflurane

$$HCFClCF_2\text{-}O\text{-}CHF_2$$

Enflurane

Figure 19. Structures of the major fluorinated anaesthetics used in clinical practice.

with different half-lives. The shorter half-lives, representative of the sites of weaker association, were the same (25–26 min) for both anaesthetics.

Burt *et al.* (1984) and Wyrwicz *et al.* (1987 a) observed a metabolite of halothane (presumed to be trifluoroacetate) as a shoulder on the halothane peak. Selinsky *et al.* (1987) also observed a trifluoroacetate peak 0.6 ppm downfield of the halothane peak at 340 MHz in rat liver. They found the half-life of halothane was decreased from 3.5 to 2.5 hours in phenobarbitone-induced rats while trifluoroacetate rapidly reached a steady state level not seen in uninduced controls. Some of these workers and others (Selinsky *et al.* 1988 a) also clearly observed methoxydifluoroacetate, the equivalent metabolite of methoxyflurane, in the whole animal *in vivo*, following methoxy-flurane exposure. Further studies (Selinsky *et al.*, 1988 b) showed that although methoxydifluoroacetate was the major metabolite, at earlier times after exposure when methoxyflurane concentrations were high, a significant fraction of methoxyflurane was metabolized via demethylation to dichloro-acetate (Figure 20) and ultimately oxalate, carbon dioxide and glycine. Fluoride ion which may have risen by enzymatic defluorination was rapidly eliminated from the liver.

The oxidative metabolite of *enflurane*, difluoromethoxy-difluoroacetate, can also be clearly seen in rat urine following enflurane exposure by ^{19}F-NMR (Preece, 1989; Figure 21).

Fluorinated anticancer drugs

Several fluorinated anticancer drugs particularly *5-fluorouracil* (5-FU) and *5'-deoxy-5-fluorouridine* (5'-dFUrd) have also been studied by ^{19}F-NMR. Malet-Martino *et al.* (1983) detected 5-FU and its metabolites (Figure 22) in the blood of a cancer patient after i.v. infusion of the prodrug 5'-dFUrd. Chemical shift values, multiplicity and H–F coupling constants for these and

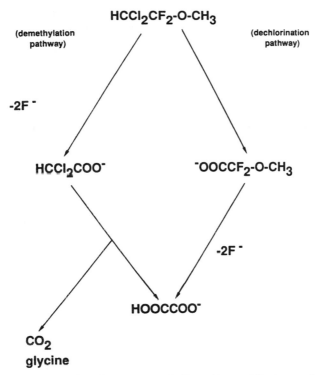

Figure 20. Pathways of methoxyfluorane metabolism. From Selinsky *et al.*, 1988, with permission.

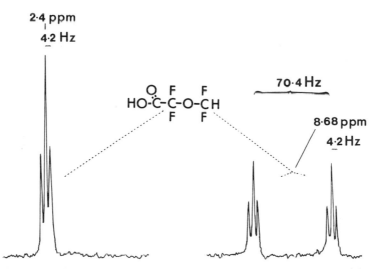

Figure 21. 19F-NMR spectrum of rat urine after exposure to enflurane (1 per cent) for 20 min. The spectrum shows the metabolite difluoromethoxy-difluoroacetate. Chemical shifts are downfield of a trifluoroacetic acid external standard. From Preece and Williams, 1990.

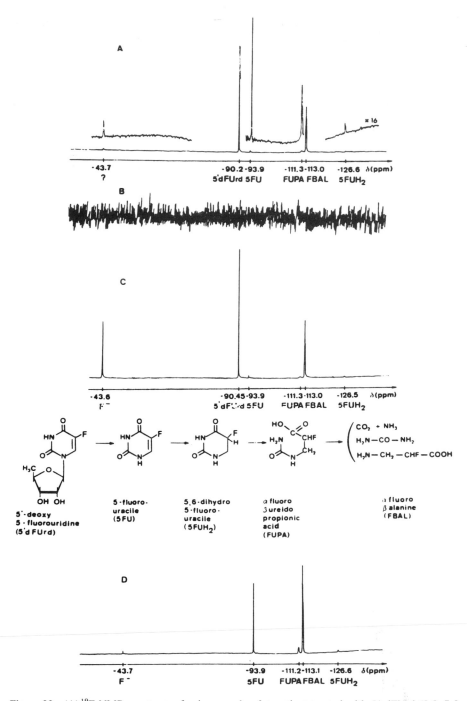

Figure 22. (A)^{19}F-NMR spectrum of urine sample of a patient treated with 5′-dFUrd (5.5–7.5 hours); (B) control urine sample; (C) as in A but after addition of HF; (D) urine sample of patient treated with 5-FU (0–3 hr). From Martino *et al.*, 1985, with permission.

known metabolites 5,6-dihydro-5-fluorouracil (5-FUH2) and α-fluoro-β-alanine (FBAL) were similar to reference standards. In addition, the initial product of ring-opening, probably α-fluoro-β-ureidopropionic acid (FUPA), was detected. Stevens *et al.* (1984) also detected the major metabolites of 5-FU in the livers of anaesthetized mice *in vivo*. Using radiolabelled 5-FU for comparison these authors estimated the minimum concentration detectable by *in vivo* NMR was 0.5 μmol/g tissue. On coadministration of thymidine which competes with 5-FU for hepatic catabolism, 5′-dFUrd was also detected in the liver. Stevens *et al.* (1984) also studied 5′-FU metabolism in implanted tumours where, in contrast to the liver, a signal was observed in the spectra which they reported was due predominantly to the major metabolic product 5-fluorodeoxyuridine monophosphate (FdUMP), although this assignment has been contested.

FdUMP is the inhibitor of thymidylate synthetase believed by some to be responsible for the antineoplastic activity of 5-FU. Others believe incorporation of 5-FU into RNA is more important for cytoxicity. The synthesis of fluorine-containing RNA species has been detected in intact bacteria (Gochin *et al.*, 1984) and cultured tumour cells (Keniry *et al.*, 1986) incubated with 5 FU. Mitomycin C, an inhibitor of RNA synthesis, suppressed 5-FU incorporation into bacterial RNA species.

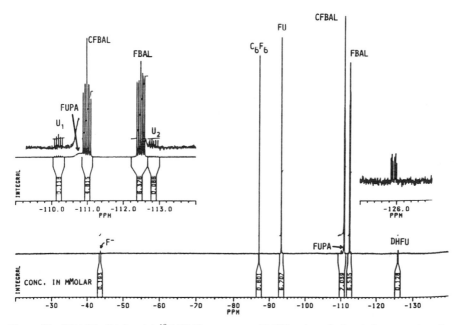

Figure 23. 470 MHz (11.8 tesla) ^{19}F-NMR spectrum of 5-FU and catabolites in human urine after a dose of 5-FU (16 mg/kg). FU = fluorouracil; FBAL = α-fluoro-β-alanine; CFBAL = N-carboxy-FBAL; FUPA = α-fluoro-β-ureidopropanoic acid; DHFU = 5-fluoro-5,6-dihydrouracil; F^- = fluoride; U_1 and U_2 = acid-labile unknowns. The expanded insets show the fine structure of the signals due to $^1H-^{19}H$ spin–spin coupling. From Hull *et al.*, 1988 a, with permission.

In further studies of 5'-dFUrd in human biofluids using NMR, Martino *et al.* (1985) and Malet-Martino *et al.* (1986) showed plasma–protein binding was appreciable (35 per cent). The authors suggested that a broad signal associated with the intense 5'-dFUrd signal was due to bound forms of the drug. As NMR does not alter the chemical state of the molecule(s) being observed, unlike many other techniques, it is possible to measure the true free concentration of a drug in the presence of protein-bound drug. Signals due to N-carboxy-α-fluoro-β-alanine (CFBAL) and fluoride ion were present in plasma. Resonances due to F^- and FBAL were the only ones observed in urine following FBAL administration to rats which indicated probable enzymatic defluorination of FBAL. Hull *et al.* (1988 a) confirmed the presence of CFBAL and FBAL in the urine of a human subject and showed the amount of F^- detected was appreciably more than could be accounted for by impurities of commercial 5-FU preparations (Figure 23). These workers have proposed that F^- is eliminated from a FBAL pyridoxal-phosphate schiff-base β-alanine transaminase-complex which results in the inhibition of FBAL transamination to α-fluoromalonic acid semialdehyde (FMAS). It is reasonable to assume that if it were formed, FMAS would be rapidly decarboxylated to fluoracetate (FA) (Figure 24). This might explain why FA and the highly neurotoxic fluorocitrate (FC) have not been detected during 5-FU or 5'-dFUrd metabolism. Indeed interference with alanine and GABA metabolism in the CNS may explain the cerebellar ataxia associated with fluorinated pyrimidine therapy. Otherwise the studies of Hull *et al.* (1988 a) in man have generally confirmed those of Malet-Martino and co-workers.

Recent studies by Wolf *et al.* (1987) in human liver *in vivo* indicate 5-FU is more rapidly metabolized to FBAL by man than rodent species. Studies by Griffiths *et al.* (1987) have shown an absence of fluoronucleotide synthesis as seen by NMR in rat prolactinomas compared to 5-FU following administration of the equally effective 5-FU analogues doxifluridin and floxuridine. Prior *et al.* (1987) also found coadministration of allopurinol, which is given to prevent chemotherapy-induced hyperuricaemia, inhibited the synthesis of fluoronucleotides. This group has also recently performed studies on fluorinated misonidazole (radiosensitizer) and methotrexate (an inhibitor of tetrahydrofolate-reductase) analogues.

Hull *et al.* (1988 a) showed that coadministration of methotrexate (MTX), in contrast to thymidine, did not effect 5-FU metabolism as observed by ^{19}F-NMR. However, the accompanying bicarbonate infusion resulted in large amounts of CFBAL in urine accompanied by smaller amounts of two unknown signals (Figure 23). The authors discounted α-fluoro-β-guanidinopropionic acid (FGPA) (Figure 24), a possible but so far NMR elusive metabolite, being the cause of these. Malet-Martino *et al.* (1988 b) have also recently shown using NMR that conjugates of FBAL with cholic, deoxycholic and chenodeoxycholic acids are the major 5-FU and 5'-dFUrd metabolites in human bile (Figure 25). These studies have shown that only the R stereoisomer at the α-carbon of these FBAL-conjugates is formed *in vivo*. Although the

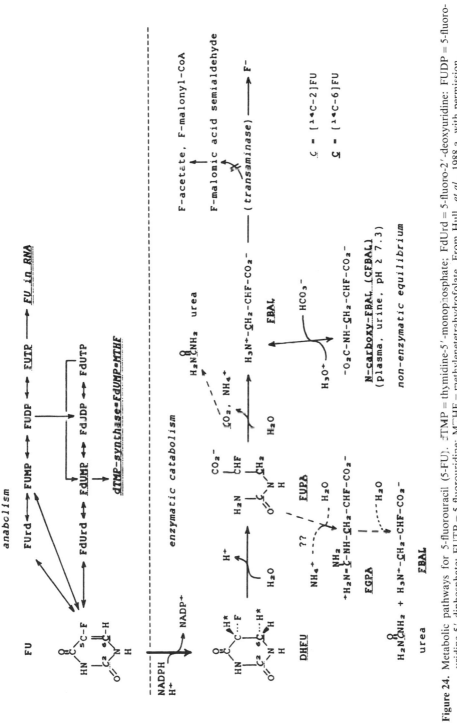

Figure 24. Metabolic pathways for 5-fluorouracil (5-FU). dTMP = thymidine-5'-monophosphate; FdUrd = 5-fluoro-2'-deoxyuridine: FUDP = 5-fluoro-uridine-5'-diphosphate; FUTP = 5-fluorouridine-5'-diphosphate; M⁻HF = methylenetetrahydrofolate. From Hull, *et al.*, 1988 a, with permission.

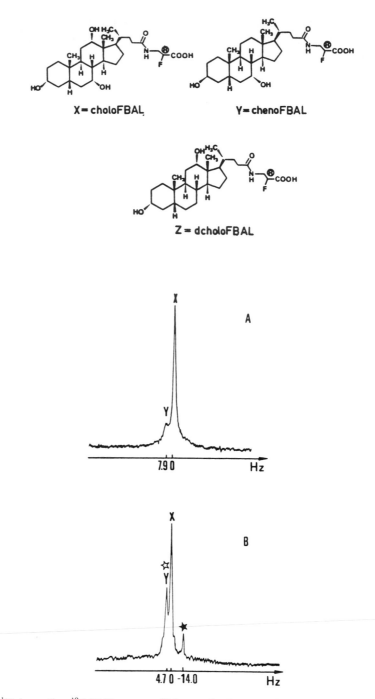

Figure 25. ^{1}H-decoupling ^{19}F-NMR spectra of bile samples from a patient treated with 5′dFUrd or 5-FU. (A) unspiked; (B) spiked with cheno-FBAL (o,*). X and Y are unknown biliary metabolites. From Malet-Martino, *et al.*, 1988, with permission.

individual fluorine signals from the bile acid-conjugates were unresolved, the conjugates were distinguishable on a 7.05-tesla spectrometer despite the fact that the differences between the structures were 11–13 bonds from their respective fluorine atoms.

5-fluorocytosine (5-FC) is used as an antifungal agent in humans because only susceptible fungi possess the cytosine deaminase activity required to convert it to 5-FU. Di Vito *et al.* (1986) used ^{19}F-NMR to study 5-FC metabolism in susceptible and resistant strains of *Candida albicans*. Interpretation of the spectra suggested one strain was resistant as a result of impaired UMP-pyrophosphorylase activity and the capacity to excrete 5-FU into the external medium. Evidence has accrued that in man, cytosine deaminase activity can be induced in the intestinal microflora following chronic exposure to 5-FC. FBAL was known to be a minor metabolite of 5-FC. Vialaneix *et al.* (1987) have shown using ^{19}F-NMR that fluoride ion, the 6-hydroxy-derivative and an uncharacterized glucuronide conjugate are also minor metabolites present in the urine and plasma of a patient with cryptococcal meningitis receiving 5-FC treatment. The glucuronide conjugate was also found to be present in cerebrospinal fluid.

Certain *fluorinated-polyamines* and *difluoromethylornithine* (DFMO), the ornithine decarboxylase inhibitor, have also been studied by ^{19}F-NMR. Digenis *et al.* (1986) found that red blood cells rapidly incorporate the polyamine analogue tetrafluoroputrescine. Joseph *et al.* (1987) found that DFMO (Figure 26), was preferentially incorporated into tumour tissue with

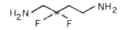

2,2 – DIFLUOROPUTRESCINE

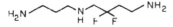

5,6 – DIFLUOROSPERMIDINE

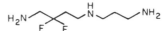

7,7 – DIFLUOROSPERMIDINE

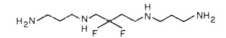

6,6 – DIFLUOROSPERMINE

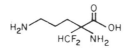

α– DIFLUOROMETHYLORNITHINE

Figure 26. Structural formulae of the geminal difluoro analogues of the natural polyamines and the ornithine decarboxylase inhibitor α-difluoromethyl-ornithine. From Hull, *et al.*, 1988 b, with permission.

respect to the surrounding muscle when administered to rats bearing metastatic prostate adenocarcinomas using ^{19}F-NMR *in vivo*. Hull *et al.* (1988 b) showed that coadministration of DFMO with 2,2-difluoroputrescine resulted in considerably increased incorporation of this polyamine analogue into implanted tumours in mice *in vivo*. It was further metabolized to 6,6-difluorospermidine and subsequently 6,6-diflurospermine although these could not be resolved *in vivo*. No 7,7-difluorospermidine could be detected in agreement with previous HPLC studies. Several unknown metabolites were detected including one which interestingly only appeared in tumour tissue and never in liver. The presence of the metabolite could be modulated by co-administration of N-methylformamide. Quantitive data obtained by *in vitro* ^{19}F-NMR agreed reasonably well with an HPLC method but was not as sensitive.

6. ^{31}P-NMR

The popularity of ^{31}P-NMR has arisen partly because of its moderate sensitivity (rs = 7 per cent) and partly because phosphorus-31 is 100 per cent naturally abundant. The biological importance of those membrane components and phosphorylated metabolites which are readily observed *in vivo* with surface coils (Ackerman *et al.*, 1980) is the main cause of interest, however.

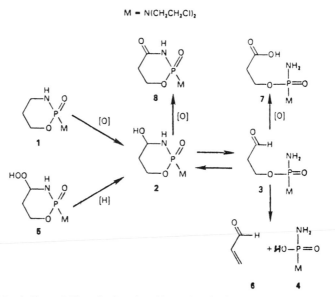

Figure 27. Metabolism of (1) cyclophosphamide to (2) 4-hydroxycyclophosphamide (4-OH-CP); (3) aldophosphamide (AP); (4) phosphoramide mustard (PM); and (6) acrolein. Structures of (5) 4-hydroperoxycyclophosphamide; (7) 4-carboxycyclophosphamide and (8) 4-ketocyclophosphamide. From Boyd *et al.*, 1986, with permission.

A considerable number of biological studies of hypoxia and disease states have been reported using ^{31}P-NMR; however, drugs containing phosphorus are fairly rare and subsequently ^{31}P-NMR studies of them have been few in number.

Compounds studied

Cyclophosphamide

Using ^{31}P NMR, Boyd *et al.* (1986) studied the uptake and transformation of metabolically activated cyclosphosphamide by human histiocytic lymphoma cells incorporated into an agarose gel thread matrix. Their studies showed that the cells were permeable to exogenous 4-hydroxycyclophosphamide (4-OH-CP, Figure 27; structure 2) and aldophosphamide (AP) but impervious to the oncostatic metabolite phosphoramide mustard (PM). Once trapped within the cells, however, the alkylating agent PM had a half-life of 125 min at 23°C. There was no evidence for the production of either 4-ketocyclophosphamide or 4-carboxycyclophosphamide (Figure 27; 7, 8). Although the levels of endogenous ^{31}P-NMR observable metabolites (Figure 28) were unaffected by

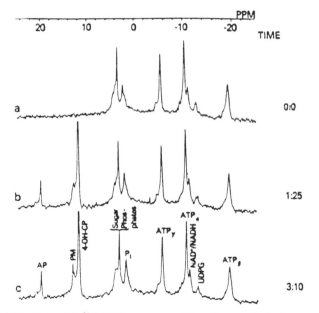

Figure 28. 161 MHz (9.4 tesla) ^{31}P-NMR spectrum of lymphoma cells in the presence of added 4-hydroxycyclophosphamide. AP = aldophosphamide, PM = phosphoramide mustard, 4-OH-CP = 4-hydroxycyclophosphamide, P_i = inorganic phosphate, UDPG = uridine diphospho-glucose (galactose). a) Spectrum of the cells prior to the introduction of metabolites, freshly prepared 4-OH-CP/AP was added to the perfusion media at time 1 hr 15 min; b) spectrum of cells aquired starting at time 1 hr 25 min; c) spectrum of cells aquired starting at time 3 hr 10 min; Reprinted with permission from Boyd *et al.*, 1986; Copyright American Chemical Society.

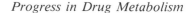

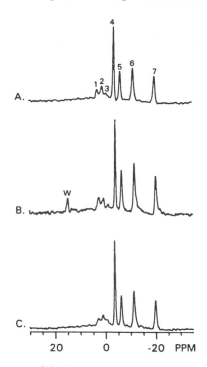

Figure 29. ^{31}P-NMR spectrum of the abdominal and hindquarter regions of a mouse. (A) Mouse prior to injection; (B) mouse after injection of WR-2721 (600 mg/kg; i.p.); (C) mouse 24 hour post injection. (1) sugar phosphates; (2) Pi (inorganic phosphate); (3) unidentified; (4) phosphocreatine: (5) γ-ATP; (6) α-ATP; (7) β-ATP; (W) phosphate of WR-2721. From Knizner *et al.*, 1986, with permission.

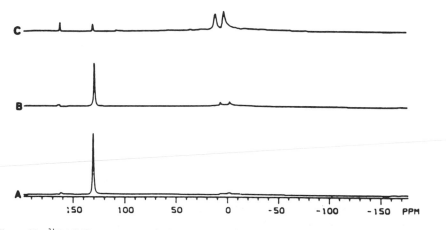

Figure 30. ^{31}P-NMR spectrum of the neck of a hen after the subcutaneous injection of 1000 mg/kg triphenylphosphite. Spectra were taken at 10 min (A), 100 min (B) or 4 hours (C) after injection. From Carrington *et al.*, 1988, with permission.

the addition of 4-OH-CP or PM, ATP levels rapidly decreased and the Pi concentration increased on incubation of the cells with 4-hydroperoxy-cyclophosphamide. Interestingly, this effect seems unrelated to the alkylating activity of this PM precursor as the same effect could be duplicated by incubating the cells with simple alkyl peroxides.

Knizner *et al.* (1986) determined the half-life of *WR-2721*, an *S-phosphorylated radiprotective-thiopolyamine* using whole-body ^{31}P-NMR in mice *in vivo* (Figure 29). The elimination of *triphenyl phosphite* (TPP) and *tri-o-cresyl phosphate* (TOCP), two organophosphorus pesticides known to produce delayed neurotoxicity, from their subcutaneous injection site was studied over several days by ^{31}P-NMR in the hen by Carrington *et al.* (1988) (Figure 30). Conversion of TPP into diphenyl phosphonate when observed *in vivo* was associated with lethality. These studies also visualized endogenous metabolites. It may be useful to study endogenous phosphorylated metabolites while simultaneously studying metabolism with another nucleus such as carbon-13 by using a double-tuned probe (Cohen, 1984).

7. ^{13}C-NMR

^{13}C, unlike the nuclei discussed above, has a low natural abundance (na = 1.1 per cent) and coupled with the relatively poor sensitivity (rs = 2 per cent), ^{13}C-NMR of unlabelled drugs and metabolites is less readily amenable for use in drug metabolism studies than proton-NMR. Despite this, spectra of drug metabolites in high concentration in biofluids are possible using non-enriched compounds and additional information about endogenous metabolites may be gained. When ^{13}C-labelled drugs are available, sensitivity is greatly improved and this is associated with spectral editing. Labelling drugs with carbon-13, and also deuterium and nitrogen-15 (see below) and performing the respective NMR experiments greatly simplifies the spectra and may identity label-incorporation into endogenous components such as acetate or urea. Carbon is, of course, as ubiquitous as hydrogen in drugs, their metabolites and endogenous compounds. In combination, proton and ^{13}C-NMR presents a powerful tool for structure elucidation. Although few studies have been performed so far there is considerable potential.

The metabolism of ^{13}C-labelled compounds has been shown to be identical to their ^{14}C-labelled counterparts in rat hepatocytes and perfused mouse liver (Cohen *et al.*, 1981). Proton decoupling will improve sensitivity through multiplet collapse and nOe enhancement of up to two-fold, but as previously explained, the power required for broad-band hetereonuclear decoupling is considerable. The internal heat generated may affect and even irreversibly damage a biological sample. This problem is particularly severe in the high field instruments in which the band width requiring irradiation is proportionally greater. The problem can be minimized by using a WALTZ-16 sequence

(Shaka *et al.*, 1983). Coupling information required for spectral interpretation can be retained without excessive loss of sensitivity by using a J-modulated spin echo (LeCocq and Lallemand, 1981) which facilitates structural elucidation by providing an 'attached proton test' (APT) (Patt and Shoolery, 1982), while the associated DEPT (distortionless enhancement by polarization transfer) sequence improves the sensitivity.

Compounds studied

Antipyrine and related compounds

Pass *et al.* (1984) observed the elimination of N,N-[$^{13}CH_3$]$_2$-aminopyrine in the perfused mouse liver with ^{13}C-NMR. Pretreatment of the animals with phenobarbitone decreased the half-life of antipyrine. Huetter *et al.* (1987) performed similar and more elaborate studies on N-[^{13}C]-methyl *antipyrine* metabolism in perfused rat liver. They utilized a DEPT sequence and APT to identify the ^{13}C-labelled inverted methyl singlets of the calcium complex and the glucuronide and sulphate conjugates of 4-hydroxy-antipyrine in the

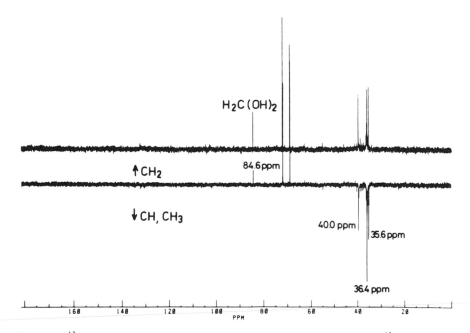

Figure 31. ^{13}C-NMR spectra of bile collected 90–120 min after the addition of ^{13}C-labelled antipyrine to the vascular perfusate (upper trace). In the lower trace the same spectrum obtained by the DEPT technique is shown. Chemical shifts: 35.6 ppm, antipyrine; 36.32 ppm, sulphate conjugate of 4-hydroxyantipyrine; 36.47 ppm, glucuronide conjugate of 4-hydroxyantipyrine; 37.5 ppm, 4-hydroxyantipyrine; 36.39 ppm, 5-hydroxyantipyrine; 36.1 ppm sulphate conjugate of 5-hydroxyantipyrine; 40 ppm, Ca^{2+} complex of 4-hydroxyantipyrine. From Huetter *et al.*, 1987, with permission.

excreted bile (Figure 31). In addition, as a result of N-demethylation they observed a singlet from the CH_2 group of formaldehyde hydrate which was phased upright. Formaldehyde hydrate would be very difficult to detect by proton-NMR in aqueous solution as its resonance position (4.8 ppm) is coincident with water.

In their studies of bacterial *formaldehyde* metabolism, Doddrell *et al.* (1984) overcame this problem by observing ^{13}C-labelled formaldehyde with ^{1}H-NMR using a reverse-POMMIE sequence. The reverse polarization transfer ensured that only those protons attached to carbon-13 were observed while sensitivity was greater than that seen with ^{13}C-NMR.

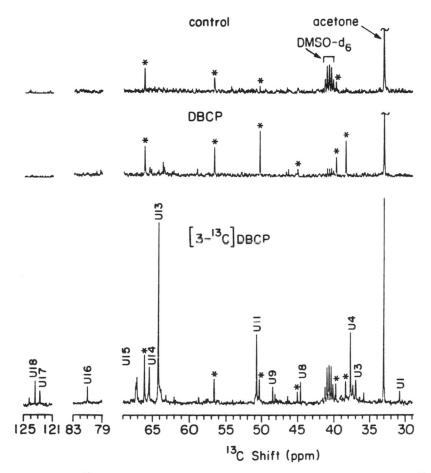

Figure 32. Partial ^{13}C-NMR spectrum of urine from control rats and those given [3-^{13}C] dibromo-chloro-propane (DBCP). Asterisks indicate substances in control urine. Signals derived from C-3 of [3-^{13}C]DBCP are designated U1, U3, U4, U8, U9, U11 and U13–U18 in order of increasing chemical shifts (see also Figure 33). Acetone was added as a chemical shift reference. From Dohn *et al.*, 1988, with permission.

Albert *et al.* (1984) used ^{13}C-NMR to study the metabolism of [^{13}C]-(ring ethoxy carbon)-labelled *phenacetin* to paracetamol (acetaminophen) in the vascular perfusate of fluorocarbon-perfused rat livers prepared from phenobarbitone treated animals.

Studies by Fennel *et al.* (1989) have identified both the 2-hydroxyethyl- and 2-cyanoethyl-N-acetyl cysteinyl conjugates in the urine of rodents given [1,2,3-^{13}C]-labelled *acrylonitrile* and thiocyanate ion using ^{13}C-NMR.

1,2-Dibromo-3-chloropropane

Dohn *et al.* (1988) used the DEPT sequence and the APT to identify the biliary and urinary glutathione-derived metabolites of the soil fumigant [3-^{13}C-labelled] 1,2-dibromo-3-chloropropane (DBCP), a potent testicular and nephrotoxin in the rat (Figure 32). These metabolites included the *cis-* and *trans-*S-1-chloropropenyl derivatives and the S-(3-chloro-2-hydroxypropyl) and the S-(2,3-dihydroxypropyl) derivatives. The latter was labelled at either end. For one of the metabolic routes described, the authors postulated that DBCP was hydroxylated at C-2 to give 1-bromo-3-chloroacetone (following loss of HBr), which was then attacked by GSH at C-1 or C-3 (Figure 33). Loss of chlorine or the second bromine atom from either glutathione-adduct explained the production of the dihydroxy derivative and the scrambling of the carbon-13 label. Another metabolic route envisioned *cis-* and *trans-*3-bromo-1-chloropropene being formed by radical-initiated dehydrobromination of DBCP and then attack by GSH at C-1 to give the S-1-chloropropenyl derivatives.

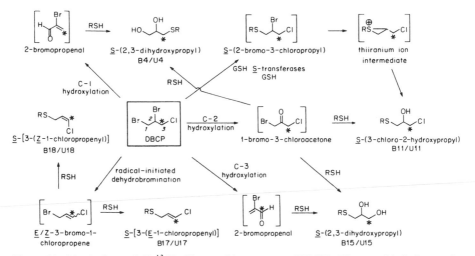

Figure 33. Metabolism of [3-^{13}C] dibromochloropropane (DBCP). The asterisk indicates the position of the label. R = glutathionyl, cysteinylglycine or cysteinyl for biliary metabolites and cysteinyl or N-acetylcysteinyl for the urinary metabolites. The letter/numbers U and B denote urinary or biliary metabolites (see also Figure 32). From Dohn *et al.*, 1988, with permission.

Tris(2,3-dibromopropyl)phosphate

Fukuoka *et al.* (1987) used ^{13}C-NMR to study the urine of rats dosed with a flame retardent, tris(2,3-dibromopropyl)phosphate (tris-BP), which is also a potent nephrotoxin. Only a trace of one metabolite, bis-BP, was identified following repeated high doses, presumably because non-enriched material was used. However, increases in lactate and glucose excretion were clearly seen by ^{13}C-NMR urinalysis analogous to changes detected by ^{1}H-NMR in studies of nephrotoxicity (Gartland *et al.*, 1989 c). However, it seems probable that proton-NMR would have readily identified these changes with more economical use of spectrometer time.

8. ^{15}N-NMR

Like ^{13}C-NMR, ^{15}N-NMR of unlabelled drugs also suffers from the low natural abundance of [15]N (na = 0.37 per cent) and the poor sensitivity (rs = 0.1 per cent). Nitrogen-15 possesses a negative magnetogyric ratio which may null some signals if broad-band decoupling is not 'inverse gated'. However, the resultant nOe enhancement factor of up to minus four-fold can be advantageous for other signals. Although many xenobiotics contain nitrogen they also usually contain carbon and hydrogen. Greater sensitivity is obtained with ^{1}H-NMR and usually with ^{13}C-NMR, and these nuclei are also more amenable to radiolabelling. Consequently ^{15}N-NMR has been little utilized for the study of the metabolism and disposition of xenobiotics. However, the use of ^{15}N-NMR does have some advantages. The metabolism of hydrazine (Figure 4), for example, is difficult to study by other methods and doubly-labelled ^{15}N-hydrazine is commercially available. A recent study by Wade *et al.* (1989) suggests ^{15}N-NMR may shed more light on the metabolism of *aniline*.

Hydrazine

Several peaks were detected by ^{15}N-NMR in urine samples from rats treated with labelled hydrazine after several hours signal accumulation (Preece and Timbrell, 1990). However in samples which had been lyophilized and concentrated, accumulation times were reduced to 1–1.5 hours (Figure 34). Ammonia was detected as a singlet at 0 ppm, coincident with the standard. Unchanged [15]N$_2$-hydrazine was present in the urine and was detectable as a singlet at 29 ppm. The unambiguous identification of free hydrazine as a urinary metabolite had not previously been shown as the assay techniques used were likely to release hydrazine from unstable metabolites, such as hydrazones. This does not occur with NMR, which is a clear advantage of the technique. A peak at 35 ppm was due to the amino-nitrogen of acetylhydrazine (Figure 35). Peaks

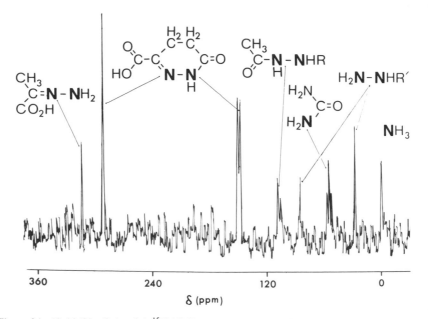

Figure 34. 40.6 MHz (9.4 tesla) ^{15}N-NMR spectrum (sweep width 16 KHz) of urine from a rat dosed with ^{15}N$_2$-hydrazine (60 mg/kg) with the structural formulae of the excreted metabolites. R = H or CH$_3$CO; R′ = H or CO$_2$; bold type N represents labelled nitrogen. From Preece and Timbrell, 1989, unpublished data.

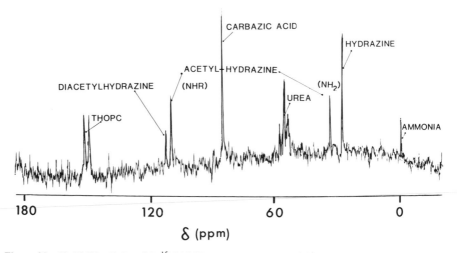

Figure 35. 40.6 MHz (9.4 tesla) ^{15}N-NMR spectrum (sweep width 8 KHz) of urine from a rat dosed with ^{15}N$_2$-hydrazine (80 mg/kg) with metabolites labelled. R = CH$_3$CO; THOPC (the cyclized hydrazone of 2-oxoglutarate). From Preece and Timbrell, 1989, unpublished data.

were also observed downfield at 110 and 113 ppm. These were identified as being due to the hydrazido-nitrogens of acetylhydrazine and diacetylhydrazine respectively. The resonance at 85 ppm was ascribed to carbazic acid, resulting from reaction of hydrazine with carbonic acid. A metabolite observed at 315 ppm was tentatively identified as pyruvate hydrazone.

The triplet observed centred at 56 ppm was found to collapse to a singlet approximately three-fold higher during proton decoupling by inverse-gated broad-band irradiation at the proton frequency indicative of a NH2 group

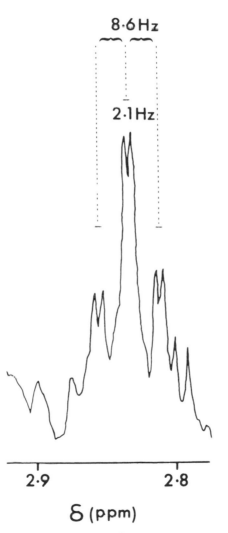

Figure 36. Expansion of the 400 MHz (9.4 tesla) ^{1}H-NMR spectrum of urine from a rat dosed with ^{15}N$_2$-hydrazine (80 mg/kg) showing additional ^{15}N splitting (2.1 Hz) of the downfield triplet (8.6 Hz) of THOPC (the cyclized hdyrazone of 2-oxoglutarate; see Figures 4 and 5). From Preece and Timbrell, 1989, unpublished data.

slowly-exchanging on the 'NMR time-scale'. A concentrated solution of standard urea gave a resonance with the same chemical shift and behaviour on decoupling. Treatment with the enzyme urease diminished the peak while simultaneously increasing the intensity of the peak (0 ppm) ascribed to ammonia. These findings confirmed the assignment of the resonance at 56 ppm as due to urea. This indicated that the N–N bond of hydrazine is cleaved *in vivo* and the resultant ammonia is probably incorporated via the urea cycle giving rise to labelled urea. A doublet centred at 150 ppm was also observed in the spectrum and also collapsed to a singlet on decoupling, indicative of a slowly exchanging NH group. This was identical with the hydrazido-nitrogen resonance from a doubly labelled synthetic standard of the metabolite tetrahydro-3-oxo-pyridazine 6-carboxylic acid (THOPC), the cyclized hydrazone of 2-oxoglutarate. Another resonance observed at 294 ppm (hydrazono-nitrogen) in the spectrum of urine was also identical with that produced from the synthetic standard of $^{15}N_2$-THOPC, confirming this as a urinary metabolite (Figures 34 and 35). In addition, the downfield triplet from THOPC seen in the proton NMR spectrum of the urine of rats given unlabelled hydrazine (Figure 5) was further split into a double triplet (Figure 36) when doubly labelled hydrazine was administered.

9. Quadrapolar nuclei

Nuclei with spin of greater than a half possess a quadrapole moment which supplies a very efficient relaxation mechanism. Consequently they produce signals with bandwidths of 100–1000 Hz and their spectra contain overlapping peaks and little fine detail reminiscent of UV and IR spectra. This is not to suggest that certain peaks cannot be sufficiently resolved to provide useful information as Balaban and Knepper (1983) and Wray and Wilkie (1987) have demonstrated with studies of tissues *in vivo*, particularly using kidney, with ^{14}N-NMR (rs = 1 per cent). Nuclei with symmetrical electron distributions, e.g. the nitrogen-14 (spin = 1, na = 99.7 per cent) in protonated amino acids, give sharper signals (30–100 Hz).

London *et al.* (1987) have studied the metabolism of *L-(methyl-$^2H_3$)-methionine* and its inhibition by coadministered ethionine in rat liver *in vivo* using ^2H-NMR (rs = 1 per cent). The deuterium nuclei (spin = 1; na = 0.02 per cent) present in the S-C$^2H_3$ unit are rapidly incorporated into sarcosine and gradually over 5 hours into several other N-methyl compounds (Figure 37). Most high field instruments require a deuterated solvent to be added to the sample for locking purposes so ^2H-NMR samples are often run unlocked unless an alternative lock is available. The 11 mM HOD present in aqueous biosamples can easily be removed by reconstitution in deuterium-depleted water. In their studies of bacterial *formaldehyde* metabolism, Hunter *et al.*

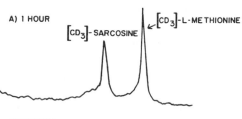

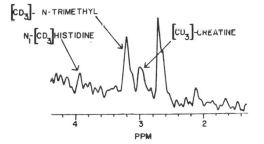

Figure 37. ^{2}H-NMR spectra of perchloric acid extracts of the livers of rats obtained at (A) 1 hour and (B) 5 hours after administration of 100 mg of L-[methyl-^{2}H$_3$]methionine (i.p.). Chemical shifts are referenced to HOD set at $\delta = 4.8$ ppm. Reprinted with permission from London *et al.*, 1987; copyright (1987) American Chemical Society.

(1984) observed the metabolism of deuteroformaldehyde to deuteroformate and deuteromethanol in a live *Escherichia coli* suspension with ^{2}H-NMR. For those elements which possess more than one NMR observable nucleus such as hydrogen (^{1}H, ^{2}H and ^{3}H) or nitrogen (^{14}N and ^{15}N), chemical shift data can be readily transferred as an aid to structural elucidation. This is because the relative chemical shift is dependent on the electronic environment of the nucleus, irrespective of its mass.

Efficient nuclear quadrapole relaxation seen with nuclei having spin greater than a half becomes advantageous because rapid pulsing of samples is possible without loss of signal strength. Therefore, transients can be accumulated more rapidly than is feasible with nuclei having a spin of a half, while relaxation rates can be measured just as easily. The relaxation rate of membrane-bound sodium-23 (spin = 3/2; na = 100 per cent) is also related to local microviscosity and therefore ultimately membrane integrity. Banni *et al.* (1987) have measured ^{23}Na-NMR (rs = 9 per cent) relaxation rates of endogenous sodium ions to study lipid peroxidation in rat liver and the protective effect of vitamin E following carbon tetrachloride administration. Other nuclei with spin > 0.5 which may be useful in drug metabolism include oxygen-17, sulphur-33 and chlorines-35 and 37.

10. Two-dimensional NMR

The rapid improvements in instrument technology seen in recent years have been paralleled by advances in multipulse sequences of which the spin-echo and polarization transfer techniques previously mentioned were forerunners. Two-dimensional NMR (2D-NMR) detects and identifies adjacent nuclei via homo- and hetereonuclear couplings. Correlated spectroscopy (COSY) or dipolar relaxation and nOe spectroscopy (NOESY) greatly enhance the information obtainable from NMR spectroscopy. 2D-NMR data are typically displayed in a grid format where the chemical shifts of the interacting nuclei can be read from the axes, signal intensity being delineated by contours (Figure 38). Spreading the individual signals in this manner theoretically enables the

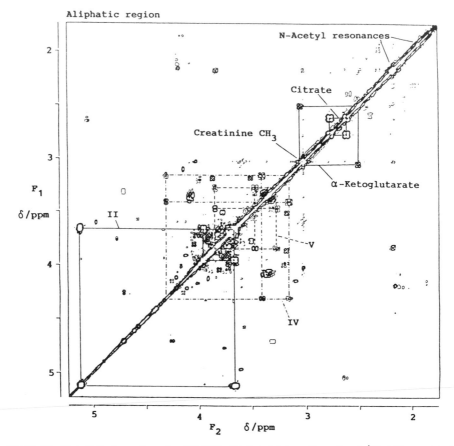

Figure 38. The aliphatic region of a 500 MHz (11.8 tesla) two-dimensional ^{1}H shift correlated (COSY) NMR spectrum of urine collected 3 hours after acetaminophen ingestion. The connectivities are shown for the side-chain protons of acetaminophen (APAP, II), N-acetylcysteinyl (APAP-NAC, IV) and cysteinyl (APAP-C, V) conjugates. From Bales *et al.*, 1985, with permission.

resolution of several thousand individual resonances even at moderate field strengths. 2D-NMR has been very successful, particularly in elucidating the structure and conformations of purified complex biomolecules in solution such as peptides, proteins, nucleic acids and polysaccharides. 2D-NMR has also recently been used to identify the components of biofluids containing drug metabolites. 2D-NMR experiments have poorer sensitivity than the analogous 1D experiments and spectra usually require several hours to acquire. It is prudent to maximize the sample concentration, estimate the magnitude of the observed couplings and minimize sweep-widths in both dimensions before embarking on a 2D-NMR experiment.

Homonuclear 2-D NMR

In their single-pulse studies of *paracetamol* metabolism discussed previously, Bales *et al.* (1984) found there was some peak overlap between the N-acetyl

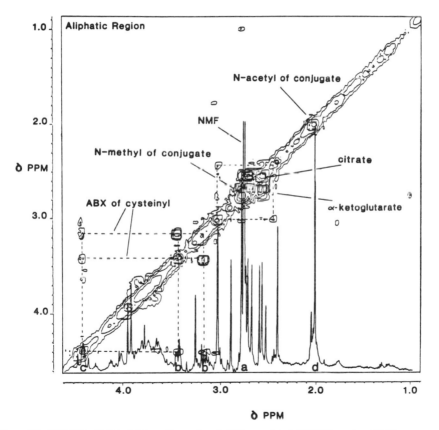

Figure 39. 400 MHz (9.4 tesla) two dimensional shift correlated (COSY) proton NMR spectrum and the corresponding one dimensional NMR spectrum of urine from a rat dosed with NMF. Resonances labelled a–d refer to the structure of the N-acetylcysteine conjugate of NMF, see Figure 9. From Tulip, Nicholson, and Timbrell, 1986, unpublished data.

resonances of the parent compound and its cysteine conjugate. However, this could be resolved by the use of ^{1}H-NMR 2D-COSY (Bales *et al.*, 1985). Specifically the paracetamol and its cysteine conjugate could be resolved on the basis of their aromatic protons in the 2D contour plot (Figure 38). Endogenous urinary components giving nearby signals such as hippurate and indoxyl sulphate were also resolved while citrate and 2-oxoglutarate gave characteristic splitting patterns upfield. Similarly ^{1}H-NMR 2D-COSY confirmed that the α-CH proton and β-methylene protons of the N$'$-acetyl-NMF conjugate found in urine samples of NMF-treated rats were spin–spin coupled (Figure 39; Tulip *et al.*, 1986).

Hetereonuclear 2D-NMR

In their studies of bacterial formaldehyde metabolism, Hunter *et al.* (1984) used ^{1}H, ^{13}C-NMR 2D-COSY to further characterize formaldehyde metabolites dissimilar to either methanol or formate. Similarly, 2D-COSY was instrumental in elucidating the biliary metabolites of carbon-13-labelled dibromochloropropane (Dohn *et al.*, 1988). Everett *et al.*, (1989) further characterized the metabolites of flucloxacillin (Figure 15) by ^{1}H, ^{19}F-NMR 2D-COSY. Those protons *ortho* and *meta* to the fluorine atoms in the parent compound and its metabolites are overlapped and covered by endogenous resonances in the single-pulse proton spectrum. However, eight signals (the *ortho* and *meta* proton for each metabolite) are clearly seen in the 2D-spectrum. Similarly, Wade and coworkers have pursued similar studies on flurbiprofen (Wade *et al.*, 1990) and *p*-fluoroacetanilide (Wade, 1990). In other recent studies these workers have characterized metabolites of ^{15}N-labelled dimethylformamide with ^{1}H, ^{15}N-NMR 2D-COSY (Wade, personal communication).

11. Quantitation

Following the identification of drug metabolites present in biofluids or *in vivo*, studies of disposition and pharmacokinetics can also be pursued with NMR. In single pulse experiments it is necessary to ensure the signals of interest are fully relaxed before comparing integrals with reference signals of known or predictable concentration for measuring purposes (Hull, 1989). When nOe are generated or more complex pulse sequences are used, quantitation by NMR becomes less reliable. Measuring metabolite concentrations *in vivo* is even more complicated because problems associated with spatial localization of the observed metabolites are compounded on the above (Tofts and Wray, 1988).

In most cases, correlation with non-resonance methods such as HPLC is recommended. Apparent underestimates of metabolite concentrations calculated by NMR compared to other methods can often be explained and can be informative. The discrepancy is often caused by macromolecular binding of the observed metabolites or exchange broadening via association with a binding site within the NMR timescale. This will broaden out the metabolites resonances in the spectrum. Alternatively, paramagnetic transition metals often found in biofluids can have the same effect by facilitating rapid relaxation of the drug metabolite signals. Appreciation of these effects can be used to generate information on the degree of protein binding of plasma metabolites for example and the kinetics of exchange between free and bound forms of the drug. When *in vitro* biofluid samples are thought to contain macromolecular components, comparing the spectra of the untreated material with an acid extract is recommended to precipitate protein. In addition, when transition metals are present, addition of chelating agents or resin is advisable so comparisons can be made. Unfortunately this cannot be performed *in vivo* but similar physical processes will certainly be modulating the final spectrum seen *in vivo*.

12. Conclusions

NMR spectroscopy is a powerful technique which has only recently found a place in the arsenal of tools employed *directly* in the study of drug metabolism. Techniques are now available to enable NMR to be used to detect and quantitate metabolites of xenobiotics both *in vivo* in whole animals and *in vitro*, in many biological fluids, in tissues and in whole organs. Observation can be performed without sample preparation in many cases. The proton is the most commonly used, sensitive, NMR observable nucleus. In addition other nuclei, with isotopic enrichment in some cases, have also proved to be particularly useful in yielding initial information about possible and in some cases unexpected drug metabolites. At the same time NMR may give information about changes in endogenous molecules resulting from exposure to xenobiotics. NMR does not significantly disturb the system under study and this makes it a uniquely useful analytical tool.

13. Appendix

Some abbreviations commonly used in NMR experiments

COSY: correlated spectroscopy
CPMG: Carr-Purcell-Meiboom-Gill
DANTE: delays alternating with nutations for tailored excitation
DEPT: distortionless enhancement by polarization transfer
INEPT: insensitive nuclei enhancement by polarization transfer
nOe: nuclear Overhauser effect
NOESY: nOe spectroscopy
SPEC: solid-phase extraction chromatography

SEFT: spin-echo Fourier transform
WEFT: water elimination by Fourier transform

Acknowledgement

The authors are grateful to Dr Jeremy K Nicholson for his critical review of the manuscript. Dr. Preece is grateful for support from the Wellcome Trust.

References

Ackerman, J. J. H., Grove, T. H., Wong, G. G., Gadian, D. G. and Radda, G. K. (1980), *Nature*, **283**, 167.

Albert, K., Kruppa, G., Zeller, K-P., Bayer, E. and Hartman, F. (1984), *Z. Naturforsch.*, **39c**, 859.

Allars, H., Coleman, M. D. and Norton R. S. (1986), *Europ. J. Drug Metab. Pharmacokin.* **10**, 253.

Balaban, R. S. and Knepper, M. A. (1983), *Am. J. Physiol.*, C439.

Bales, J. R., Sadler, P. J., Nicholson, J. K. and Timbrell, J. A. (1984), *Clin. Chem.*, **30**, 1631.

Bales, J. R., Nicholson, J. K. and Sadler, P. J. (1985), *Clin. Chem.* **31**, 757.

Bales, J. R., Bell, J. D., Nicholson, J. K., Sadler, P. J., Timbrell, J. A., Hughes, R. D., Bennett, P., Williams, R. (1988), *Magnetic Resonance in Medicine*, **6**, 301.

Banni, S., Canu, M., Corangin, F. P., Devi, M. A., Lai, A. and Meloni C. (1987), *Chem. Biol. Interact.* **63**, 207.

Bell, J. D., Gadian, D. G. and Preece, N. E. (1990), *Euro. J. Drug Metab. and Pharmacokinet.*, **15**, 127.

Boyd, V. L., Robbins, J. D., Egan. W. and Ludeman, S. M. (1986), *J. Med. Chem.*, **29**, 1206.

Brindle, K. M., Brown, F. F., Campbell, I. D., Grathwol, C. and Kuchel, P. W. (1979), *Biochem. J.*, **180**, 37.

Brown, F. F., Campbell, I. D., Kuchel, P. W. and Rabenstein, D. L. (1977), *FEBS Lett.*, **82**, 12.

Burt, C. T., Eisemann, A., Schofield, J. C. and Wyrwicz, A. M. (1982), *J. Magnet. Reson.*, **46**, 176.

Burt, C. T., Moore, R. P., Roberts, M. F. and Brady, T. J. (1984), *Biochim. Biophys. Acta*, **805**, 375.

Calder, I. C. (1979), *Prog. Drug Metab.*, **3**, 303.

Carrington, C. D., Tyler Burt, C. and Abou-Donia, M. B. (1988), *Drug Metab. Dispos.*, **16**, 104.

Case, D. E. (1973), *Xenobiotica*, **3**, 451.

Cass, A. E. G., Ribbons, D. W., Rossiter, J. T. and Williams, S. R. (1987), *FEBS Lett.*, **220**, 353.

Clore, G. M., Kimber, B. J, and Groneborn, A. M. (1983), *J. Magnet. Reson.*, **54**, 170.

Cohen, S. M. (1984), *Fed. Proc.*, **43**, 2657.

Cohen, S. M., Rogmtad, R., Shulman, R. G. and Katz, J. (1981), *J. Biol. Chem.*, **256**, 3423.

Coleman, M. D. and Norton, R. G. (1986), *Xenobiotica*, **16**, 61.

Connor, S., Everett, J. and Nicholson, J. K. (1987 a), *Magnet. Reson. Med.*, **4**, 461.

Connor, S., Nicholson, J. K. and Everett, J. R. (1987 b), *Analyt. Chem.*, **59**, 2885.

Di Vito, M., Podo, F., Torosantucci, A., Carpinelli, G., Whelan, W. L., Kerridge, D. and Cassone, A. (1986), *Antimicrob., Agents Chemother.*, **29**, 303.

Digenis, G. A., Hawi, A. A., Yip, H. and Layton, W. J. (1986), *Life Sci.*, **38**, 2307.

Doddrell, D. M., Nicholls, K. M. and Sanders, J. K. M. (1984), *FEBS Lett.*, **170**, 73.

Dohn, R. D., Graziano, M. J. and Canida, J. E. (1988), *Biochem. Pharmacol.*, **37**, 3435.

Eads, T. M., Kennedy, S. D. and Bryant, R. G. (1986), *Analyt. Chem.*, **58**, 1752.

Everett, J. R., Jennings, K. R., Woodnutt, G. and Buckingham, M. J. (1984), *J. Chem. Soc. Chem. Commun.*, **84**, 894.

Everett, J. R., Jennings, K. and Woodnut, G. (1985), *J. Pharmacy and Pharmacol.*, **37**, 869.

Everett, J. R., Tyler, J. W. and Woodnutt, G. (1989) *J. Pharm. Biomed. Anal.*, **7**, 391.

Evers, A. S., Berkowitz, B. A. and d'Avignon, D. A. (1987), *Nature*, **328**, 157.

Fennel, T. R., Held, S. D. and Kedderis, G. L. (1989), *Proc. Vth International Congress Toxicology*, p. 110, Taylor & Francis, London.

Foxall, P. J. D., Bending, M. R., Gartland, K. P. R. and Nicholson, J. K. (1989), *Human Toxicology.*, **9**, 491.

Fukuoka, M., Takahashi, T., Tanaka, A., Yamaha, T., Naito, K., Nakaji, Y., Kobayashi, K. and Tobe M., (1987), *J. Appl. Toxicol.*, **7**, 23.

Gartland, K. P. R., Bonner, F. W., Timbrell, J. A. and Nicholson, J. K. (1989 a), *Arch. Toxicol.*, **63**, 97.

Gartland, K. P. R., Eason, C. T., Bonner, F. W. and Nicholson, J. K. (1990), *Arch. Toxicol.*, **64**, 14.

Gartland, K. P. R., Bonner, F. W. and Nicholson, J. K. (1989 c), *Molec. Pharmacol.*, **35**, 242.

Gartland, K. P. R., Eason, C. T., Wade, K. E., Bonner, F. W. and Nicholson J. K. (1989 b), *J. Pharm. Biomed. Anal.*, **7**, 699.

Gochin, M., James, T. L. and Shafer, R. H. (1984), *Biochim. Biophys. Acta*, **804**, 118.

Griffiths, J. R., Bhujwalla, Z., Coombes, R. C., Maxwell, R. J., Midwood, C. J., Morgan, R. J., Nias, A. H. W., Perry, P., Prior, M., Prysor-Jones, R. A., Rodrigues, L. M., Stubbs, M. and Tozer, G. M. (1987), *Ann. NY Acad. Sci.*, **508**, 183.

Hore, P. J. (1983), *J. Magnet. Reson.*, **55**, 283.

Huetter, P., Albert, K., Bayer, E., Zeller, K. P. and Hartmann, F. (1987), *Biochem. Pharmacol.*, **36**, 2724.

Hull, W. E. (1989), *JEOL News*, 15.

Hull, W. E., Rudinger, E. P., Herrmann, R., Brilsch, F. and Kunz, W. (1988 a), *Cancer Res.*, **48**, 1680.

Hull, W. E., Kunz, W., Port, R. E. and Seiler, N. (1988 b), *NMR in Biomed.*, **1**, 11.

Hunter, B. K., Nicholls, K. M. and Sanders J. K. M. (1984). *Biochemistry*, **23**, 508.

Jacobson, R. A. and Gerig, J. T. (1988), *Chem. Res. Toxicol.*, **1**, 304.

Joseph, A., Davenport, C., Kwock, L., Burt, C. T. and London, R. E. (1987), *Magnet. Reson. Med.*, **4**, 137.

Keniry, M., Benz, C., Shafer, R. H. and James, T. L. (1986), *Cancer Res.*, **46**, 1754.

Kestell, P., Gill, M. H., Threadgill, M. D., Gescher, A., Howarth, O. W. and Curzon, E. H. (1986), *Life Sci.* **38**, 719.

Knizner, S. A., Jacobs, A. J., Lyon, R. C. and Swenberg, C. E. (1986), *J. Pharmacol. Exp. Therap.*, **236**, 37.

Laude, D. A. and Wilkins, C. L. (1987), *Analyt. Chem.*, **59**, 546.

Le Cocq, C. and Lallemand, J. Y. (1981), *J. Chem. Soc. Chem. Commun.*, 150.

London, R. E., Gabel, S. A. and Funk, A. (1987), *Biochemistry*, **26**, 7166.

Malet-Martino, M. C. and Martino, R. (1989), *Xenobiotica*, **19**, 583.

Malet-Martino, M. C., Martino, R., Lopez, A., Beteille, J. P., Bon, M., Bernadou, J. and Armand, J. P. (1983), *Biomed. Pharmacother.*, **37**, 357.

Malet-Martino, M. C., Armand, J. P., Lopez, A., Bernadou, J., Beteille, J. P., Bon, M. and Martino, R. (1986), *Cancer Res.*, **46**, 2105.

Malet-Martino, M. C., Martino, R., Bernadou, J. and Chevreau, P. (1988 a) in *Liver Cells and Drugs* (A. Guillouzo, ed.) p. 113, INSERM, Paris.

Malet-Martino, M. C., Benadon, J., Martino, R. and Armand, J. P. (1988 b), *Drug Metabol. Dispos.*, **16**, 78.

Martino, R., Lopez, A., Malet-Martino, M. C., Bernadon, J. and Armand, J. P. 1985, *Drug Metab. and Dispos.*, **13**, 116.

Nakada, T. and Kwee, I. L. (1987), *Magnet. Reson. Med.* **4**, 366.

Nakada, T., Kwee, I. L. and Conboy, C. B. (1986), *J. Neurochem.*, **46**, 198.

Nicholson, J. K. and Wilson, I. D. (1987), *Prog. Drug. Res.*, **31**, 427.

Nicholson, J. K., Buckingham, M. J. and Sadler, P. J. (1983), *Biochem. J.*, **211**, 605.

Nicholson, J. K., Timbrell, J. A., Bales, J. R. and Sadler P. J. (1985 a), *Molec. Pharmacol.*, **27**, 634.

Nicholson, J. K., Timbrell, J. A. and Sadler, P. J. (1985 b), *Molec. Pharmacol.*, **27**, 644.

Pass, M. A., Geoffrion, Y., Deslauriers, R., Butler, K. W. and Smith, I.C.P. (1984), *J. Biochem. Biophys. Methods*, **10**, 135.

Patt, S. L. and Shoolery, J. N. (1982), *J. Magnet. Reson.*, **46**, 535.

Preece, N. E. and Timbrell, J. A. (1990) in: Progress in Pharmacology and Clinical Pharmacology (Hlavica, P., Darnani, L. and Gorrod, J. W., eds) in press.

Preece, N. E. and Williams, S. C. R. (1990) *Proc. VIIth European Congress of NMR Med. Biol.*, p. 70, GRAMM, Strasbourg.

Preece, N. E., Ghatineh, S. and Timbrell, J. A. (1989); *Human Toxicol.*, **8**, 156.

Prior, M. J. W., McSheehy, P. M. J., Maxwell, R. J. and Griffiths, J. R. (1987), *Proc. VIth Ann. Meet. Soc. Magnet. Reson. Med.*, **1**, 502.

Rabenstein, D. L. and Fan, S. (1986). *Analyt. Chem.*, **58**, 3178.

Rabenstein, D. L. and Nakashima, T. L. (1979), *Analyt. Chem.*, **51**, 1465A.

Roth, K., Kimber, B. J. and Feeney, J. (1980), *J. Magnet. Reson.*, **41**, 302.

Sanders, J. K. and Hunter, B. K. (1987), *Modern NMR Spectroscopy. A Guide for Chemists*, Oxford University Press, Oxford.

Sanins, S. M., Timbrell, J. A., Elcombe, C. and Nicholson, J. K. (1988), in *Bioanalysis of Drugs and Metabolites. Methodological, Surveys in Biochemistry and Analysis* (E. Reid and I. D. Wilson, eds), p. 375 Plenum Press, New York.

Selinksy, B. S., Thompson, M. and London, R. E. (1987), *Biochem. Pharmacol.*, **36**, 413.

Selinsky, B. S., Perlman, M. E. and London, R. E. (1988 a), *Molec. Pharmacol.*, **33**, 559.

Selinsky, B. S., Perlman, M. E. and London, R. E. (1988 b), *Molec. Pharmacol.*, **33**, 567.

Shaka, A. J., Keeler, J. and Freeman, R. (1983), *J. Magnet. Reson.*, **53**, 313.

Stevens, A. N., Morris, P. G., Iles, R. A., Sheldon, P. W. and Griffiths, J. R. (1984), *Br. J. Cancer*, **50**, 113.

Tofts, P. S. and Wray, S. (1988), *NMR in Biomed.*, **1**, 1.

Tulip, K., Timbrell, J. A., Nicholson, J. K., Wilson, I. D. and Troke, J. (1986), *Drug Metab. Dispos.*, **146**, 746.

Tulip, K., Nicholson, J. K. and Timbrell, J. A. (1989), *J. Pharmaceut. Biomed. Anal.*,, **7**, 499.

Vialaneix, J. P., Malet-Martino, M. C., Hoffman, J. S., Pris, J. and Martino, R. (1987), *Drug Metab. Dispos.*, **15**, 718.

Wade, K. E., Troke, J., Macdonald, C. M., Wilson, I. D. and Nicholson, J. K. (1988), in *Bioanalysis of Drugs and Metabolites* (E. Reid., J. D. Robinson and I. Wilson, eds), p. 383, Plenum Publishing Corporation, New York.

Wade, K. E., Wilson, I. D. and Nicholson, J. K. (1989), *Proc. Vth International Congress on Toxicology*, p. 114, Taylor & Francis, London, NY, Philadelphia.

Wade, K. E. (1990). PhD Thesis, University of London.

Wade, K. E., Wilson, I. D., Troke, J. A. and Nicholson, J. K. (1990), *J. Pharm. Biomed. Anal.* in press.

Walsh, C. (1983), *Adv. Enzymol.*, **55**, 197.

Wilson, I. D. and Ismail, J. M. (1986), *J. Pharmaceut. Biomed. Anal.*, **45**, 663.

Wilson, I. D. and Nicholson, J. K. (1987), *Analyt. Chem.*, **59**, 2830.

Wilson, I. D., Fromson, J., Ismail, I. M. and Nicholson, J. K. (1987), *J. Pharmaceut. Biomed. Anal.*, **5**, 157.

Wolf, W., Albright M. J., Silver, M. S., Weber, H., Reichardt, U. and Sauer, R. (1987), *Magnet. Reson. Imaging*, **5**, 165.

Wray, S. and Wilkie, D. R. (1987). *Proc. VIth Ann. Meet. Soc. Magnet. Reson. Med.*, **2**, 597.

Wyrwicz, A. M., Pszenny, M. H., Schofield, J. C., Tillman, P. C., Gordon, R. E. and Martin, P. A. (1983), *Science*, **222**, 423.

Wyrwicz, A. M., Conboy, C. B., Nichols. B. G., Ryback, K. R. and Eisele, P. (1987 a), *Biochim. Biophys. Acta*, **929**, 271.

Wyrwicz, A. M., Ryback, K., Nichols, B. G., Corboy, C. B. and Eisele, P. (1987 b), *Biochim. Biophys. Acta*, **927**, 86.

CHAPTER 5

MO-QSARs: a review of molecular orbital-generated quantitative structure-activity relationships

David F. V. Lewis

Department of Biochemistry, University of Surrey, Guildford, Surrey, GU2 5XH, England, UK

1. Introduction

Over the last thirty-five years there has been a large number of studies undertaken to reveal molecular structural features responsible for various types of biological activity. The search for meaningful structure-activity relationships (SARs) within groups of compounds naturally progressed, with the advent of computer technology, to the formulation of quantitative structure-activity relationships (QSARs) in series of compounds of known biological activity. Although less publicized, the use of calculated quantum-mechanical parameters as structure descriptors for QSARs has continued in parallel with the more widespread employment of experimentally measurable (and often additive) physicochemical parameters (such as log P) in QSAR analysis.

It is both helpful and timely to reflect on and collate the many examples where structural parameters obtained from molecular orbital (MO) calculations have been successfully correlated with varieties of biological data and to attempt some degree of rationalization and classification of MO-QSARs. However, it is useful and necessary to delineate the way in which the QSAR technique has developed, to outline the concurrent advance of molecular orbital procedures, to explore the possible ways in which theoretically derived features of electronic structure can be related to various types of intermolecular forces encountered in biological systems and to illustrate the statistical methods which have been derived to assist in the formulation and discovery of QSARs in particular instances. First of all, it is logical to trace the development of QSARs in general.

The development of QSARs

About thirty years ago Hansch *et al.* (1962) suggested that the work on linear-free energy relationships (LFERs) by Hammett (1940) and Taft (1956) could be extended to encompass the sphere of biological activity. The application of LFERs lies in the use of substituent parameters for electronic (using the Hammett σ values) and steric (using the Taft E_S values) effects in relating chemical structure with reactivity (Chapman and Shorter, 1972). Hansch's great contribution to QSAR analysis has been the introduction (Hansch and Leo, 1979; Leo *et al.*, 1971) of the hydrophobic substituent parameter, π, based on the logarithm of experimental octanol/water partition coefficients (log P values), where:

$$\pi_{\text{substituent}} = \log\ P_{\substack{\text{substituted}\\ \text{compound}}} - \log\ P_{\substack{\text{parent}\\ \text{compound}}}$$

The additivity of π values and log P fragments, which enables one to produce partition coefficients for compounds where the experimental data have not been measured, coupled with a large data base of determined values and fragments (MEDCHEM data base, available from C. Hansch, Pomona College, Claremont, California 91711) considerably enhances the applicability of the Hansch method. Furthermore, Hansch and others have been able to extend their scheme to incorporate non-linear analysis, usually involving quadratic expressions in log P or π (Hansch *et al.*, 1963) and to include the Hammett and Taft substituent constants so that electronic and steric effects can be assessed (Hansch and Fujita, 1964). The success of the Hansch method with its enhancements cannot be overestimated: the extensive literature on QSARs contains a large proportion of studies showing correlations between hydrophobic parameters and biological activity in many systems, and the contribution that Corwin Hansch has made to this branch of science is reflected in the number of publications which bear his name.

The rationalization of the Hansch approach lies in the fact that partition coefficients between organic and aqueous phases provide some measure of the relative ease with which compounds are able to be transported through cell membranes and across other biological barriers. When coupled with the employment of the statistical methods of regression analysis, the Hansch method gives rise to a very powerful technique for biological correlations, the application of which has been reviewed by Gould (1972).

Although the hydrophobic effect (Tanford, 1980) is clearly an important factor in pharmacological and toxicological activity, in many cases the major one, it became clear that there were certain limitations to the initial Hansch approach of employing either partition coefficients or their derived substituent parameter, π. For simple biological systems, such as bacteria, Hansch analysis was widely applicable but in more complicated life forms, for example mammalia, other effects than hydrophobicity were clearly important. The Hansch group developed modifications such as π-σ-E_S analysis and the π^2-π-σ

equation to include steric and electronic parameters, and to incorporate transport through multicompartmental systems, respectively. These improvements produced notable successes and were in line with current views on substrate–receptor binding interaction energies and in agreement with theories of the contributions to overall biological activity of a compound based on dose concentration, rate of response and ability to reach the site of action. A mathematical treatment of these considerations yields the general linear equation of a QSAR and it is useful to show how such an equation may be derived.

Formulation of a QSAR using Hansch analysis

It is generally assumed that the rate of a biological response (dR/dt) can be equated with the product of three factors relating to the concentration of the effector (C_x), the probability of the chemical reaching the site of action (P_x) and its reactivity (K_x). Mathematically, this can be expressed as follows:

$$\frac{dR}{dt} = P_x \cdot C_x \cdot K_x \tag{1}$$

Hansch derived an expression for the probability P_x in terms of an exponential Gaussian function in π, thus:

$$P_x = ae^{-(\pi - \pi_0)^2/b} \tag{2}$$

where a and b are constants, e is the exponential constant, π is the hydrophobic substituent parameter (defined previously) and π_0 is the optimum π value for transport to the active site.

Combining (1) with (2) gives the following:

$$\frac{dR}{dt} = ae^{-(\pi - \pi_0)^2/b} C_x \cdot K_x \tag{3}$$

If C_x is the dose concentration required to elicit a unit response in a given time, then:

$$\frac{dR}{dt} = 1 \tag{4}$$

Using this condition and taking the logarithm of both sides of equation (3), we get:

$$0 = \log a - \frac{(\pi - \pi_0)^2}{b} + \log C_x + \log K_x \tag{5}$$

Then rearrangement of the expression, gives:

$$-\log C_x = \log a - \frac{(\pi - \pi_0)^2}{b} + \log K_x \tag{6}$$

Expansion of the term in brackets produces a quadratic equation as follows:

$$-\log C_x = k_1\pi - k_2\pi^2 + \log K_x + k_3 \tag{7}$$

where k_1, k_2 and k_3 are constants (as π_0 is a constant).

Now from the Hammett equation, we get:

$$\log K_x = \rho\sigma \tag{8}$$

where ρ is a constant and σ is the Hammett substituent parameter. Combining (8) with (7) produces a quadratic in π which equates with dose concentration as shown below:

$$-\log C_x = k_1\pi - k_2\pi^2 + \rho\sigma + k_3 \tag{9}$$

The constant terms in (9) can be arrived at from regression analysis of the appropriate substituent parameters in a series of compounds of known biological activity, measured by concentrations, C_x, required to produce a known response. It is, therefore, usual to employ the logarithmic values of dose concentrations as activity data in QSAR analysis. This is a natural consequence of the origin of the technique in LFER analysis due to the fact that the logarithmic form of an exponential equation gives rise to a linear expression which then becomes more amenable to statistical methods.

2. Receptor binding and QSARs

The generally accepted theory of drug action is that an effector molecule interacts with some intracellular receptor macromolecule in a specific way at a particular part of the receptor, usually referred to as an active site, or binding site. Apart from a few particular examples, little is known about the mode of this substrate–receptor interaction with respect to the nature of functional groups on the receptor involved in the interaction and conformational changes in the effector species. However, it is thought that the determining step in the production of a biological response is the formation of the drug–receptor complex. Mathematically, this may be expressed as follows:

$$S + R \overset{k_1}{\rightarrow} SR \overset{k_2}{\rightarrow} \text{biological response}$$

where S and R refer to substrate and receptor, respectively.

There is some controversy as to whether k_1 or k_2 is the rate constant for the response-determining step, but it is valid to equate drug activity, A, with the free energy of formation of the drug-receptor complex, ΔG_{RS}. Assuming that electronic, solvent and steric interactions between drug and receptor, and conformational changes in the receptor are of the 1st order and separable, it is possible to write the following expression for the activity, A_n, of a compound n in a series of N compounds tested against a common receptor:

$$A_n = \Delta G_{RS} = \Delta G_n^e + \Delta G_n^d + \Delta G_n^s + \Delta G_n^p + k \qquad (10)$$

where k is a constant and the ΔG_n terms refer to electronic, desolvation, steric and conformational contributions to the overall free energy change, respectively.

If such a series of compounds differ only by substitution at various positions in a parent species, then one can logically show that the change in A_n through the series is paralleled by changes in substituent properties as follows:

$$\delta A_n = \delta(\Delta G^e)_n + \delta(\Delta G^d)_n + \delta(\Delta G^s)_n + \delta(\Delta G^p)_n \qquad (11)$$

Assuming that conformational changes are constant within the series, it is possible (Cammarata, 1968) to equate the above expression with the following linear free energy equation:

$$\delta A_n = a\sigma + b\pi + cE_s + k \qquad (12)$$

where a, b, c and k are constants, σ is the Hammett (electronic) substituent constant, π is the Hansch (lipophilic) substituent constant relating to desolvation events occurring during the formation of the substrate–receptor complex, and E_s is the Taft (steric) substituent constant. This equation enables one to account for biological activity within a series of compounds in terms of the linear-free energy parameters derived by Hansch analysis.

For the purposes of a theoretical rationale for the use of quantum-chemical parameters in QSARs, Cammarata (1970) found it convenient to express (10) in terms of contributions from electronic, desolvation and steric effects of interacting atoms on the substrate (s) and receptor (r) as shown below:

$$A_n = \sum_r \sum_s (E_{rs} + L_{rs} + V_{rs})_n + k \qquad (13)$$

where E_{rs} is the electronic component, L_{rs} is the lipophilic (or desolvation) component, V_{rs} is the volume (or steric) component and k is a constant. The summations are over all atoms comprising the receptor (r) and the substrate (s).

For a series of structurally related molecules, E_{rs}, L_{rs} and V_{rs} can be assumed to be constant for atoms that are common to each compound, leading to the following modification:

$$A_n = \sum_g a_{ng} + \mu \qquad (14)$$

where μ is a constant and $a_{ng} = \sum_{r'} \sum_{s'} (E_{r's'} + L_{r's'} + V_{r's'})$. The primes indicate that specific interactions are identified with a given atom or group, *g.* Equation (14) is the basis of the Free and Wilson (1964) approach to structure–activity correlations.

It is possible to express the E_{rs} term from (13) in terms of theoretical parameters obtained from MO calculations using the equation of Klopman and Hudson, if one assumes that interactions between the substrate and receptor are conveyed via electron transfer. The quantum-chemical formulation of the electronic contribution then becomes:

$$E_{rs} = \frac{-q_r q_s e^2}{\varepsilon_{rs} D_{rs}} + \sum_m^{occ} \sum_n^{unocc} \frac{2C_{mr}^2 C_{ns}^2 \beta^2}{E_m - E_n} \tag{15}$$

where q_r and q_s are net electronic charges on the receptor and substrate atoms, respectively, separated by a distance D_{rs} in a medium of dielectric constant ε_{rs}; e is the charge on the electron and C_{mr}, C_{ns} are molecular orbital coefficients for receptor and substrate molecules, respectively, with orbital energies F_m and E_n. These are equated with the energies of the LEMO and HOMO, respectively, and the summations are over occupied and unoccupied MOs. β is the resonance integral obtained from MO calculation.

When $E_m > E_n$, the second term in (15) becomes negligible compared with the Coulombic (first) term and the overall interaction is largely dependent on the charges q_r and q_s. This leads to what is known as a charge-controlled interaction and (15) can be rewritten as:

$$E_{rs} - \frac{-q_r q_s e^2}{\varepsilon_{rs} D_{rs}} + 2\left(\sum_m C_{mr}^2\right)\left(\sum_n C_{ns}^2\right)\gamma \tag{16}$$

where $\gamma = \beta^2/(E_m - E_n)$.

However, when $E_m \cong E_n$ the second term in (15) becomes predominant giving rise to a frontier-controlled interaction because it is the so-called frontier electrons (i.e. those associated with the HOMO and LEMO) that are involved. In this instance, the expression for E_{rs} becomes:

$$E_{rs} = 2C_{mr} C_{ns} \beta \tag{17}$$

and the electronic reactivity is thus determined by the frontier orbital electron density, f_{ns}. Cammarata has reported instances where either net atomic charges or frontier electronic densities correlate with biological activity, thus indicating that electronic effects can make a major contribution to substrate-receptor binding (Cammarata, 1969). Furthermore, he showed that an orbital-weighted electron density parameter, known as superdelocalizability (S_E) could also be incorporated into the frontier orbital term of (15), which then can be rewritten as:

$$E_{rs} = \frac{-q_r q_s e^2}{\varepsilon_{rs} D_{rs}} + \tfrac{1}{2} q_r S_E \beta \tag{18}$$

The electrophilic superdelocalizability, S_E, is a term coined by Fukui *et al.* (1954) and is a so-called reactivity index, derived as follows:

$$S_E = 2 \sum_{m}^{occ} \frac{C_{ms}^2}{E_m} \qquad (19)$$

and is a parameter readily calculable by MO procedures. If electronic changes within the receptor are negligible but overall electronic changes within a series of structurally related substrates relate to activity differences, it is feasible to simplify (18) to the following expression:

$$A_n = \sum_{s} (aq_s + bS_E) + c \qquad (20)$$

where a, b and c are constants obtained from statistical analysis. Cammarata was able to show quite convincingly that the use of such parameters derived from MO calculations can produce significant QSARs in certain cases. He went on (Cammarata, 1969) to investigate a theoretical representation of the lipophilic parameter, π, which he first equated in a simple way with the electric polarizability, α, a parameter which may be either calculated via MO procedures or obtained from experimental measurements. Recently, it has been shown that log P values for structurally diverse compounds can be calculated from first principles by MO methods (Lewis, 1989 b). Interestingly, Cammarata found that π and log P values related well with a linear combination of net atomic charge, Q_T, and superdelocalizability, S_E, summed over all atoms in the molecule, using equations of the type:

$$\log P \ (\text{or } \pi) = a \sum_{s} Q_T + b \sum_{s} S_E \qquad (21)$$

In some cases, either or both of these electronic factors correlated well with activity data in a variety of biological systems (Cammarata and Rogers, 1971).

The important work of Cammarata gives a physical rationalization for the use of substituent parameters in QSAR analysis and also provides a link between the Hansch approach and the use of MO methods in structure–activity correlations. Before we consider the development of MO calculations of electron structure, it will be of use to consider the factors involved in the manifestation of biological activity by chemicals.

The physicochemical basis of bioactivity

A biological reaction may involve the making or breaking of covalent bonds and/or one or more of the other varieties of intermolecular interactions listed in Table 1. QSAR analysis attempts to rationalize the effect of structural modification on the biological activity of a group of compounds. As we have seen previously, 'classical' QSAR analysis utilizes physicochemical parameters

Table 1. Various types of interaction found in biological systems (from: Nogrady, 1988; Simon, 1976; Gabler, 1978; Kollman, 1980).

Type of interaction	Energy expression	Energy range (kJ.mole^{-1})	Distance range (Å)	Example
Covalent bond	—	200–400	1–2	C-C
Electrostatic	$\dfrac{q_1 q_2 e^2}{\varepsilon d}$	4–8 (much higher in chemical systems)	5–8	$H^+...Cl^-$
Ion–dipole	$\dfrac{q\ \mu\ \cos\theta}{\varepsilon(d^2 - r^2)}$	4–8 (higher in chemical systems)	2.5–3	$F^-...H_2O$
Hydrogen bond	—	8–32	2.5–3.5	$H_2O...H_2O$
Charge transfer	$\dfrac{E^2}{I - A - q^2/d}$	8–32	3–3.5	$C_2(CN)_4...H_2O$
Dipole–dipole	$\dfrac{\mu_1\mu_2\ \cos\theta}{\varepsilon d^3}$	3–5	2–2.5	$R_3N \rightarrow R_2CO$
Ion-induced dipole	$\dfrac{q^2\alpha}{\varepsilon^2 d^4}$	2–3	2–2.5	$F^-...C_6H_6$
Dipole-induced dipole	$\dfrac{\mu^2\alpha(1 + 3\cos^2\theta)}{\varepsilon^2 d^6}$	2–3	2 2.4	$H_2CO...C_6H_6$
Hydrophobic	—	3–5	2–2.3	$C_6H6...C_6H_6$
Van der Waals	$\dfrac{3\alpha^2 I_1 I_2}{4d^6(I_1 + I_2)}$	1–4	2–2.2	Xe...Xe

q = charge on species
e = charge on the electron
ε = dielectric constant
d = distance
θ = angular separation
α = polarizability

I = ionization energy
A = electron affinity
r = radial separation
E = interaction energy
μ = dipole moment

(which are often composed from additive substituent parameters) in its explanation of activity differences within a congeneric series of chemicals. However, MO-QSAR analysis makes use of electronic structural descriptors and/or other molecular structural measures obtained from quantum-chemical calculations to probe biochemical interactions at the submolecular level. Although there is some degree of comparability between physicochemical and quantum-chemical parameters, as can be seen from an inspection of Table 2, which illustrates the parallelism between the two types, it is found in practice that the former are often crude or incomplete estimations of the likely biological situation due to their empirical nature. The reason for the preference for MO parameters is also due to the fact that it is possible to relate the

Table 2. Physical rationalization of quantum chemical parameters (from: Cammarata, 1970).

Physicochemical property/parameter	Quantum chemical expressions
π, log P, hydrophobicity	ΣS_E, $\Sigma S_E + \Sigma Q_T$, $\Sigma \alpha_N$
σ, electronic energy	Q_N, localization energy, L_E
E_S, steric interaction energy	ΣS_E, van der Waals volume, V
Charge transfer energy	Q_H, Q_L, S_E, S_N
Solvation energy	Q_N^2
Dispersion energy	α^2. ΔE, $\alpha.E_H$
Rate constant, ionization energy	I, E_H, interaction energy
Activation energy	ΔE

different types of intermolecular forces likely to be involved in biochemical events to quantum-mechanical quantities.

Factors which contribute to an overall biological response may be summarized as transport, binding and metabolism (or reactivity). All of these processes can be satisfactorily explained in terms of the molecular and electronic structure of the effector species itself. First of all, the above factors will be discussed in relation to the processes involved. It is generally regarded that passive diffusion, as expressed by Fick's Law (Fick, 1855), through cellular barriers and biological fluids, is effected by a compound's ability to exert a partitioning between different phases. Active transport is mediated by some biological carrier process involving either an enzyme system or ionophores, though this can be a combination of the two. The lipid nature of cell membranes and the aqueous nature of extra and intracellular phases has led to the employment of the octanol/water partition coefficient as a measure of a compound's hydrophobicity and, consequently, an estimate of the degree of its transport across cellular barriers. There is, of course, a considerable volume of published evidence to suggest that, in many instances, the overall range of biological potencies in series of chemicals can be successfully related to a hydrophobic (lipophilic) parameter such as log P, π, or f, the hydrophobic fragmental constant (Rekker, 1977). Some recent examples of such studies are those of Lipnick in correlation of fish toxicity (Lipnick, 1985; Lipnick *et al.*, 1985), induction of cytochrome P450 by alcohols and pyrazoles (Sinclair *et al.*, 1986) and drug toxicity (Cassidy *et al.*, 1987). Compilations of earlier QSAR involving hydrophobic parameters may be found in the publications of Hansch (1969, 1971, 1973 and 1976), Gould (1972) and Kubinyi (1979), whereas van de Waterbeemd and Testa (1987) have reported an extensive analysis of the parameterization of lipophilicity and other structural properties. Although it is generally regarded that ease of biological transport is adequately explained in terms of partition coefficients, it is possible to describe cellular transport in quantum-mechanical terms as has been shown by Hosur using a modification of the Schrödinger equation (Hosur, 1978).

Binding may be reversible or irreversible (covalent), specific or non-specific, although all of these varieties are a result of structural features of the substrate molecule concerned. The intermolecular forces involved in substrate–receptor interactions can be classified as ionic, ion–dipole, dipole–dipole and van der Waals, or dispersion forces. Hydrogen bonding is a special case of dipole–dipole interaction, whereas covalent bonding is not usually regarded as an intermolecular force because it involves the formation of a chemical bond which is not reversible. The overall binding process is likely to be a combination of two or more of these basic types, although one component may be more significant than another and other forces, although almost certainly present, may be relatively insignificant. It is one of the aims of QSAR analysis to seek to establish the relative magnitude of each contribution from these forces in describing the total activity of a group of chemicals and MO-QSARs are, in general, more applicable than those involving purely substituent parameters in facilitating a true understanding of the biological situation. In a way which is, at present, little understood, binding to a receptor effects some form of biological response which can involve a conformational change in a macromolecule and/or transmission of electric charge via the movement of ionic species.

The metabolism of a compound can be a complex process involving a number of enzyme systems. Essentially, the extent of metabolism is a result of a compound's reactivity towards one or more of the metabolizing enzymes and thus can be related to particular structural features of the molecule itself. The process is further complicated by the fact that metabolites can also effect a biological response which may exert a (positive or negative) feedback on the initial activity. It is also possible that the chemical may have undergone some degree of metabolism prior to receptor interaction with its pharmacophore.

Although the above events are going to contribute in varying degrees to the overall manifestation of a response to a given chemical, one should also consider the dose, route of administration, rate of absorption and possible structural changes brought about by variations in pH of the appropriate medium before interaction with a receptor occurs. Of course, the actual concentration of the active material at the receptor site (which may be a protein, enzyme or nucleic acid) will be affected by the extent of absorption, metabolism and elimination. The effect of pH on the partition coefficient can be quantified if the dissociation constant, K_a, of the substance is known; this is expressed in the following equation:

$$\log \frac{(P_N - 1)}{P_0} = \mathrm{pH} - pK_a \tag{22}$$

where P_0 is the overall (observed) partition coefficient, P_N is the unionized (normal) partition coefficient, pH is the measurable acidity of the medium and pK_a is the negative logarithm of the dissociation constant, K_a. If the K_a value of the substance is not known, then it is useful to have some means of estimation and MO calculations leading to QSARs can assist in the computation of acidity constants.

Kier has shown that it is possible to rationalize biological activity in terms of MO-calculated quantities (Kier, 1971) whereas Barlow has demonstrated how physicochemical parameters can explain different events in a biological response (Barlow, 1980). It can be seen from the expressions in Table 1 that certain electronic quantities, such as atomic charges and energy levels, should be capable of being related to different types of interactions encountered in receptor binding. Some of these properties such as dipole moments and ionization energies can be measured experimentally but it is invariably easier to calculate these, and other quantities, by MO methods, the latter having a wider applicability than experimental determinations which often involve specialist equipment and, inevitably, a greater time scale. Table 2 indicates the degree of comparability between MO parameters and physicochemical factors found in QSAR expressions. It is thus possible to demonstrate that, in many instances, there is an equivalence between the two sources of structural descriptors for QSAR and SAR analysis.

It is well established that biological transport is a function of compound hydrophobicity and the logarithm of the (octanol/water) partition coefficient (log P) is a good measure of this effect. However, Cammarata and Rogers have shown that a combination of total superdelocalizability and total net atomic charge provides a measure of log P in several aromatic and hetero-aromatic systems (Cammarata and Rogers, 1971); it is also apparent that molecular polarizability can be equated with log P in some instances (Hansch and Coats, 1970) although the inclusion of polarity (μ) and electron availability, E(HOMO), takes other contributions into account (Lewis, 1989 a). Furthermore, within certain essentially homologous series, the total superdelocalizability, S_E, is sufficient to establish a parallelism with log P (Lewis, 1987 a, 1989 b).

As far as receptor binding is concerned there are a number of types of interaction which have to be considered as shown in Table 1. Taking these intermolecular forces in turn and excluding covalent binding for the moment, it can be seen from an inspection of Table 2 that the energies roughly match the order of distance dependency. It is likely that there are a number of stages involved in molecular recognition and interaction with the receptor site whereby different forces come into play during the time taken from when the substrate enters the receptor environment until actual binding takes place, and this is reflected in their distance dependencies and ranges respectively. Thus, the electrostatic forces initiate a long range attraction and dipolar interactions produce an alignment of substrate with the receptor from where the short range forces can exert a 'fine-tuning' effect to complete the binding process.

Electrostatic forces are likely to be determined by overall molecular charges and, as such, are readily calculable by MO methods, although formal charges may be estimated by inspection of the molecular formula of the compound concerned. However, the extent to which a charge is distributed around adjacent atoms would require an MO calculation and such information can often assist in the explanation of molecular interactions, as can a consideration of the effect of counter ions on biological events. Dipolar interactions are a function of the distribution of partial electronic charges within a molecule as this is responsible for overall polarity as the vectorial summation of charges results in the dipole moment quantity. Thus, the dipole moment and its components as obtained from MO calculation can be employed in structure-activity studies, such as the correlation of anti-inflammatory activity with dipole moment for H_2-antagonists (Young *et al.*, 1986). In some varieties of dipole interaction, it is possible for the polarizability of the molecule to be involved, thus showing the propensity for a dipole to be induced due to polarization of the molecule by an external field.

Hydrogen bonding is a special type of dipole dipole interaction which is usually of higher energy than normal. As such it is a quantity that has always been difficult to evaluate by MO procedures, but recent developments indicate that estimations are improving and some of the latest molecular modelling systems are able to identify potential hydrogen bonds with a fair degree of accuracy.

Molecular association brought about by charge transfer has been thoroughly studied giving rise to an empirical expression (Table 1) which may be verified experimentally. Quantum-mechanical derivations for this type of interaction involve frontier orbital terms such as electron population in the HOMO and LEMO, energies of the respective orbitals or the difference between them, in particular the reciprocal of ΔE. The matching of complementary frontier orbitals between interacting molecules is a prerequisite for electron transfer, and for a treatment of frontier orbitals and reactivity the reader is recommended to refer to an excellent monograph by Fleming (1980).

Van der Waals forces of attraction are associated with an energy term composed of the square of the molecular polarizability together with ionization energy terms of the respective interacting species. The corresponding MO description of this interaction involves the product of polarizability and E(HOMO) because one is only concerned with the effect on one of the two interacting entities. However, it is possible to quantify this effect experimentally from determinations of ionization energies and polarizabilities (Agin *et al.*, 1965; Handa *et al.*, 1983).

Molecular size and dimensions, which can be calculated as well as being measurable from crystallographic data, can determine whether a substrate is capable of being accommodated within the confines of a receptor site on grounds of the substrate's bulk and shape. Complementarity between chemical groups on the substrate and amino acid residues at the receptor site play an important role in the docking process.

A number of electronic factors are likely to be involved in metabolism and general reactivity of compounds. The precise description depends on the nature of the metabolic process in question. Moreover, for example, the magnitude of the bond energy would be expected to reflect the potential for bond fission during a biological reaction. The ease of metabolic activation relates to the energy difference between frontier orbitals, E(LEMO) and E(HOMO), if the promotion of electrons is involved. This probably explains the correlation between nitrosamine carcinogenicity and ΔE (Parke *et al.*, 1988). Electrophilic and nucleophilic reactivity of compounds has been shown to be dependent on atom superdelocalizabilities, S_E and S_N (Fukui *et al.*, 1954). Some MO procedures are able to calculate the standard enthalpy of formation, Hf, of a compound and it can be expected that this quantity will give an indication of the chemical or, more precisely, thermodynamic stability of the compound which could be of importance in direct-acting substrates. If a compound is capable of being ionized under biological conditions then its pK_a will enable the assessment of the extent of ionization. It is of interest, therefore, to obtain structural descriptors of pK_a using MO techniques. Some of the earlier successes of MO calculation involved the correlation of basicity with nitrogen atomic charge (Pullman and Pullman, 1960; Collin and Pullman, 1964) and the pK_a values of aliphatic mono carboxylic acids appear to be governed by net charge on the hydroxyl oxygen (Lewis, unpublished results).

There is increasing interest in the calculation of the molecular electrostatic potential (MEP) energy as a means of gaining an understanding of the way in which substrate molecules react in many biological processes. The results of an MO calculation are utilized for evaluation of MEP energies based on net atomic charges. Electrostatic isopotential (EIP) contour maps and surfaces are produced by successive computation of the potential energy value between a unitary point positive or negative charge and the array of net atomic charges resulting from electronic distribution in molecules. The appearance of the overall electrostatic potential energy profile of a molecule and the associated electric field are thought to be intimately related with the way in which biological activity is expressed. However, it is often difficult to correlate actual values with activity data because the MEP is a global quantity, though the COMFA (comparative molecular field analysis) method of Marshall and Cramer (1988) could provide a satisfactory solution to this problem.

Although there is, in many cases, a clear rationale for the use of an MO-derived quantity in explaining an aspect of bioactivity, it can also be seen that some parameters are involved in differing areas of interaction: the only simple way of separating the effects is from the type of expression which most successfully relates to the QSAR equation and its individual terms. In the most recent developments in theoretical methods it is possible to include consideration of the effect of solvent as this will moderate the magnitude of the interaction energy. For instance, it is feasible to introduce changes in dielectric constant to model solvent effects or to perform a calculation where a substrate molecule is placed in a three-dimensional array of solvent molecules, although such investigations are highly computationally intensive.

Further discussions on substrate–receptor interactions and on the role of theoretical investigations can be obtained from accounts by Kollman (1980) and Cammarata (1970), in monographs by Kier (1971), Korolkovas (1970),

Korolkovas and Birkhalter (1976) and Simon (1976) and in a recent publication by Nogrady (1988). Detailed analyses of MO calculations and their use in correlations with biological activity, together with treatments of substrate–receptor interactive forces are presented in theses by Blair (1979) and Lewis (1981).

3. Molecular orbital methods for the calculation of structural indices

Molecular orbital (MO) methods for the calculation of the electronic structure of molecules have arisen out of the perceived need to find approximate solutions to the Schrödinger equation (Schrödinger, 1926) for many electron systems. There are, therefore, out of necessity, varying degrees of approximation in all existing methods of MO calculation. Essentially, these are based on an LCAO (linear combination of atomic orbitals) approach which assumes that electrons reside in orbitals that subsist over the entire molecule and are made up of contributions from individual atomic orbitals (AOs) on each atom. These so-called molecular orbitals each have a corresponding energy associated with them which can be calculated to varying degrees of accuracy as compared with experimental data, such as ionization energies, electron affinities and electronic transition energies obtained from spectroscopic measurements. Photoelectron spectroscopy, in particular, is proving to be extremely useful in providing experimental values for electronic energy levels in molecules.

The major types of MO method are shown in Table 3 and these have been listed in chronological order. As a general rule, the degree of approximation involved in an MO procedure is related to the accuracy of the various parameters calculated. For the most widely used MO methods the series HMO, CNDO, INDO, MINDO, MNDO and *ab initio* represent an order of increasing accuracy roughly consistent with the year of their origin. However, accuracy is not the only criterion with which to judge the relative merits of these techniques; time taken to execute a calculation is also an important factor and the relative speeds of computation are presented in Table 4. It can be seen that the time of processing is approximately inversely proportional to the supposed accuracy of the result. A comparison between speed and accuracy with respect to experimental data is shown in Table 5, which only considers some of the more recent MO procedures. Table 6, however, shows the level of agreement between some of the earlier MO methods and experimentally measured ionization energies for nucleic acid bases (Lewis, 1986). Virtually all of the methods presented in Table 3 can be obtained as computer programs from QCPE (Quantum Chemistry Program Exchange at the University of Indiana, Bloomington, Indiana, USA) though the latest molecular modelling packages contain several of the most important and widely used MO procedures, interfaced with graphics software and also QSAR routines. Such integrated systems, which have only become available over the last five years, greatly facilitate MO-QSAR studies on large numbers of compounds.

The aim of an MO method is to obtain approximate solutions to the eigen-

Table 3.   Various types of molecular orbital calculation.

Molecular orbital method	Comments/limitations	Reference
Hückel	π-systems	Hückel, 1931
SCF	common to most MO methods	Roothaan, 1951
PPP	π-systems	Pople, 1953; Parizer and Parr, 1953
Del Re*	charge calculation, empirical	Del Re, 1958
CNDO/2	up to 150 atoms	Pople *et al.*, 1965
INDO	can take 3rd row parameters	Pople *et al.*, 1967
PCILO*	uses localized orbitals	Diner *et al.*, 1969
MINDO	development for MINDO/3	Baird and Dewar, 1969
MINDO/2	development for MINDO/3	Dewar and Haselbach, 1970
MINDO/3	up to 80 atoms	Bingham *et al.*, 1975
MNDO	parameters for *S* and *P*	Dewar *et al.*, 1978
AM1	up to 90 atoms	Dewar *et al.*, 1985
STO-3G	up to 40 atoms	Clark, 1985
Gaussian 86	up to 40 atoms	Hehre *et al.*, 1986

* Not strictly MO methods
SCF   = Self-consistent field
PPP   = Pople–Parizer–Parr
CNDO   = Complete neglect of differential overlap
INDO   = Intermediate neglect of differential overlap
PCILO = Perturbed configurational interaction using localized orbitals
MINDO = Modified intermediate neglect of differential overlap
MNDO   = Modified neglect of differential overlap
AM1   = Austin method, 1st version
STO-3G = Slater-type orbitals—3 Gaussians

Table 4.   Comparisons between speed of MO calculations (from Fernandez-Alonso, 1976).

Method or Basis	Type of calculation	Relative time[+]
EHT	semi-empirical; independent electrons	1
CNDO/2	semi-empirical; no electron interaction	3
INDO	semi-empirical; electron interaction with ZDO	5
MINDO/3	semi-empirical; electron interaction	10
STO-3G	*ab initio*; minimal Slater-type basis	150
4-31G	*ab initio*; split-valence basis	1000
6-31G*	*ab initio*; split-valence basis and d polarization	6000

[+] Absolute time (seconds) for a single calculation on ethanol

Table 5. Comparison between speed and accuracy of MO methods for propane (from Clark, 1985).

Parameter	MINDO/3	MNDO	3-21G	6-31G*	Expt.
Computer time(s)	9.75	10.32	550	4702	—
C-C distance(Å)	1.495	1.530	1.541	1.528	1.526
CCC bond < (°)	121.5	115.4	111.6	112.7	112.4
ΔHf (kcal. mole^{-1})	− 26.5	− 24.9	—	—	− 25.0

* Lewis, 1986

Table 6. Comparison between MO results for the calculation of ionization energies (eV) for DNA and RNA bases.

	CNDO[+]	SCF[+]	MINDO/3*	Expt[++]
Adenine	10.08	7.92	7.60	8.00
Cytosine	10.78	8.16	8.70	8.90
Thymine	—	8.80	9.31	9.43
Guanine	9.06	7.59	7.66	7.80
Uracil	11.88	9.15	9.59	9.82

[+] Pullman and Pullman, 1969
* Lewis, 1986
[++] Lifschitz *et al.*, 1967; Machmer and Duchesne, 1965

value equation:

$$H\psi - E\psi \qquad (23)$$

where H is the Hamiltonian operator, ψ is the electron wave function and E is the energy of the molecular orbital. MO energies are the eigenvalues obtained from solving the set of equations contained in the secular determinant of the Fock matrix (Hartree, 1928; Fock, 1930). The various MO procedures have the capability of solving the eigenvalue equation in different ways, and via differing levels of approximation, to achieve a self-consistent field (SCF) by an iterative process (Roothaan, 1951).

There is a widely held misconception that *ab initio* methods are, by their very nature, always 'better' than the other semi-empirical methods of MO calculation. This notion that *ab initio* methods are preferable to, and more desirable than, semi-empirical ones and are, by definition, more accurate is simply not the case, as has been shown in an important paper by Dewar (1983). Dewar has pointed out, very rightly, that many of the *ab initio* procedures contain as many approximations and parameterizations as some semi-empirical methods.

The main reason why *ab initio* methods are, in fact, often undesirable is that they involve a considerable amount of computer time and memory space for the execution of MO calculations on relatively small molecules as can be seen from Tables 4 and 5. However, the fact that the run-times of such processes are longer does not necessarily mean that they are bound to be more accurate. Indeed with the inevitable degree of parameterization that is present in the *ab initio* methods, there is some merit in their description as being semi-empirical even though the extent of approximation is not as great as in the NDO procedures.

The yardstick for determining the relative accuracy of MO methods has been their ability to reproduce experimental data such as molecular geometries obtained from crystallographic or microwave spectroscopic measurements, ionization energies, dipole moments, heats of formation, etc. There are often quite substantial errors involved in such physical determinations, however, whereas computational calculations can reproduce structural parameters to many decimal places. The choice of MO calculation depends very much on the particular problem under consideration. For example, the Hückel method would be perfectly satisfactory if one was intending to calculate the electronic structures of π systems; whereas for small molecules it would be advantageous to employ one or more of the *ab initio* techniques. Of the existing armoury of MO methods at the computational chemist's disposal, the techniques comprising the AMPAC package probably represent the best compromise between accuracy and time. However, if time is at a premium, CNDO/2 is perfectly adequate for, say, correlating structural differences within a series of structurally related analogues, such as histamine receptor antagonists (Young *et al.*, 1986). This study involved the calculation of dipole moments by the CNDO/2 method and, since the calculated dipole moment is the resultant of the vectorial summation of MO partial charges, the generally good agreement between CNDO/2-calculated and observed dipole moment values gives confidence in the charge calculation, even though the geometry agreement is not as good as MINDO/3, MNDO or *ab initio*. In fact, depending on the compound under consideration, CNDO/2 can provide better results than the more rigorous MO treatments. Similar arguments can also be used for the use of MINDO/3, which is not recommended for certain classes of compound (Clark, 1985) but is actually better than MNDO or even *ab initio* in other cases. These procedures have been reviewed by Dewar (1983) and by Clark (1985) whereas the published literature on the use of MINDO/3 calculations has been reviewed recently (Lewis, 1986). Furthermore, a recent study (Boyd *et al.*, 1988) of the three methods in AMPAC provides a good comparison between MINDO/3, MNDO and AM1, showing the effect of the small, but significant, enhancements to the MINDO/3 technique.

Of the methods presented in Table 1 that are still in general use, it is fair to say that PPP and HMO perform well for π systems but would not be recommended otherwise unless modifications for the inclusion of σ electrons have been made. PCILO is a quantum-chemical method for structure calculation which differs from the MO techniques but is useful for the fast computation of global and local conformational energy minima in conformationally flexible molecules. The INDO procedures are generally more accurate than

CNDO and all of the NDO methods are substantially faster than the *ab initio* techniques. Furthermore, until very recently many molecules of importance in biological systems have been too large to permit *ab initio* calculation within a reasonable time scale, whereas the semi-empirical methods have found a wide application in many areas of biological interest mainly due to their relative speed and, hence, low cost. For a very readable and informed account of quantum mechanics and its applications to pharmacology, the reader is referred to an excellent book by Richards (1983). Comparisons between different MO methods can be obtained from works by Pople and Beveridge (1970), Segal (1977), Murrell and Harget (1972), Heilbronner and Bock (1976), Boyd *et al.* (1988), Yates (1978), Streitwieser (1961), Pullman (1970, 1976), Dewar and Dougherty (1975) and from Lewis *et al.* (1989 a).

4. Statistical methods in QSAR analysis

The aim of the MO-QSAR is to form an intuitive bridge between quantum-chemical parameters and biological activity which can be used both as a predictive tool and as a means to gain an understanding of biological processes at the submolecular level. It is an inevitable necessity, arising out of the nature of the experimental techniques involved in both systems of measurement (i.e. biological and quantum-mechanical) that statistical methods of analysis and correlation are employed in the formulation of MO-QSARs and, indeed, QSARs in general. Consequently, analytical procedures have evolved concurrently with the development of MO methods and appropriate computer modelling software to aid the investigator in rationalization of relationships between molecular structure and biological function.

A summary of the different types of correlative techniques employed in QSAR analysis is shown in Table 7. Probably the most widely used of these methods is that of regression analysis which utilizes a least squares approach to assess the degree of correlation between potential structural descriptors and activity data. Single linear regression analysis can be readily achieved on a programmable hand-held calculator, but multiple regression analysis involving a set of independent variables as descriptors requires the facilities of a computer for its execution. An introduction to this method of QSAR analysis can be found in a useful monograph by Shorter (1973). It should be noted that great care has to be exercised in using statistics in the search for significant and meaningful relationships between sets of data.

Regarding publications of results, some journals lay down quite rigid criteria for the assessment of QSAR expressions and it would be helpful to potential authors if a standard set of guidelines could be universally adopted. In general, the number of descriptors should be small compared with the total number of observations, ideally a ratio of about 1:6 would be considered acceptable. The error limits of each independent variable coefficient should also be small compared with the regression coefficient, something like 16 per

Table 7. Methods for QSAR and SAR analysis

Correlative technique	Type	Reference
Linear regression analysis	Computational	Daniel and Wood, 1971
Linear-free energy relationship	Manual	Leffler and Grunwald, 1963
Hansch analysis	Computational	Hansch et al., 1963
Non-linear regression analysis	Computational	Kubinyi, 1976
De Novo or Free–Wilson approach	Computational	Free and Wilson, 1964
Decision-free approach	Manual	Cramer et al., 1978
Discriminant analysis	Computational	Martin, 1978
Fragment analysis	Computational	Enslein, 1984
Principal components (SIMCA)	Preprocessing	Wold, 1976
Factor analysis	Computational	Cammarata and Menon, 1976
Cluster analysis (CLUSTAN)	Computational	Hansch and Leo, 1979
Combined multivariate analysis	Computational	Lewi, 1976
Pattern recognition (ADAPT)	Computational	Stuper and Jurs, 1975
Topological method	Manual	Kier and Hall, 1976
Topliss scheme	Manual	Topliss, 1972
Craig plot	Manual	Craig, 1971
Simplex analysis	Manual	Darvas, 1974
Fibonacci search	Manual	Deming, 1976
Partial least squares	Computational	Haskuldsson, 1987
Comparative molecular field analysis	Computational	Marshall and Cramer, 1988
CASE programme	Computational	Klopman, 1985

General References: Chu, 1980; Martin, 1978; Blankley, 1983.

cent is usually admissible. Furthermore, the autocorrelation between supposedly independent variables should be less than 50 per cent and the standard error should be small compared with the variation in the biological data itself. The correlation coefficient should be as close to unity as possible but, in multiple regressions, this rises with inclusion of more variables and, in such instances, the magnitude of the variance ratio (F-value) indicates whether there has been an increase in statistical significance. The percentage of the data points which lie outside the F-distribution enable a confidence index to be formulated, corresponding to the likelihood of a correlation appearing by chance.

Methods to reduce the required minimum number of variables under consideration have arisen out of the concern that the possibility of chance correlations increases with the size of the independent variables set (Topliss and Costello, 1972). The analysis of principal components (Wold, 1976) is one example of such a method. Also, the technique of partial least squares is becoming an acceptable alternative to stepwise multiple regression analysis (Hoskuldsson, 1987). A detailed description of cluster analysis, topological methods, pattern recognition and other techniques are beyond the scope of this article but the interested reader is referred to a number of general publications (Martin, 1978; Chu, 1980; Blankley, 1983). However, an example of the use of pattern recognition can be found in a paper by Jurs et al. (1979) whereas, in a recent publication, cluster analysis has been compared with other QSAR methods (McFarland and Gans, 1987). Klopman and co-workers have developed a computer-automated structure evaluation (CASE) technique (Klopman and Frierson, 1984; Klopman, 1985; Klopman and Macina, 1985; Klopman *et al.*, 1985) and Enslein and colleagues have formulated a toxicity evaluation package (TOPKAT) which involves fragment analysis (Enslein, 1984; Enslein *et al.*, 1986; Enslein *et al.*, 1987 a and b). There are a number of computer packages available which contain a variety of the currently used QSAR and SAR techniques. Apart from those mentioned above, ADAPT is a stand-alone system which uses the pattern recognition techniques pioneered by Jurs, whereas integrated molecular modelling packages such as Chem-X (available from Chemical Design Ltd, Oxford) and Sybyl (available from Evans and Sutherland Ltd) have QSAR modules as add-on options. The decision regarding which QSAR to employ depends on the particular situation being investigated. For example, cluster analysis would be used for the differentiation between substrates of different isozymes or between agonists and antagonists of a receptor type, whereas regression analysis might be employed in the determination of structural factors responsible for potency differences within a series of related analogues. It should be noted that an improvement in the understanding of a particular biological process is more important than obtaining high correlations in QSAR analysis. The following example shows a typical QSAR equation with the relevant statistical data: this relates hallucinogenic activity, A, with the magnitude of the HOMO energy in a series of mescaline derivatives (Snyder and Merril, 1965):

$$\log A = -10.26 \ \text{E(HOMO)} + 5.96 \quad n = 6; \ s = 0.33; \ R = 0.97; \ F = 68.8 \quad (24)$$
$$(\pm 1.24) \qquad\qquad (\pm 0.57)$$

where n is the number of compounds, s is the standard error, R is the correlation coefficient and F is the variance ratio.

5. *MO-generated QSARs and related topics*

Inasmuch as it is true that a QSAR can aid drug design by extrapolation (or interpolation) of activity values, the more important aspect from a scientific viewpoint is one of gaining an understanding of effector processes. Therefore, MO descriptors are potentially of greater benefit than substituent parameters since there is a clearer rationale for their explanation of real biological events. Indeed, Corwin Hansch has stated that gaining an insight into effector-receptor pathways is more important than achieving good correlations in QSAR analysis. Having considered the types of interactions which may relate to various structural parameters calculable by MO procedures, there is value in attempting to analyse MO-generated QSARs in terms of the interactive forces involved.

The literature concerning MO-QSARs commences around 1960 with the work of the Pullmans, some of which is collated in their volume on *Quantum Biochemistry* (Pullman and Pullman, 1963) and in a book by Pullman on *Electronic Aspects of Biochemistry* (Pullman, 1962). Furthermore, the literature up to 1970 has been reviewed by Purcell *et al.* (1970) and by Kier (1971). Subsequently, Blair has summarized publications in this area up to 1978 (Blair, 1979). Other useful compilations may be found in reports of a conference on MO studies in chemical pharmacology (Kier, 1970) and in an excellent book by Richards on quantum pharmacology (Richards, 1983). The use of MO calculations in QSARs and in other areas of drug research has also been noted by Tute (1971), Green *et al.* (1974), Bergmann and Pullman (1974), Joyner and Purcell (1976) and by Kaufman (1977). In the previous year, the application of molecular connectivity to drug research was the subject of a book by Kier and Hall (1976). Descriptions of MO indices and their correlations with chemical and biochemical phenomena have been reported by Schnaare and Martin (1965), de Broglie (1966), Greenwood and McWeeney (1966), Schnaare (1971), Wohl (1971), Kier (1972 and 1973), Richards and Black (1975) and by Carbo *et al.* (1977).

Other useful accounts of QSARs in general have been given by Goodford (1973), Cavallito (1973), Tichy (1976), Saxena and Ram (1979), Seydel and Schaper (1982), Dearden (1982), Goldberg (1983), Seydel (1985), Tichy (1985), Hopfinger (1985), Ganellin and Young (1986), Lewis *et al.* (1987 a), Hadzi and Jerman-Blazic (1987) and by Turner *et al.* (1987), the latter having been published previously as an ECETOC report. Also, the application of SARs in chemoreception has been the subject of a book by Betts (1978). The advent of molecular graphics has had a considerable impact on the processing of SAR information as can be seen from recent reports by Li *et al.* (1982), Hansch *et al.* (1985), Kende *et al.* (1985), Cairns *et al.* (1985), Miyamoto and Yoshimoto (1987), Parke (1987) and by Schwalbe *et al.* (1987). QSARs have an important position in the sphere of computer-aided drug design (CADD) and the interested reader is referred to the following publications in CADD (Olsen and Christoffersen, 1979; Marshall, 1983; Cavalla, 1983; Boyd, 1983; Marshall *et al.*, 1985; Cohen, 1985; Burgen *et al.*, 1986; Fauchere, 1986; Thornton *et al.*, 1986; Marshall, 1987; Upton and Gasking, 1988; Boyd and Lipkowitz, 1988; Howard and Kollman, 1988; Marshall and Cramer, 1988).

The present review concentrates on material published since 1974 as this represents the bulk of previously uncatalogued literature on MO-QSARs. This work has been assisted by computer searches of *Chemical Abstracts* and *Biological Abstracts* data bases in addition to regular bibliographic updates appearing in the *Journal of Molecular Graphics* from the Richards group at Oxford (Taylor and Durant, 1985; Smith *et al.*, 1986; and Stedman *et al.*, 1987). The material summarized in Table 8 is probably not completely exhaustive and has been collated in order to illustrate certain techniques and to represent areas of current interest. In certain instances non-MO-QSARs and SARs have been included for comparison (Barlow, 1979; Martin, 1979).

Although the information presented in Table 8 has been arranged chronologically, and this is to highlight the change in MO methods, it has been felt necessary and, indeed, helpful to discuss the use of MO calculations in QSAR analysis from the point of view of topic areas in the form of receptors and biological effects.

Inspection of the material shown in Table 8 enables a number of trends to be observed. For example, it can be seen that the type of MO method gradually changes with time from the Hückel technique, through CNDO/2 to the rather more accurate MINDO/3 and associated methods, together with a number of *ab initio* studies. One noticeable trend is the increased use of EIP calculations to describe substrate-receptor interactions. In fact, the employment of EIPs is becoming so common that they warrant a separate review in themselves. Although difficult to correlate by QSARs, EIP calculations can also be used to predict metabolism; for example, the metabolites of aflatoxin B1 can be correctly estimated from the EIP maxima and minima of the original molecule (Lewis, unpublished results). However, it would probably be more straightforward to use an expert system such as METABOLEXPERT (available from Compudrug, Ltd) to predict metabolites.

The following sections, which have been collated from the literature presented in Table 8, arrange the various MO-QSAR and associated studies by topic, relating to the type of biological activity expressed by the chemicals involved. There is, however, some degree of overlap between biological activities because some compounds possess activity in more than one area; for example, dihydrofolate reductase (DHFR) inhibitors are used in the treatment of cancer, though they would be regarded as enzyme inhibitors for the purposes of the present review provided that DHFR inhibition is the activity being related to structure.

Anaesthetic activity

The minimum blocking concentration of local anaesthetics has been related to the product of polarizability and ionization potential (Agin *et al.*, 1965) using Hückel MO calculations for the determination of ionization potentials for about forty compounds. In this study, molecular polarizabilities were obtained from atomic refraction constants. The London interaction energy (dispersion or van der Waals interaction energy) can be simplified to $\alpha I/8r^3$ (see Table 1) when one considers the interaction between a neutral molecule and a conducting wall, which is a reasonable first approximation for membrane active anaesthetics. Agin and co-workers showed that the greater the product of α and I, the smaller the concentration of anaesthetic required.

In 1973, Pullman and Courriere used PCILO calculations to investigate conformational energy minima of acetylcholine and number of its analogues. They found that the preferred conformation in choline derivatives is gauche-gauche but reported that conformational preferences alone do not account for the fine details of parasympathomimetic activity. In the following year, a novel approach by Lin (1974) involved the utilization of a quantum statistical

Table 8. MO-generated relationships between structure and activity

Compound	Property	Activity	MO Method	Authors	Year
Purine and pyrimidines	Q_N	Acidity	HMO	Pullman and Pullman	1960
Antifolates	Q_N	Acidity	HMO	Collin and Pullman	1964
Phenylethylamine	E(HOMO)	Psychotropic	HMO	Snyder and Merril	1965
Anaesthetics	α, IE	Anaesthetic	HMO	Agin *et al.*	1965
Carbamates	Q_N	Anticholinergic	HMO	Neely	1965
N-alkyl amides	Q_N	Anticholinergic	HMO	Purcell	1966
Indolealkylamines	E(HOMO)	Tryptaminergic	HMO	Kang and Green	1969
Amphetamines	E(HOMO)	Psychotropic	INDO	Kang and Green	1970
Benzothiadiazines	E(HOMO)	Antihypertensive	EHT	Wohl	1970
Coumarins	ΔE	AHH	IEHT	Wald and Feuer	1971
Tetracyclines	Q_N	Antibacterial	Del Re	Peradejordi	1971
Piperidines	Q_N	Anticholinergic	HMO, Del Re	Milner and Purcell	1971
Cholines	Structure	Anaesthetic	PCILO	Pullman and Courriere	1973
Phenylethylamines	Structure	Adrenergic	CNDO,INDO	Katz *et al.*	1973
Lysergic acids	Structure	Tryptaminergic	HMO	Kumber and Sankar	1973
Naphthoquinones	E(LEMO)	Antimalarial	HMO	Martin *et al.*	1973
Cephalosporins	Q_N	Antibiotic	CNDO,INDO	Boyd	1973
Chloramphenicols	$E_{interaction}$	Antibacterial	CNDO/2	Holtje and Kier	1974
β-blockers	Structure	Adrenergic	CNDO/2	Germer	1974
Nitrogen mustards	Q_N	Alkylating	CNDO/2	Berges and Peradejordi	1974
Aromatic hydrocarbons	Bond orders	Carcinogenic	HMO,CNDO/2	Herndon	1974
Local anaesthetics	$E_{vibrational}$	Anaesthetic	Quantum statistics	Lin	1974
Aminobutyric acids	Structure	Gabanergic	EHT	Kier *et al.*	1974
Serotonins	Structure	Tryptaminergic	HMO	Sankar and Kumber	1974
Tryptamines	Q_N, Q_H	5-HT binding	CNDO/2	Johnson and Green	1974
Pyridazines	Q_N	Antihypertensive	CNDO/2	Kulkarni	1975
Cyclopropylamines	E binding	MAO inhibition	CNDO/2	Holtje	1975
Phenylethylamines	EIP, structure	Adrenergic	Semi-empirical	Martin *et al.*	1975
Tryptamines	Q_H	Tryptaminergic	PPP	Glennon and Gessner	1975
Indolealkylamines	E_{occ}	Tryptaminergic	CNDO/2	Kumber *et al.*	1976
Oxazines	EIP	Tryptaminergic	CNDO/2	Daudel *et al.*	1976
Phenylethylamines	μ	Tryptaminergic	EHT	Lukovits *et al.*	1976
Hydroxybenzoic acids	E(HOMO),μ	Antirheumatoid	CNDO/2	Catalan and Fernandez-Alonso	1976

Compound class	MO parameter	Property	Method	Author	Year
Parabens	Q_N, structure	Preservative	IEHT	Alexander et al.	1976
Imidazolines	Structure	Antihypertensive	CNDO/2	Timmermans and van Zweiten	1977
Thyroxines	Structure	Hormonal	CNDO/2	Dietrich et al.	1977
Benzodiazepines	μ, Q_N	Tranquillizing	CNDO/2	Blair and Webb	1977
Oxymorphones	Structure	Analgesic	PCILO	Loew and Berkowitz	1978
Phthalides	Structure	Gabaergic	CNDO/2	Steward and Lowe	1978
Phenylisopropylamines	E(HOMO)	Psychotomimetic	CNDO/2	Anderson et al.	1978
Carboxylic acids	E(LEMO)	Antiallergic	ab initio	Cheney et al.	1978
Benzylamines	$\Delta E, \alpha$	N-methyl transferase	CNDO/2	Otto et al.	1979
Polyaromatics	Reactivity indices	Carcinogenic	INDO, MINDO/3	Loew et al.	1979
Polyaromatics	Reactivity indices	Carcinogenic	HMO	Pullman	1979
Prostaglandins	EIP	Hormonal	EHT	Rusu et al.	1979
Quinazolines	α	Antineoplastic	CNDO/2	Abdul-Ahad et al.	1980
Secondary amines	E(HOMO)	P450 binding	CNDO/2	LePage et al.	1980
Benzanthracenes	ΔE	Carcinogenic	INDO, IEHT	Loew et al.	1980
β-lactams	$E_{transition}$	Antibacterial	CNDO/2	Boyd et al.	1980
Purines	Q_N	Phosphoribosyl transferase	HMO, Del Re	Olaru and Simon	1981
Pyrimidines	Structure	DHFR inhibition	Semi-empirical	Hopfinger	1981
Sulphanilamides	Q_N	Antibacterial	CNDO/2	De Benedetti et al.	1981
Alcohols	E(LEMO)	P450 inhibition	MNDO	Testa	1981
Methyl histamines	$E_{tautomer}$	H2-receptor agonism	CNDO/2	Xiau-Yuan and Shu-Jun	1981
β-lactams	ΔE	Antibacterial	CNDO/2	Boyd	1981
Pyrimidines	ΔE, E(HOMO)	Analgesic	CNDO/2	Miyashita et al.	1982
Triazines	Q_H, Q_L	DHFR inhibition	CNDO/2	Abdul-Ahad and Webb	1982 a
Diacridines	Q_H	Antitumour	CNDO/2	Abdul-Ahad and Webb	1982 b
Prostaglandins	EIP	Muscle stimulation	CNDO/2	Kothekar and Dutta	1982
Semicarbazones	α, Bond energy	Anticarcinogenic	CNDO/2	Blair & Webb	1982
Pyrimidines	EIP	DHFR inhibition	Semi-empirical	Hopfinger	1983
Nitrosamines	ΔH	Carcinogenicity	MNDO	Loew et al.	1983
Polyaromatics	ΔE	Mutagenicity	MINDO/3	Mohammed and Hopfinger	1983
Local anaesthetics	α, IE	Anaesthetic	HMO	Handa et al.	1983
Sulphones	Q_N	Antibacterial	CNDO/2	De Benedetti and Frassinetti	1983
Benzodiazepines	EIP	Antianxiety	MNDO	Lukovits	1983
β-lactams	Q_N	Antibiotic	MINDO/3	Boyd	1983

(continued)

Table 8. (*Continued*)

Compound	Property	Activity	MO Method	Authors	Year
Oxanilic acids	E(LEMO)	Antiallergic	*ab initio*	Cheney and Christoffersen	1983
Benzodiazepines	EIP	Antianxiety	MNDO	Loew *et al.*	1984
Steroids	EIP	Digitalis receptor	CNDO/2	Bohl *et al.*	1984
Indoles	S_E, Q_N	Tryptaminergic	CNDO/2	Gomez-Jeria and Morales-Lagos	1984
Polyaromatics	Reactivity indices	Carcinogenicity	MINDO/3	Mohammed	1985
Sulphonamides	Structure	CAB inhibition	Connolly surface	Hansch *et al.*	1985
Tryptamines	Q_N	5-HT receptor affinity	CNDO/2	Loew *et al.*	1985
Tryptamines	Q_N	Tryptaminergic	CNDO/2	Gomez-Jeria *et al.*	1985
5-HT blockers	EIP	Tryptaminergic	Semi-empirical	Humber *et al.*	1985
Phenothiazines	μ, Q_N	Neuroleptic	CNDO/2	Buydens *et al.*	1986
H₂-antagonists	μ	Anti-inflammatory	CNDO/2	Young *et al.*	1986
Captoprils	$E_{binding}$	ACE inhibition	INDO	Saunders	1986
Amidines	EIP	Trypsin inhibition	CNDO/2	Recanatini *et al.*	1986
Pyrimidines	Structure	DHFR inhibition	Semi-empirical	Selassie *et al.*	1986
Polychlorobiphenyls	Structure	EROD inhibition	MINDO/3	Parke *et al.*	1986
Alkyl benzenes	S_E	P450 binding	MINDO/3	Lewis *et al.*	1986
Cis-platins	$E_{interaction}$	Toxicity	*ab initio*	Barnett	1986
Nitroarenes	E(LEMO)	Mutagenicity	*ab initio*	Maynard *et al.*	1986
Polyaromatics	Q_L	Carcinogenicity	MINDO/3	Mohammed *et al.*	1986
H₂-agonists	EIP	Histaminergic	AMPAC, *ab initio*	Luque *et al.*	1987
Alcohols	E(LEMO)	P450 inhibition	MINDO/3	Lewis	1987 b
Benzamides	EIP	Dopaminergic	*ab initio*	Testa *et al.*	1987
Phthalates	S_N	Peroxisomal proliferation	MINDO/3	Lake *et al.*	1987
Clofibrates	S_E	Peroxisomal proliferation	MINDO/3	Lewis *et al.*	1987
Sulphonamides	Q_N	Carbonic anhydrase	CNDO/2	De Benedetti *et al.*	1987
DNA bases	S_E, S_N	Methylation	MINDO/3	Lewis and Griffiths	1987
TCDDS	α	Ah receptor binding	CNDO/2	Long *et al.*	1987
Phenols	E(HOMO)	Antibacterial	MINDO/3	Esaki	1987
Polyaromatics	S_E	Carcinogenicity	MINDO/3	Lewis	1987 a

Benzamides	EIP	Dopaminergic	*ab initio*	Hogberg *et al.*	1987
Barbiturates	Structure	Anticonvulsant	Semi-empirical	Jones and Andrews	1987
H$_2$-agonists	EIP	Histaminergic	*ab initio*	Luque *et al.*	1988
Nitrosamines	ΔE	Carcinogenicity	CNDO/2	Parke *et al.*	1988
Nitrosoureas	S_E	Anticarcinogenic	MINDO/3	Lewis	1988
Orthopramides	Structure	Dopaminergic	*ab initio*	El Tayar *et al.*	1988
Acrylic acids	EIP	Toxicity	*ab initio*	Osman	1988
Phenytoins	α	Toxicity	CNDO/2	Brown *et al.*	1989
Phenylaziridines	S_E	Antineoplastic	MINDO/3	Lewis	1989 b
Aniline mustards	S_E	Antineoplastic	MINDO/3	Lewis	1989 c
α-adrenergic agonists	E(LEMO)	Adrenergic	CNDO/2	Mitchell *et al.*	1989
Benzanthracenes	E(LEMO)	Mutagenicity	CNDO/2	Lewis *et al.*	1989 b
Aliphatic amines	S_E	P450 binding	MINDO/3	Lewis	1990
Indolealkylamines	α,E(HOMO)	Melatonin receptor	CNDO/2	Lewis *et al.*	1989 d

Key:

'Structure': a combination of conformational and electronic characteristics

'Property': the major structural parameters calculated by MO techniques, although there may be other parameters involved

Q_N: net atomic charge(s) on unspecified atoms

$Q_{H,L}$: frontier electron densities in H(OMO) and L(EMO)

S_E, S_N: electrophilic (S) and nucleophilic (N) superdelocalizabilities

EIP: electrostatic isopotential energies

μ: dipole moment

α: polarizability

E(HOMO): energy of the Highest occupied MO

E(LEMO) energy of the Lowest Empty MO

ΔE: E(LEMO)-E(HOMO)

E$_{binding}$: binding energy

E$_{interaction}$: interaction energy

E$_{tautomer}$: tautomerization energy

IE: ionization energy

ΔH: enthalpy change

E$_{occ}$: total energy of occupied MO

E$_{transition}$: transition energy

E$_{vibration}$: vibrational energy

method for calculating the vibrational energy of anaesthetics from their infrared spectra. In eleven compounds it was found that there was a very good correlation ($r = 0.99$) between anaesthetic activity and energy of the carbonyl stretching vibration. It was proposed that the reason for this relationship was a result of the binding between the carbonyl moiety of the ester group in the substrates being dependent upon a coupling between vibrational energy levels. Although not an MO method, this is an example of the application of quantum chemistry to biological activity.

More recently, Handa and co-workers (Handa *et al.*, 1983) used the same data as Agin *et al.* in a re-examination of the relationship between the product of polarizability and ionization potential and local anaesthesia. Although it was shown that a high degree of correlation ($r = 0.99$) existed between structural data and activity, these workers reported that the individual components of the product also related to anaesthesia but with reduced significance. The authors further presented evidence to show that the total van der Waals volume (based on the summation of van der Waals radii of component atoms) was closely related to molar polarizability. It is worth noting here that the product of polarizability and ionization potential (which is measured by E(HOMO) in MO terminology) has been used in other areas of bioactivity, such as in a study of angiotensin-converting enzyme (ACE) inhibitors by Saunders (1986).

Analgesic activity

Kier (1971) has shown that the analgesic activity of imidazolines can be related to a quadratic in the hydrophobic fragmental constant and the Hückel-calculated energy of the highest occupied MO, E(HOMO), with a correlation coefficient of 0.98. The conclusion drawn from this study was that analgesia in these compounds was partly due to their favourable partitioning (transport term) and to the ability to form a charge transfer complex with a receptor feature as reflected by the E(HOMO) index.

In 1978, Loew and co-workers investigated a series of oxymorphone opiates using PCILO to estimate conformational barriers to inversion of the C_{14}-OH group. The observed potencies and binding data could be explained in terms of the availability of low energy equatorial conformations of N-substituents and in their interactions with the C_{14} hydroxy group through a common receptor site (Loew *et al.*, 1978). The most recent study on analgesic pyrazoles and pyrimidines (Miyashita *et al.*, 1982) involved the use of CNDO/2 calculations for the generation of QSARs, including fragmentally calculated log P values. These co-workers reported correlations involving quadratics in log P with either E(HOMO), giving a correlation coefficient of 0.8, or with nitrogen atom charges, with improved correlation ($r = 0.89$) for eighteen compounds. Essentially, this result parallels the finding of Kier mentioned previously and indicates that the interaction with the relevant receptor involves the formation of a charge transfer complex, and that the transport of the compounds to the site of action is an important factor.

Adrenergic activity

The application of MO techniques in the area of α- and β-adrenoreceptor research has been mainly concerned with conformational energy minima and their relation to receptor binding interactions. This is due to the fact that, generally, specific and different conformations are thought to be required for the expression of activity towards different receptor subtypes (α_1, α_2, β_1 and β_2). For example, Katz and co-workers (1973) employed CNDO/2, INDO and PCILO to study the conformational energy minima of noradrenaline and 3, 4-dihydroxyphenylamine. It was found that the energy minima for the trans and gauche forms were of similar magnitude but it was regarded that conformational effects and charge distributions are likely to be important for receptor interaction.

In the following year, Germer reported a CNDO/2 study on eight β-blockers including propranolol and practolol (Germer, 1974). Although charge distributions were presented, this study was mainly concerned with interatomic distances between the protonated nitrogen and hydroxyl oxygen atoms of the side chain and the phenyl ring, because these are thought to represent potential receptor-binding points. It was apparent that the position of phenyl ring substituents affected the conformation of the side chain which was regarded as being crucial for β-selectivity.

In 1975, Martin *et al.* published findings based on *ab initio* (STO-3G) and semi-empirical (EHT, CNDO, INDO and PCILO) calculations of phenyl-ethylamine in its neutral and protonated forms. The charge calculations were used to generate EIP maps for these two structures and it was found that there was a correlation between E(HOMO) and EIP minima for different conformers, indicating which would be likely to present a favourable interaction with the adrenoreceptor.

In the same year, Holtje found that MAO inhibition by phenoxyethyl cyclopropylamines correlated well with their binding energy of interaction between the substituted anisole moiety and n-propyl guanidine, representing an arginine residue on the receptor protein (Holtje, 1975).

More recently, Mitchell presented the results of an extensive MO-QSAR study on α-adrenoceptor agonists and antagonists (Mitchell, 1988). Using *ab initio* (STO-3G) calculations, he found that E(LEMO) exhibited a parallelism with α_2-adrenoceptor binding for twenty clonidine-like imidazolines. One of the more significant correlations ($r = 0.96$) in this work involved the inclusion of the parachor, which is a hydrophobic parameter similar to log *P*. The QSAR combining a quadratic expression for the parachor with E(LEMO) indicates that the nature of the receptor binding is likely to be due to a combination of desolvation and charge transfer effects as has been suggested by modelling of the adrenoceptor interaction (Mitchell *et al.*, 1989).

Antiallergic activity

In two separate studies on oxanilic acids, oxoquinaldic acids and benzopyran carboxylic acids mediating the allergic response, Cheney and co-workers showed that *ab initio* (SCF) calculated E(LEMO) values correlated with activity in thirteen (Cheney *et al.*, 1978) and later, in fifty-one chemicals (Cheney and Christoffersen, 1983). Although other structural factors were thought to be involved, the fact that antiallergic activity was negatively dependent on E(LEMO) indicates that charge transfer interactions stabilize the drug–receptor complex.

Antibiotic, antibacterial and antimalarial activity

Evidence for a charge-transfer mechanism for the interaction between antimalarial drugs related to quinine and malarial parasitic DNA, thus blocking the synthesis of nucleic acids, has been indicated by the low LEMO energy of chloroquine and quinacrine which facilitates electron acceptance from quanine via the 2-amino group (Kier, 1971). Further, the *in vitro* bacteriostatic activity of twenty tetracyclines has been related to Del Recalculated charges on a number of oxygen atoms on the phenol diketone moiety (Peradejordi, 1971). This study shows that the inhibition of *Escherichia coli* by tetracyclines involves a charge-controlled interaction with a ribosomal receptor.

Martin and co-workers employed the HMO technique in a QSAR study of 1, 4-naphthoquinones. It was found that E(LEMO) and a quadratic expression in log P correlated with antimalarial activity in a series of ten compounds (Martin *et al.*, 1973). These authors also showed that there was a good relationship between redox potentials, E_0, and E(LEMO) values, and found that the latter was a better predictor of antimalarial activity than E_0 values.

In the same year, Boyd reported that EHT charge calculations on cephalosporins and penicillins indicated that requirements for antibacterial activity in β-lactams involved the ease of acylation of the amide group (Boyd, 1973). A publication in the following year involved the utilization of CNDO/2 calculations in a study of chloramphenicols and N-acetyl amino acid methyl esters (Holtje and Kier, 1974). These authors formulated an expression for the interaction energy between these compounds and the acylase binding site based on electric polarization and dispersion components.

In a number of publications, Boyd and co-workers studied the antibiotic activity of cephalosporins using CNDO/2 calculations. It was found that the transition state energy related well with minimum inhibitory concentrations of the β-lactams (Boyd *et al.*, 1980). Using the hydroxyl ion as a model nucleophile, the transition state energy, TSE, is a measure of the ease of formation of an initial complex which relates to the ease of amide hydrolysis. For fourteen β-lactam antibiotics, a quadratic in TSE successfully explains the antibacterial activity with a correlation coefficient of 0.85 (Boyd, 1981), and the same author went on to show that alkaline hydrolysis depends on the charge on the oxygen atom of the β-lactam moiety, indicating that the reaction is charge-controlled (Boyd, 1983).

De Benedetti and co-workers reported CNDO/2 studies on sulphanilamides (De Benedetti et al., 1981) and diaryl sulphones (De Benedetti and Frassinetti, 1983) where antibacterial activity was found to be related to the total charge on the oxygen atoms of the SO_2 group. These authors modified the CNDO/2 procedure to include sulphur d orbitals which probably assisted in the obtainment of good correlations ($r = 0.94$) for twenty-six compounds. These results give evidence for a charge-controlled reaction in the expression of antibacterial activity of sulphanilamides.

More recently, Esaki has presented the results of a QSAR study on phenols using MINDO/3 calculations and principal components analysis (Esaki, 1987). In a similar expression to that found previously by Martin et al. (1973), Esaki shows that E(LEMO) and a quadratic in log P explains the antibacterial potency of these compounds. This result is consistent with the hypothesis of a charge-transfer interaction involving electron acceptance from the receptor macromolecule, thought to involve a tryptophan residue as these are good electron donors.

Antirheumatoid activity

Assuming a planar geometry for the substrates, Catalan and Fernandez-Alonso (1976) carried out CNDO/2 calculations on seven hydroxybenzoic acids. It was found that antirheumatic activity depended on E(HOMO) and dipole moment with a correlation of 0.92; thus it would appear that receptor interaction involves charge-transfer together with dipolar alignment.

Anticancer activity

Berges and Peradejordi used CNDO/2 and HMO calculations to investigate the alkylating activity of aromatic nitrogen mustards and to find structural descriptors relating to ease of hydrolysis. These workers found that alkylation correlated with the π electron charge on nitrogen and on nucleophilic superdelocalizability, whereas hydrolysis was dependent on the nitrogen atomic charge and on ΔE, the energy difference between frontier orbitals (Berges and Peradejordi, 1974). Using more recent biological data and employing MINDO/3 calculations, it has been found that antitumour activity in aniline mustards is dependent on the electron population in the HOMO frontier orbital of the nitrogen atom (Lewis, 1989 a). The balance between therapeutic activity and toxicity, as measured by the chemotherapeutic index, correlates with total electrophilic superdelocalizability and total net atomic charge within the same group of compounds. The overall expression of activity of aniline mustards is thus determined by their transport characteristics and by a frontier-controlled interaction with the receptor.

The Webb group have reported MO-QSARs in series of diacridines (Abdul-Ahad and Webb, 1982 b) and isoquinoline thiosemicarbazones (Blair and Webb, 1982) using CNDO/2 calculations. For twenty-seven diacridines, which act as bi-intercalators of DNA, the binding energy together with other electronic factors correlates fairly well ($r = 0.74$) with antitumour activity. In thiosemicarbazones, anticancer activity was found to be dependent on bond energy and upon polarization energy, which relates to the electrostatic potential energy. It is probable that receptor interaction involves the isoquinoline ring atoms in a charge-transfer process.

In an *ab initio* (STO-3G) study of eighteen cis-platin analogues, Barnett reported that the energy of interaction with a guanine-cytosine pair correlates weakly ($r = 0.61$) with LD_{50} data (Barnett, 1986). Lewis has used MINDO/3 calculations to investigate the antineoplastic activity of nitrosoureas (Lewis, 1988) and phenyl aziridines (Lewis, 1989 c). It was found that similar expressions gave correlations with alkylating and carbamoylating activity of CCNU derivatives, whereas therapeutic activity relates to the urea group nitrogen and oxygen atoms in nitrosoureas. The nucleophilic reactivity of phenylaziridines correlated with protonation energy and with E(HOMO), whereas toxicity exhibits a parallelism with the HOMO frontier electron density on the aziridine moiety. Furthermore, chemotherapeutic activity was found to be dependent on a combination of total electrophilic superdelocalizability and total net atomic charge, thus showing a similarity to the expression of aniline mustard antitumour activity (Lewis, 1989 b).

Antifolate activity

The basicity of antifolates such as pteridines, purines and pyrimidines has been related to HOMO-calculated atomic charge and free valence on the 2-amino group nitrogen atom (Collin and Pullman, 1964). The relevance of this early success of MO calculations is that binding to dihydrofolate reductase (DHFR) is known to be related to basicity and this also correlates well with the inhibition data (Kier, 1971).

The Webb group have studied DHFR-inhibitory quinazolines (Abdul-Ahad *et al.*, 1980), pteridines and triazines (Abdul-Ahad and Webb, 1982 a) using CNDO/2 calculations. In a series of twenty-five antineoplastic quinazolines, it was found that inhibition was well correlated ($r = 0.96$) with atom polarizabilities and bond energy, and this was thought to indicate van der Waals contributions to the interaction energy. For nineteen pteridines and triazines, the nitrogen atom frontier electron density (LEMO) was related to DHFR inhibition ($r = 0.87$) when combined with a bond energy term. This result implied that there was also a charge-transfer interaction at the enzyme binding site and this is likely on the grounds of crystallographic evidence for methotrexate-bound DHFR.

Hopfinger (1981; 1983) has investigated the steric requirements for DHFR inhibition in a series of 2,4-diamino-5-benzylpyrimidines, finding that a quadratic expression in steric volume together with hydrophobicity of substituents accounted for antifolic activity in twenty-three compounds ($r = 0.93$). This relationship was thought to measure the effect of desolvation and transport processes within the series (Hopfinger, 1981). By incorporating molecular electrostatic potential energy fields in a novel procedure called molecular shape analysis (MSA), Hopfinger was able to improve the correlation with activity ($r = 0.96$) using a quadratic expression for the electrostatic field together with hydrophobic fragmental constants (Hopfinger, 1983).

More recently, Selassie and co-workers (1986) obtained a good description of the antifolic activity of 2,4-diamino-pyrimidines using a combination of Hansch analysis and molecular graphics based on X-ray data for the enzyme binding site.

Anticholinergic activity

For a series of nine phenols, Neely has shown that pKa correlates with electron deficiency at the C–O group from the results of MO calculations via the Hückel method (Neely, 1965). He also found that cholinesterase inhibition was related to phenyl-oxygen bond stretching frequencies in the infrared spectra of organophosphates.

In the following year, Purcell reported the results of an HMO study on N-alkyl substituted amide cholinesterase inhibitors. He reported that there was a relationship between inhibition and net atomic charge on the amide nitrogen, though the dipole moment of the amide group and hydrophobicity were also important factors in anticholinergic activity expressed by this series of compounds (Purcell, 1966).

Purcell later collaborated with Millner in an HMO study of 1-decyl-piperidines. These workers found that butyryl cholinesterase inhibition was related to the net atomic charge on the piperidine ring nitrogen atom (Millner and Purcell, 1971). This finding indicates that the interaction with cholinesterase is a charge-controlled process and this is in agreement with previous work reviewed by Kier (1971).

Antihypertensive activity

In 1970, Wohl reported a study of thirty-six antihypertensive benzothiadiazines using extended Hückel theory (EHT). He obtained a very good correlation ($r = 0.96$) using a combination of E(HOMO), nucleophilic superdelocalizabilities and group charges. The conclusion from this result was that the interaction involved a frontier-controlled charge transfer to the receptor with some degree of electron acceptance at key atoms on the benzene ring, presumably by back-donation (synergic effect).

Kulkarni has employed CNDO/2 calculations to investigate a small series of pyridazines and phthalazines (Kulkarni, 1975). Although not quantitative, this study related antihypertensive activity with nitrogen atomic charge and with conformational preferences.

In a series of twenty-five chloridine-like imidazolines, Timmermans and Van Zweiten presented a significant relationship ($r = 0.97$) between activity and E(HOMO), together with a variety of substituent parameters (Timmermans and Van Zweiten, 1977). It was thought that receptor binding was brought about by charge-transfer with some contribution from hydrogen-bonding.

Antipsychotic, anticonvulsant and anti-anxiety activity

Blair and Webb used the CNDO/2 method for a QSAR study of thirty-nine 1,4-benzodiazepin-2-ones exhibiting CNS depressant activity. Although they found that sedative and anti-anxiety effects could not be differentiated, there was a good correlation between tranquillizing activity and a combination of dipole moment and net atomic charge on the carbonyl oxygen atom (Blair and Webb, 1977). This result shows that features on the diazepine ring, in particular the carbonyl group, are responsible for receptor interaction. Lukovits subsequently used principal component analysis to produce an improved correlation with CNS depressant activity with the same data set (Lukovits, 1983). In the following year, Loew and co-workers compared MNDO, INDO and CNDO procedures in a study of benzodiazepine analogues (Loew *et al.*, 1984). Although there were no QSARs presented, this work used EIP maps to show the importance of the carbonyl group (as reported by Blair and Webb) and the ring nitrogen as indicators of potential receptor binding interaction points.

More recently, Jones and Andrews have compared the molecular structures of fourteen anticonvulsant barbiturates to show conformational preferences for activity (Jones and Andrews, 1987). These workers used the results of crystallographic determinations to provide an SAR, and crystal packing environments suggest a receptor interaction model. This study augments earlier work by Andrews who employed CNDO/2 calculations in an unsuccessful attempt to generate QSARs in series of anticonvulsants, and his interesting concept of hydrogen-bonding interaction with the receptor is discussed by Kier (1971).

Benzodiazepine receptor affinity and antagonist activity of β-carbolines has been investigated using EIP energies generated from MNDO calculations (Loew *et al.*, 1985). This study provides an indication of the structural requirements for compounds fitting the benzodiazepine receptor.

Gabanergic activity

Kier and co-workers have studied γ-aminobutyric acid (GABA) analogues using EHT calculations (Kier *et al.*, 1974). Their results indicate that compounds related to GABA preferentially adopt a fully extended conformation which is at variance with the solid state structure of GABA where a gauche conformation is adopted. In later studies, Steward and colleagues have shown that CNDO/2-calculated conformations of GABA agonists give rise to structural parameters which correlate with GABA activity (Steward and Clarke, 1975; Steward and Lowe, 1978). Apparently, the distance between centres of positive and negative charge on these zwitterions provide indications of the steric requirements for fitting the GABA receptor binding site.

Dopaminergic activity

Buydens and co-workers used CNDO/2 calculations to generate molecular electrostatic potential (MEP) energies for neuroleptic butyrophenones and phenothiazines exhibiting dopaminergic activity (Buydens *et al.*, 1986). By the method of principal components, these authors have shown that proton affinity and net charge on the nitrogen atom gives rise to a good correlation ($r = 0.91$) with activity.

The optimum substituent characteristics for dopamine D-2 receptor affinity were revealed by an *ab initio* (STO-3G) study of substituted benzamides (orthopramides) involving a comparison of MEP energies (Testa *et al.*, 1987). It was found that there was a good correlation ($r = 0.93$) between steric and electronic substituent parameters and dopaminergic activity. In the same year, another *ab initio* study at the STO-3G level using Gaussian 80 was reported on D-2 antagonists (Hogberg *et al.*, 1987). It was shown that low energy conformers, calculated using the molecular mechanics procedure, could be superimposed defining the structural requirements for activity in a series of 2,6-alkoxybenzamides. A QSAR was reported which employed the partial least squares method for correlating dopaminergic activity with partial charges and other structural factors that explained 83 per cent of the variance. In the following year, El Tayar and colleagues published findings on neuroleptic benzamides and phenothiazines (El Tayar *et al.*, 1988). Using cluster analysis, it was possible to establish structural and electronic requirements for differentiation between D-1 and D-2 receptors. A pharmacophoric model was proposed on the basis of QSARs obtained from EIP calculations and additive substituent constants.

A recent publication employed AM1 and MNDO calculations for a conformational study on benzocyclohepten-6-ylamine where the analysis of excluded volumes defined the D-2 receptor pharmacophore (Karlen *et al.*, 1989).

Miscellaneous activity

The Pullmans have shown that the Hückel method can be used to calculate atomic charges which enable an estimation of the basicity of purines in terms of electron availability on the nitrogen atom. This result represents an early success of MO calculations in their determination of molecular electronic properties (Pullman and Pullman, 1960).

Alexander and co-workers utilized an extension of the Hückel technique (IEHT) in a study of the preservative action of para-hydroxybenzoic acids. It was found that conformational energy minima, frontier orbital energies and atomic charges could be related to preservative activity suggesting that the receptor interaction involved a frontier-controlled reaction (Alexander *et al.*, 1976).

More recently, Osman has looked at the toxicity of acrylic acids using *ab initio* (STO 6-31G) calculations within the Gaussian 82 program (Osman, 1988). From the results of MEP calculations, using the fluoride ion as a probe species, it was suggested that the toxic effect of these compounds could be described in terms of electrostatic attraction, polarization and charge-transfer interactions.

Hormonal activity

The thyromimetic activity of thirty-one thyroxine analogues has been investigated using CNDO/2 calculations and a receptor binding model has been proposed (Dietrich *et al.*, 1977). The interaction energies relating to the free energies of conformational changes within these compounds, in addition to other structural parameters, were found to correlate well ($r = 0.96$) with binding to rat hepatic nuclear protein and thyroxine-binding globulin.

Rusu and co-workers have used the EHT method to calculate EIP maps for prostaglandin E_1 and its analogues (Rusu *et al.*, 1979). They have demonstrated that there is a similarity between the electrostatic isopotential fields of active analogues which are different from prostaglandins that exhibit a different physiological activity. Kothekar and Dutta generated EIP maps for prostaglandins (PGE_1 and PGE_2) using the results of CNDO/2 calculations (Kothekar and Dutta, 1982). Apparently, the differences in charge distribution, EIP minima and conformation correlate with smooth muscle stimulatory activity in these compounds. More recently, it has been shown that the receptor binding affinity for a series of ten melatonin analogues is dependent upon the product of molar polarizability and E(HOMO), as calculated by the CNDO/2 procedure (Lewis *et al.*, 1989 a). The results of EIP calculations and QSAR analysis were used to construct a model peptide thought to represent part of the melatonin receptor binding site.

Psychotropic activity

In an early study, Snyder and Merril showed that E(HOMO) values, calculated by the Hückel method, exhibit a parallelism with the hallucinogenic activity of six known hallucinogens (Snyder and Merril, 1965). Together with other evidence, this finding points to a charge transfer mechanism for the interaction between hallucinogens and their receptor (Kier, 1971).

Kang and Green have reported an INDO study on fourteen amphetamine analogues where E(HOMO) correlates with hallucinogenic potency ($r = 0.74$) thus supporting earlier work, and strengthening the charge-transfer receptor interaction hypothesis (Kang and Green, 1970).

Kumber and Sankar, however, have shown that hallucinogenic activity in forty-two lysergates correlates with HMO-calculated total orbital energy (Kumber and Sankar, 1973).

Tryptaminergic activity

In a study using the Hückel method, Kang and Green have shown that the contraction of stomach muscle correlates with resonance constants in a small number of 5-substituted tryptamines (Kang and Green, 1969). Johnson and Green used CNDO/2 calculations to investigate a series of seventeen tryptamines acting on the LSD receptor of rat fundus strip (Johnson and Green, 1974). These co-workers found that tryptaminergic activity could be related to frontier electron density and net charge on the indole nitrogen atom, together with substituent fragmental constants ($r = 0.93$). Also, in a separate study, Sankar and Kumber found that the antiserotonin activity of twenty derivatives of LSD depended on total orbital energy as calculated by the Hückel method (Sankar and Kumber, 1974). In the following year, Glennon and Gessner published the results of an MO study using the Pople-Parizer-Parr (PPP) method on eight dimethyltryptamines (Glennon and Gessner, 1975). Intrinsic 5-HT activity correlated well ($r = 0.96$) with frontier electron density in the 4 position of the indole moiety.

Electrostatic isopotential energies, calculated via the CNDO/2 method, enabled Daudel and co-workers to demonstrate the structural similarity between oxazines and 5-HT leading to a rationalization of tryptaminergic activity (Dandel *et al.*, 1976). In the same year, the Kumber group established that HMO-calculated total orbital energy was related ($r = 0.89$) to the inhibition of 5-HT uptake by tryptamine analogues (Kumber *et al.*, 1976).

Lukovits has reported that the tryptaminergic activity of phenylethylamines is related to their dipole moment, as calculated by the EHT method (Lukovits *et al.*, 1976). Although this finding points to a dipolar interaction with the receptor, there is a possibility that the magnitude of the dipole moment influences solvation effects in these compounds.

A combination of CNDO/2 and PCILO procedures was employed in an investigation of phenylisopropylamines (Anderson *et al.*, 1978) in which E(HOMO) was found to correlate weakly ($r = 0.65$) with hyperthermic potencies. It is of interest to record that log P did not produce any significant relationship with activity, thus providing an example of a situation where the Hansch approach is not applicable. CNDO/2 calculations have also been used by Gomez-Jeria and co-workers in QSAR studies on the binding of tryptamines to the 5-HT receptor (Gomez-Jeria and Morales-Lagos; 1984; Gomez-Jeria *et al.*, 1985). For about twenty compounds a good correlation ($r = 0.97$)

was achieved between a combination of reactivity indices, atomic charges and steric factors, and 5-HT binding, leading to the proposal of a receptor-binding site model.

An investigation of serotonin uptake blockers using EIP maps and excluded volume characteristics enabled a rationalization of tryptaminergic activity in terms of shape and potential field similarities (Humber *et al.*, 1985). In an, as yet, unpublished study the present author has employed MINDO/3 calculations to explore structure-activity relationships in a series of twenty tryptamines. This work confirms the findings of Gomez-Jeria *et al.*, although a slightly different set of structural descriptors provide an improved correlation with 5-HT binding data (Lewis, unpublished results). Furthermore, computer modelling of the 5-HT receptor indicates a similarity with the β-adrenoreceptor binding site.

Histaminergic activity

MO calculations have assisted in the recognition of two preferred conformations of the histamine monocation that are thought to be relevant to the expression of two types of receptor selectivity, designated as H_1 and H_2 which give rise to ileum and gastric stimulation, respectively (Kier, 1971).

In 1981, Xiao-Yuan and Shu-Jun reported a CNDO/2 study on methyl histamines showing that protonation energies related to basicity, and that the energy required to form the preferred tautomer correlated well with H_2 agonism (Xiao-Yuan and Shu-Jun, 1981). An important QSAR investigation on thirteen cimetidine analogues involved the use of CNDO/2 calculations for the estimation of dipole moment components (Young *et al.*, 1986). A good correlation ($r = 0.91$) was reported between H_2 receptor antagonism and a combination of log P and the dipole moment orientation: this indicated the optimum dipole moment orientation for alignment of the hydrogen-bonding moiety on the antagonist species, whereas the desolvation effects were determined by log P.

Recently, Luque and colleagues have employed *ab initio* (STO-3G) and AMPAC procedures for the calculation of molecular electrostatic potential energies of histamine analogues (Luque *et al.*, 1987, 1988). It was reported that the activation energy for proton transfer between the neutral and cationic species relates to H_2 agonism, and that this was also characterized by electrostatic potential minima at the imidazole ring nitrogen atom where the histamines are in the trans–trans conformation.

Enzymic activity

The results of CNDO/2 calculations on twenty-two phenylethanolamines have provided a good correlation ($r = 0.88$) between x and y components of dipole moment and N-methyl transferase activity (Otto *et al.*, 1979). Sklenar and Jaeger used the same MO method to show that the inhibition of thymidine phosphorylase by uracils correlates well ($r = 0.97$) with charges on ring carbon atoms (Sklenar and Jaeger, 1979).

Olaru and Simon (1981) have shown that HMO and Del Re electronic parameters can be related to the phosphoribosyl transferase activity of purine derivatives, whereas CNDO/2 calculations on cardiotonic steroids provide evidence that EIP energies correlate with the inhibition of heart ATPase (Bohl *et al.*, 1984). By performing calculations on different conformers, the QSARs generated indicate that the digitalis receptor binding energy compensates for overcoming the conformational energy barrier in these compounds.

The inhibition of carbonic anhydrase (CAB) has been studied by Hansch and co-workers using molecular graphics to highlight the effect of hydrophobic interactions at the enzyme binding site (Hansch *et al.*, 1985). It was found that a combination of log P and Hammett constants related to inhibitory activity, whereas electronic effects were good descriptors of substrate basicity.

In the following year, Saunders reported the results of INDO calculations on angiotensin-converting enzyme (ACE) inhibitors (Saunders, 1986). He found that dipole moment and electric field components were important for activity in addition to expressions involving binding energy and the product of polarizability and E(HOMO). This extensive study involved the calculation of solvation effects using a solvent dielectric constant of 4, thought to reflect the ACE receptor environment.

A molecular graphics study of fifty-five amidines exhibiting trypsin inhibitory activity showed the importance of hydrophobic and hydrophilic regions at the binding site (Recanatini *et al.*, 1986). It was also found that enzyme inhibition could be related to a combination of electronic and hydrophobic substituent parameters

The CNDO/2 method was employed by De Benedetti and co-workers in a QSAR investigation of sulphonamides inhibiting carbonic anhydrase (De Benedetti *et al.*, 1987). It was shown that net atomic charges on the sulphonamide group were responsible for binding site interactions, implying a charge-controlled interaction. More recently, the AM1 procedure was used to obtain correlations between electronic structure and activity in carbonic anhydrase inhibitors (Menziani *et al.*, 1989). This study reported that E(HOMO) and binding energy were important descriptors of the binding interaction.

Cytochrome P450 activity

In view of the fact that cytochromes P450-mediated oxygenations account for about 95 per cent of all oxidative metabolism and, being mindful of this publications readership, it is appropriate to separate MO-QSARs on P450 substrates from those of other enzymes.

Wald and Feuer reported a QSAR investigation of coumarins exhibiting aryl hydrocarbon hydroxylase (AHH) activity (Wald and Feuer, 1971). They found that activity was related to the activation energy (ΔE) and net atomic charges on the pyran ring. This good correlation ($r = 0.91$) suggested that the interaction with AHH (comprising one or more of the P450 proteins) involved a charge-transfer mechanism.

CNDO/2 calculations on eleven secondary amines show that there is a correlation ($r = 0.87$) between E(HOMO), the highest occupied frontier orbital energy, and binding affinity to phenobarbital-induced microsomal cytochrome P450 (LePage *et al.*, 1980). The results of this work imply that hydroxylation involves an electrophilic mechanism or that the binding interaction to cytochrome P450 is frontier-controlled.

Testa employed the MNDO procedure in a QSAR study of alcohols inhibiting the N-hydroxylation of aniline, which involves one of the cytochrome P450 isozymes (Testa, 1981). He found that the inhibitory activity could be explained in terms of frontier orbital energy and other structural factors.

The modulation of cytochrome P450 spin state equilibria by alkyl benzenes has been correlated with MINDO/3-generated electrophilic superdelocalizabities (Lewis *et al.*, 1986) and MINDO/3 calculations were used for the determination of conformational minima in a number of polychlorinated biphenyls (PCBs) binding to the TCDD receptor (Parke *et al.*, 1986). It was found that the degree of planarity of PCBs related fairly well ($r = 0.83$) with ethoxyresorufin O-deethylase (EROD) activity. Furthermore, a MINDO/3 study of alcohols (Lewis, 1987 b) showed that the inhibition of aniline N-hydroxylation could be related to the HOMO frontier orbital energy together with other frontier electron indices.

Lake and co-workers have demonstrated the applicability of MO techniques to QSAR investigations of peroxisomal proliferating agents (Lake *et al.*, 1987; Lewis *et al.*, 1987 b). Electronic structural parameters, calculated by the MINDO/3 method, were shown to be important in the description of potency differences in a series of phthalate esters and clofibrate analogues.

The activity of polychlorinated dibenzofurans have been described by Long and colleagues using MO calculations to generate QSARs for EROD and AHH induction (Long *et al.*, 1987). It was demonstrated that enzyme induction exhibited a parallelism with molecular polarizability, which is a component in the expression for van der Waals interaction, and is thus thought to be involved in the desolvation contribution to binding free energy. More recently, it has been found that the binding characteristics of primary aliphatic amines with respect to phenobarbital-induced microsomal cytochrome P450 can be rationalized in terms of total electrophilic superdelocalizability calculated by the MINDO/3 method (Lewis, 1990).

Carcinogenic and mutagenic activity

The understanding of carcinogenesis at the molecular level has been, and still is, a major challenge for quantum chemists. The pioneering work of the Pullmans has been reviewed by Kier (1971) who has explained the importance of the K and L region reactivities for the expression of carcinogenesis in poly-aromatic hydrocarbons (PAHs).

Herndon has shown that the bond orders of the K and L regions relate to the Iball index of carcinogenicity in ten compounds from the results of Hückel calculations (Herndon, 1974). However, there were instances where the predicted activity was not found, implying that the K—L theory could not be universally applied to the carcinogenicity of PAHs. It was subsequently found that the bond reactivity in the K region was related to carcinogenicity of seventeen PAHs using iterative extended Hückel theory (IEHT) calculations (Loew *et al.*, 1979). Furthermore, INDO calculations yielded energy values for the formation of carbocations from the corresponding diols which related in a qualitative manner to carcinogenicity. In the same year, Pullman reviewed the current theories of carcinogenesis involving the reactivity of K and L regions, together with the formation of diol epoxides via triol carbonium ions (Pullman, 1979). In the following year, an IEHT study on twelve methyl benzanthracenes indicated that the activation energy required for the formation of triol carbocations relates to carcinogenicity in PAHs (Loew *et al.*, 1980). The Loew group went on to employ MNDO calculations to investigate the carcinogenicity of dialkylnitrosamines (Loew *et al.*, 1983). These workers found that nitrosamine carcinogenicity depended on their relative ease of activation and transformation to hydroxyalkylnitrosamines.

Mohammed and Hopfinger have reported that the MINDO/3-calculated activation energy of polyaromatics may be related to their mutagenicity provided that an overlap volume term is incorporated in the expression (Mohammed and Hopfinger, 1983). Mohammed went on to use MINDO/3 calculations in an investigation of fifteen polyaromatics (Mohammed, 1985). It was found that it was possible to explain the rank order of carcinogenic potencies of these compounds in terms of their frontier orbital energies and bond reactivities.

In the following year, the results of an *ab initio* (STO-3G) study on nitroarenes were reported (Maynard *et al.*, 1986). Mutagenicity in a variety of bacterial strains was shown to be related to E(LEMO) values and this was explained in terms of electron-acceptance from DNA for ability to form a nitrene intermediate via nitro group reduction by nitro reductase. A further study by Mohammed was published in the same year where the carcinogenicity and metabolic activation of polyaromatic hydrocarbons was shown to correlate with reactivity indices calculated by the MINDO/3 procedure (Mohammed, 1986). It was thought that the appearance of expressions involving the lowest empty molecular orbital (LEMO) indicated that the electrophilicity of the hydrocarbon was important to its carcinogenic potential.

Lewis and Griffiths used the MINDO/3 method to explain the pattern of methylation of DNA bases relating to the manifestation of carcinogenicity by alkylation of DNA (Lewis and Griffiths, 1987). The percentage of DNA methylation at different sites exhibited a parallelism with the charge and nucleophilic superdelocalizability of electronegative atoms. Electrostatic isopotential (EIP) energy minima provided evidence for a free radical mechanism of DNA methylation.

In a MINDO/3 study on a small number of polyaromatic hydrocarbons, mutagenicity and AHH activity were found to be related to the electrophilic reactivity due to the appearance of LEMO qualities in QSAR expressions (Lewis, 1987 a). However, protein binding correlated with electrophilic super-delocalizability and net atomic charge, indicating the importance of transport capabilities. The likely formation of epoxides and diol epoxides was suggested by LEMO terms for ring carbon atoms 8 and 9.

More recently, CNDO/2 calculations have been employed in a study of dialkylnitrosamines where carcinogenicity increases concomitantly with activation energy as measured by the difference in frontier orbital energies (Parke *et al.*, 1988). Furthermore, the importance of frontier orbitals in rationalization of potency differences in carcinogenic and mutagenic polyaromatic hydrocarbons has been underlined in a CNDO/2 investigation of mutagenic benzanthracenes. For fourteen compounds, the mutagenicity was found to be directly proportional to the magnitude of the LEMO energy ($r = 0.82$) which supports the theory that mutagenesis involves electron transfer from nucleophilic DNA bases to empty frontier orbitals on polyaromatic hydrocarbons (Lewis *et al.*, 1989 b).

Finally, Brown and co-workers have demonstrated that CNDO/2 calculated molar polarizability can be related to the teratogenicity of phenytoins (Brown *et al.*, 1989). This study made use of a previous finding that polarizability appears to be a major component of the hydrophobic parameter, log P (Lewis, 1989 a).

6. Conclusions

The formulation of Quantitative Structure-Activity Relationships represents a major field of endeavour in the biological sciences in which there is increasing interest and confidence. The search for parameters linking chemical structure with biological activity has been an important area for many years and has produced a vast number of structure-activity expressions spanning a wide range of chemicals and biological properties. Indeed, computer-assisted drug design (CADD) is already giving rise to new pharmaceuticals and agrochemicals (Hopfinger, 1985).

MO and other quantum-chemical calculations are now becoming universally accepted as the most sophisticated techniques for investigating and explaining chemical and biochemical phenomena at the submolecular level. The MO approach in QSAR analysis should eventually provide a realization of the goal of toxicologists, biochemists, pharmacologists and medicinal chemists in completely describing, and hence predicting, the mode of action of biologically active compounds.

The important developments within the current decade have been the critical assessment, refinement and redetermination of QSAR studies, in the improvement of methods for data capture and retrieval, and in the way in which data is processed and used for the description and rationalization of activity differences between congeners in structurally related series of compounds.

What was once regarded as a theoretical and abstract curiosity is now being employed in many areas of biological research such as in the design and development of novel chemicals, notably pharmaceutical products. With the advancing technological developments in computer hardware and integrated molecular modelling software systems, which can include QSAR modules, there is a bright future for the design and development of novel agents for the control, alleviation and treatment of diseases and other medical conditions.

Appendix

Abbreviations used in molecular orbital studies

MO:	molecular orbital
QSAR:	quantitative structure-activity relationship
HMO:	Hückel MO
PCILO:	perturbed configuration interaction using localized orbitals
CNDO:	complete neglect of differential overlap
INDO:	intermediate neglect of differential overlap
MINDO:	modified intermediate neglect of differential overlap
MNDO:	modified neglect of differential overlap
AM1:	Austin method version 1
STO:	Slater-type orbitals
Q_N:	electron density/net atomic charge on atom N
E(HOMO):	energy of the highest occupied MO
E(LEMO):	energy of the lowest empty MO
α:	molecular polarizability
μ:	dipole moment
S_E:	electrophilic superdelocalizability
S_N:	nucleophilic superdelocalizability
IE:	ionization energy
EIP:	electrostatic isopotential energy
log P:	common logarithm of the octan-1-ol/water partition coefficient
π:	Hansch hydrophobic parameter (or substituent constant) which is the difference between log P for a derivative and log P for the parent compound
ΔE:	the difference between E(HOMO) and E(LEMO)
LFER:	Linear Free Energy Relationship
σ:	the Hammett substituent constant
E_S:	the Taft steric substituent constant
QSPR:	quantitative structure–property relationship

Acknowledgements

The financial support of the University of Surrey, the Humane Research Trust, and Food and Veterinary Laboratory Ltd is gratefully acknowledged.

References

Abdul-Ahad, P. G. and Webb, G. A. (1982 a), *J. Molec. Struct. (Theochem.)*, **88**, 15.
Abdul-Ahad, P. G. and Webb, G. A. (1982 b), *Int. J. Quantum Chem.*, **21**, 945.
Abdul-Ahad, P., Blair, T. and Webb, G. A. (1980), *Int. J. Quantum Chem.*, **17**, 821.
Agin, D., Hersh, L. and Holtzman, D. (1965), *Proc. Nat. Acad. Sci. USA*, **53**, 952.
Alexander, K. S., Peterson, H., Turcotte, J. G. and Paruta, A. N. (1976), *J. Pharmaceut. Sci.*, **65**, 851.
Anderson, G. M., Castagnoli, N. and Kollman, P. A. (1978), *NIDA Res. Monog.*, **22**, 199.
Baird, N. C. and Dewar, M. J. S. (1969), *J. Chem. Phys.*, **50**, 1262.
Barlow, R. B. (1979), *Trends Pharmaceut. Sci.*, **1**, 109.
Barlow, R. B. (1980), *Quantitative Aspects of Chemical Pharmacology*, Croom Helm, London.
Barnett, G. (1986), *Molec. Pharmacol.*, **29**, 378.
Berges, J. and Peradejordi, F. (1974), *Molecular and Quantum Pharmacology* (E. D. Bergmann and B. Pullman, eds), p. 549, Reidel, Dordrecht.
Bergmann, E. D. and Pullman, B. eds (1974), *Molecular and Quantum Pharmacology*, D. Reidel, Dordrecht.
Betts, M. G. J. (1978), *Structure-Activity Relationships in Human Chemoreception*, Applied Science, London.
Bingham, R. C., Dewar, M. J. S. and Lo, D. H. (1975), *J. Am. Chem. Soc.*, **97**, 1285.
Blair, T. (1979), Ph.D. Thesis, University of Surrey, England, UK.
Blair, T. and Webb, G. A. (1977), *J. Med. Chem.*, **20**, 1206.
Blair, T. and Webb, G. A. (1982), *J. Molec. Struct. (Theochem.)*, **89**, 35.
Blankley, C. J. (1983), *Quantitative Structure-Activity Relationships of Drugs* (J. G. Topliss, ed), p. 1, Academic Press, New York.
Bohl, M., Ponsold, K. and Reck, G. (1984), *J. Steroid Biochem.*, **21**, 373.
Boyd, D. B. (1973), *J. Med. Chem.*, **16**, 1195.
Boyd, D. B. (1981), *Ann. N. Y. Acad. Sci.*, **367**, 531.
Boyd, D. B. (1983), *Drug Inform. J.*, **17**, 121.
Boyd, D. B. and Lipkowitz, K. B. (1988), *Supercomputing Mag.* (Spring), 23.
Boyd, D. B., Herron, D. K., Lunn, W. H. W. and Spitzer, W. A. (1980), *J. Am. Chem. Soc.*, **102**, 1812.
Boyd, D. B., Smith, D. W., Stewart, J. J. P. and Wimmer, E. (1988), *J. Comput. Chem.*, **9**, 387.
Burgen, A. S. V., Roberts, G. C. K. and Tute, M. S. (1986), *Molecular Graphics and Drug Design*, Elsevier, Amsterdam.
Buydens, L., Massart, D. L. and Geerlings, P. (1986), *Europ. J. Med. Chem.*, **21**, 35.
Cairns, H., Cox, D., Gould, K. J., Ingal, A. H. and Suschitzky, J. L. (1985), *J. Med. Chem.*, **28**, 1832.
Cammarata, A. (1968), *J. Med. Chem.*, **11**, 1111.
Cammarata, A. (1969), *J. Med. Chem.*, **12**, 314.
Cammarata, A. (1970), *Molecular Orbital Studies in Chemical Pharmacology* (L. B. Kier, ed), p. 156, Springer-Verlag, New York.
Cammarata, A. and Menon, G. K. (1976), *J. Med. Chem.*, **19**, 739.
Cammarata, A. and Rogers, K. S. (1971), *J. Med. Chem.*, **14**, 269.
Carbo, R., Martin, M. and Pons, V. (1977), *Afinidad*, **34**, 348.

Cassidy, S. L., Lympany, P. A. and Henry, J. A. (1987), *J. Pharmacy Pharmacol.*, **40**, 130.

Catalan, J. and Fernandez-Alonso, J. I. (1976), *Experientia* (Suppl. 23), 177.

Cavalla, J. F. (1988), in *Decision Making in Drug Research* (F. Gross, ed), p. 165, Raven Press, New York.

Cavallito, C. J. (1973), *Structure-Activity Relationships*, Pergamon, Oxford.

Chapman, N. B. and Shorter, J. (1972), *Advances in Linear Free Energy Relationships*, Plenum, London.

Cheney, B. V. and Christofferson, R. E. (1983), *J. Med. Chem.*, **26**, 726.

Cheney, B. V., Wright, J. B., Hall, C. M., Johnson, H. G. and Christofferson, R. E. (1978), *J. Med. Chem.*, **21**, 936.

Chu, K. C. (1980), *The Basis of Medicinal Chemistry* (M. E. Wolff, ed), p. 393, Wiley, New York.

Clark, T. (1985), *A Handbook of Computational Chemistry*, Wiley, New York.

Cohen, N. C. (1985), *Adv. Drug Res.*, **14**, 42.

Collin, R. and Pullman, B. (1964), *Biochim. Biophys. Acta*, **89**, 232.

Craig, P. N. (1971), *J. Med. Chem.*, **14**, 680.

Cramer, G. M., Ford, R. A. and Hall, R. L. (1978), *Fd Cosmet. Toxicol.*, **16**, 255.

Daniel, C. and Wood, F. S. (1971), *Fitting Equations to Data*, Wiley, New York.

Darvas, F. (1974), *J. Med. Chem.*, **17**, 799.

Daudel, R., Esnault, L., Labil, C., Busch, N., Moleyre, J. and Lambert, J. (1976), *Europ. J. Med. Chem.*, **11**, 443.

De Benedetti, P. G. and Frassinetii, C. (1983), *J. Molec. Struct. (Theochem.)*, **92**, 191.

De Benedetti, P. G., Quartieri, S. and Rastelli, A. (1981), *J. Molec. Struct. (Theochem.)*, **85**, 45.

De Benedetti, P. G., Menziani, M. C. and Cocchi, M. (1987), *Quantitative Structure-Activity Relationships*, **6**, 51.

De Broglie, L. (1966), *Wave Mechanics and Molecular Biology*, Reidel, Dordrecht.

Dearden, J. C. (1982), *Quantitative Approaches to Drug Design*, Elsevier, Amsterdam.

Del Re, D. (1958), *J. Chem. Soc.*, 4031.

Deming, S. (1976), *J. Med. Chem.*, **19**, 977.

Dewar, M. J. S. (1983), *J. Mol. Struct.*, **100**, 41.

Dewar, M. J. S. and Dougherty, R. C. (1975), *The PMO Theory of Organic Chemistry*, Plenum, New York.

Dewar, M. J. S. and Haselbach, E. (1970), *J. Am. Chem. Soc.*, **92**, 590.

Dewar, M. J. S., McKee, M. L. and Rzepa, H. S. (1978), *J. Am. Chem. Soc.*, **100**, 3607.

Dewar, M. J. S., Zoebisch, E. G., Kealy, E. F. and Stewart, J. J. P. (1985), *J. Am. Chem. Soc.*, **107**, 3902.

Dietrich, S. W., Bolger, M. B., Kollman, P. and Jorgensen, E. C. (1977), *J. Med. Chem.*, **20**, 863.

Diner, S., Malrieu, J. P. and Claverie, P. (1969), *Theoret. Chim. Acta.*, **13**, 1.

El Tayar, N., Kilpatrick, G. J., van de Waterbeemd, H., Testa, B., Jenner, P. and Marsden, C. D. (1988), *Europ. J. Med. Chem.*, **23**, 173.

Enslein, K. (1984), *Pharmacol. Rev.*, **36**, 131.

Enslein, K., Blake, B. W., Tomb, M. E. and Borgstedt, H. H. (1986), *In Vitro Toxicol.*, **1**, 33.

Enslein, K., Borgstedt, H. H., Blake, B. W. and Hart, J. B. (1987 a), *In Vitro Toxicol.*, **1**, 129.

Enslein, K., Borgstedt, H. H., Tomb, M. E., Blake, B. W. and Hart, J. B. (1987 b), *Toxicol. Indust. Hlth.*, **3**, 267.

Esaki, T. (1987), *Chem. Pharmaceut. Bull.*, **35**, 3105.

Fauchere, J.-L. (1986), *Adv. Drug Res.*, **15**, 29.

Fernandez-Alonso, J. I. (1976), in *Quantum Mechanics of Molecular Conformations* (B. Pullman, ed), p. 110, Wiley, New York.

Fick, A. (1855), *Annalen Physik*, **94**, 59.

Fleming, I. (1980), *Frontier Orbitals and Organic Chemical Reactions*, Wiley, New York.

Fock, V. (1930), *Z. Phys.*, **61**, 126.

Free, S. and Wilson, J. (1964), *J. Med. Chem.*, **7**, 395.

Fukui, K., Yonezawa, T. and Nagata, C. (1954), *Bull. Chem. Soc. Japan*, **27**, 423.

Gabler, R. (1978), *Electrical Interactions in Molecular Biophysics*, Academic Press, New York.

Ganellin, C. R. and Young, R. C. (1986), *Neuropharmacology and Pesticide Action* (M. G. Ford, ed), Ch. 5. p. 86, Ellis Horwood, Chichester.

Germer, H. A. (1974), *J. Pharmacy Pharmacol.*, **26**, 799.

Glennon, R. A. and Gessner, P. K. (1975), *Pharmacology.*, **17**, 259.

Goldberg, L. (1983), *Structure-Activity Correlation as a Predictive Tool in Toxicology*, Hemisphere, Washington.

Gomez-Jeria, J. S. and Morales-Lagos, D. R. (1984), *J. Pharmaceut. Sci.*, **73**, 1725.

Gomez-Jeria, J. S., Morales-Lagos, D. R., Rodriguez-Gatica, J. I. and Saavedra-Aguilar, J. C. (1985), *Int. J. Quantum Chem.*, **28**, 421.

Goodford, P. J. (1973), *Adv. Pharmacol. Chemother.*, **11**, 51.

Gould, R. F. (1972), *Biological Correlations—The Hansch Approach*, American Chemical Society, Washington.

Green, J. P., Johnson, C. L. and Kang, S. (1974), *Ann. Rev. Pharmacol.*, **14**, 319.

Greenwood, H. H. and McWeeney, R. (1966), *Adv. Phys. Org. Chem.*, **4**, 73.

Hadzi, D. and Jerman-Blazic, B. (1987), *QSAR in Drug Design and Toxicology*, Elsevier, Amsterdam.

Hammett, L. P. (1940), *Physical Organic Chemistry*, McGraw-Hill, New York.

Handa, A., Bindal, M. C., Prabhakar, Y. S. and Gupta, S. P. (1983), *Indian J. Biochem. Biophys.*, **20**, 318.

Hansch, C. (1969), *Acc. Chem. Res.*, **2**, 232.

Hansch, C. (1971), *Drug Design*, **1**, 270.

Hansch, C. (1973), *Structure-Activity Relationships.*, **1**, 75.

Hansch, C. (1976), *J. Med. Chem.*, **19**, 1.

Hansch, C. and Coats, E. (1970), *J. Pharmaceut. Sci.*, **59**, 743.

Hansch, C. and Fujita, T. (1964), *J. Am. Chem. Soc.*, **86**, 1616.

Hansch, C. and Leo, A. (1979), *Substituent Constants for Correlation Analysis in Chemistry and Biology*, Wiley, New York.

Hansch, C., Maloney, P. P., Fujita, T. and Muir, R. M. (1962), *Nature*, **194**, 178.

Hansch, C., Muir, R. M., Fujita, T., Maloney, P., Geiger, E. and Streich, M. (1963), *J. Am. Chem. Soc.*, **85**, 2817.

Hansch, C., McLarin, J., Klein, R. and Langridge, R. (1985), *Molec. Pharmacol.*, **27**, 493.

Hartee, D. R. (1928), *Proc. Camb. Phil. Soc.*, **24**, 89.

Hehre, W. J., Radom, L., Schleger, P. V. R. and Pople, J. A. (1986), *Ab Initio Molecular Orbital Theory*, Wiley, New York.

Heilbronner, E. and Bock. H. (1976), *The HMO Model and its Application*, Wiley, New York.

Herndon, W. C. (1974), *Int. J. Quantum Chem., Quantum Biol. Symp.*, **1**, 123.

Hogberg, T., Ramsby, S., Ogren, S.-O. and Norinder, U. (1987), *Acta Pharmaceut. Suecica.*, **24**, 289.

Holtje, H. D. (1975), *Arch. Pharmacol.*, **308**, 438.

Holtje, H. D. and Kier, L. B. (1974), *J. Med. Chem.*, **17**, 814.

Hopfinger, A. J. (1981), *J. Med. Chem.*, **24**, 818.

Hopfinger, A. J. (1983), *J. Med. Chem.*, **26**, 990.

Hopfinger, A. J. (1985), *J. Med. Chem.*, **28**, 1133.

Hoskuldsson, A. (1987), *J. Chemometrics.*, **2**, 211.

Hosur, R. V. (1978), *Int. J. Quantum Chem.*, **13**, 411.

Howard, A. E. and Kollman, P. A. (1988), *J. Med. Chem.*, **31**, 1669.

Hückel, E. (1931), *Z. Phys.*, **70**, 204.

Humber, L. G., Lee, D., Rakhit, S. and Treasurywala, A. M. (1985), *J. Molec. Graphics*, **3**, 84.

Johnson, C. L. and Green, J. P. (1974), *Int. J. Quantum Chem.*, *Quantum Biol. Symp.*, **1**, 159.

Jones, G. P. and Andrews, P. R. (1987), *J. Chem. Soc. Perkin Trans.*, **II**, 415.

Joyner, J. C. and Purcell, W. P. (1976), *Experientia* (Suppl. 23), 13.

Jurs, P. C., Chou, J. T. and Yuan, M. (1979), *J. Med. Chem.*, **22**, 476.

Kang, S. and Green, J. P. (1969), *Nature*, **222**, 794.

Kang, S. and Green, J. P. (1970), *Nature*, **226**, 645.

Karlen, A., Helander, A., Kenne, L. and Macksell, U. (1989), *J. Med. Chem.*, **32**, 765.

Katz, R., Heller, S. R. and Jacobson, A. E. (1973), *Molec. Pharmacol.*, **9**, 486.

Kaufman, J. J. (1977), *Int. J. Quantum Chem.*, *Quantum Biol. Symp.*, **4**, 375.

Kende, A. S., Ebetino, F. H., Drendel, W. B., Sundaralingam, M., Glover, E. and Poland, A. (1985), *Molec. Pharmacol.*, **28**, 445.

Kier, L. B. (1970), *Molecular Orbital Studies in Chemical Pharmacology*, Springer-Verlag, New York.

Kier, L. B. (1971), *Molecular Orbital Theory in Drug Research*, Academic Press, New York.

Kier, L. B. (1972), *Adv. Chem. Series.*, **113**, 278.

Kier, L. B. (1973), *Experientia* (Suppl. 23), 151.

Kier, L. B. and Hall, L. H. (1976), *Molecular Connectivity in Chemistry and Drug Research*, Academic Press, New York.

Kier, L. B., George, J. M. and Holtje, H. D. (1974), *J. Pharmaceut. Sci.*, **63**, 1435.

Klopman, G. (1985), *Environ. Hlth Perspect.*, **61**, 269.

Klopman, G. and Frierson, M. R. (1984), *Croatica Chemica Acta.*, **57**, 1411.

Klopman, G. and Macina, P. T. (1985), *J. Theoret. Biol,*, **113**, 637.

Klopman, G., Namboodiri, K. and Kalos, A. N. (1985), in *Molecular Basis of Cancer, Part A*: *Macromolecular Structure, Carcinogens and Oncogenes*, p. 287, Alan R. Liss Inc., New York.

Kollman, P. A. (1980), in *The Basis of Medicinal Chemistry* (M. E. Wolff, ed), p. 313, Wiley, New York.

Korolkovas, A. (1970), *Essentials of Molecular Pharmacology*, Wiley, New York.

Korolkovas, A. and Burckhalter, J. M. (1976), *Essentials of Medicinal Chemistry*, Wiley, New York.

Kothekar, V. and Dutta, S. (1982), *Indian J. Biochem. Biophys.*, **19**, 266.

Kubinyi, H. (1976), *Arzneimittel—Forsch.*, **26**, 1991.

Kubinyi, H. (1979), *Prog. Drug Res.*, **23**, 97.

Kulkarni, V. M. (1975), *Indian J. Biochem. Biophys.*, **12**, 367.

Kumber, M. and Sankar, D. V. (1973), *Res. Commun. Chem. Path. Pharmacol.*, **6**, 65.

Kumber, M., Cusimano, V. and Sankar, D. V. (1976), *J. Pharmaceut. Sci.*, **65**, 1014.

Lake, B. G., Gray, T. J. B., Lewis, D. F. V., Beamand, J. A., Hodder, K. D., Purchase, R. and Gangolli, S. D. (1987), *Toxicol. Indust. Hlth*, **3**, 165.

Leffler, J. E. and Grunwald, E. (1963), *Rates and Equilibria of Organic Reactions*, Wiley, New York.

Leo, A., Hansch, C. and Elkins, D. (1971), *Chem. Rev.*, **71**, 525.

LePage, C., Schaefer, M., Batt, A. M. and Siest, G. (1980), in *Biochemistry*

Biophysics and Regulation of Cytochrome P450 (J. A. Gustafsson, J. Carlstedt-Duke, A. Mode and J. Rafter, eds), p. 363, Elsevier, Amsterdam.

Lewi, P. J. (1976), *Arzneimittel—Forsch.*, **26**, 1295.

Lewis, D. F. V. (1981), Ph.D. Thesis, University of Surrey, England, UK.

Lewis, D. F. V. (1986), *Chem. Rev.*, **86**, 1111.

Lewis, D. F. V. (1987 a), *Xenobiotica.*, **17**, 1351.

Lewis, D. F. V. (1987 b), *Chem.-Biol. Interactions*, **62**, 271.

Lewis, D. F. V. (1988), *Int. J. Quantum Chem.*, **33**, 305.

Lewis, D. F. V. (1989 a), *Journal of Computational Chemistry*, **10**, 145.

Lewis, D. F. V. (1989 b), *Xenobiotica.*, **19**, 243.

Lewis, D. F. V. (1989 c), *Xenobiotica.*, **19**, 341.

Lewis, D. F. V. (1990), *Xenobiotica*, in press.

Lewis, D. F. V. and Griffiths ʼ. S. (1987), *Xenobiotica.*, **17**, 769.

Lewis, D. F. V., Tamburini, P. P. and Gibson, G. G. (1986), *Chem.-Biol. Interactions*, **58**, 289.

Lewis, D. F. V., Gray, T. J. B. and Lake, B. G. (1987 a), *Drug Metabolism—from Molecules to Man* (D. J. Benford, J. W. Bridges and G. G. Gibson, eds), p. 369, Taylor and Francis, London.

Lewis, D, F. V., Lake, B. G., Gray, T. J. B. and Gangolli, S. D. (1987 b), *Archives of Toxicology*, Suppl., **11**, 39.

Lewis, D. F. V., Arendt, J. and English, J. (1989 a), *J. Pharmacol. Exp. Therap.*, **252**, 370.

Lewis, D. F. V., Ioannides, C. and Parke, D. V. (1989 b), *Xenobiotica*, in press.

Lewis, D. F. V., Ioannides, C. and Parke, D. V. (1989 c), *Toxicology Letters*, **45**, 1.

Li, R.-L., Hansch, C., Mathews, D., Blaney, J. M., Langridge, R., Delcamp, J. J., Susten, S. S. and Freisheim, (1982), *Quantitative Structure-Activity Relationships.*, **1**, 1.

Lifschitz, C., Bergmann, E. D. and Pullman, B. (1967), *Tetrahedron Lett.*, **46**, 4583.

Lin, T. K. (1974), *J. Med. Chem.*, **17**, 151.

Lipnick, R. L. (1985), in *Aquatic Toxicology and Hazard Assessment* (R. C. Bacher and D. J. Hansen, eds), p. 78, ASTM, Philadelphia.

Lipnick, R. L., Johnson, D. E., Gilford, J. H., Bickings, C. K. and Newsome, L. D. (1985), *Environ. Toxicol. Chem.*, **4**, 281.

Loew, G. H., Berkowitz, D. S. and Burt, S. K. (1978), *NIDA Res. Monograph Series*, **22**, 278.

Loew, G. H., Sudhindra, B. S. and Ferrel, J. E. (1979), *Chem.-Biol. Interact.*, **26**, 75.

Loew, G., Poulsen, M., Ferrel, J. and Chaet, D. (1980), *Chem.-Biol. Interact.*, **31**, 319.

Loew, G. H., Poulsen, M. T., Spangler, D. and Kirkjian, E. (1983), *Int. J. Quantum Chem., Quantum Biol. Symp.*, **10**, 201.

Loew, G. H., Nienow, J. R. and Poulsen, M. (1984), *Molec. Pharmacol.*, **26**, 19.

Loew, G. H., Nienow, J. T., Lawson, J. A., Toll, L. and Uyeno, E. T. (1985), *Molec. Pharmacol.*, **28**, 17.

Long, G., McKinney, J. D. and Pedersen, L. G. (1987), *Quantitative Structure Activity Relationships.*, **6**, 1.

Lukovits, I. (1983), *J. Med. Chem.*, **26**, 1104.

Lukovits, I., Biczo, G. and Pataki, I. (1976), *Experientia* (Suppl. 23), 165.

Luque, F. J., Illas, F. and Pouplana, R. (1987), *Molec. Pharmacol.*, **32**, 557.

Luque, F. J., Sauz, F., Illas, F., Pouplana, R. and Smeyers, Y. G. (1988), *Europ. J. Med. Chem.*, **23**, 7.

Machmer, P. and Duchesne, J. (1965), *Nature*, **206**, 618.

Marshall, G. R. (1983), in *Quantitative Approaches to Drug Design* (J. C. Dearden, ed), Elsevier, Amsterdam.

Marshall, G. R. (1987), *Ann. Rev. Pharmacol. Toxicol.*, **27**, 193.

Marshall, G. R. and Cramer, R. D. (1988), *Trends Pharmaceut. Sci.*, **9**, 285.

Marshall, G. R., Naruta, D., Motoc, I., Nelson, R., Schneider, C., Nukes, T. and Mearn, T. (1985), in *QSAR and Strategies in the Design of Bioactive Compounds* (J. K. Seydel, ed), VCH, Weinheim.

Martin, M., Carbo, R., Petrongolo, C. and Tomasi, J. (1975), *J. Am. Chem. Soc.*, **97**, 1338.

Martin, Y. C. (1978), *Quantitative Drug Design. A Critical Introduction*, Dekker, New York.

Martin, Y. C. (1979), *Drug Design*, **8**, 5.

Martin, Y. C., Bustard, T. M. and Lynn, K. R. (1973), *J. Med. Chem.*, **16**, 1089.

Maynard, A. T., Pederson, L. G., Posner, H. S. and McKinney, J. D. (1986), *Molec. Pharmacol.*, **29**, 629.

McFarland, J. W. and Gans, D. J. (1987), *J. Med. Chem.*, **30**, 46

Menziani, M. C., De Benedetti, P. G., Gago, F. and Richards, W. G. (1989), *J. Med. Chem.*, **32**, 951.

Millner, O. E. and Purcell, W. P. (1971), *J. Med. Chem.*, **14**, 1134.

Mitchell, T. (1988), Ph.D. Thesis, University of Surrey, England, UK.

Mitchell, T., Tute, M. S. and Webb, G. A. (1989), *J. Computer-Aided Molec. Design*, in press.

Miyamoto, S. and Yoshimoto, M. (1987), *Chem. Pharmaceut. Bull.*, **35**, 4510.

Miyashita, Y., Seki, T., Yotsui, Y., Yamazaki, K., Sano, M., Abe, H. and Sasaki, S. (1982), *Bull. Chem. Soc. Japan*, **55**, 1489.

Mohammed, S. N. (1985), *Indian J. Biochem. Biophys.*, **22**, 56.

Mohammed, S. N. (1986), *Indian J. Biochem. Biophys.*, **23**, 45.

Mohammed, S. N. and Hopfinger, A. J. (1983), *J. Theoret. Biol.*, **102**, 323.

Murrell, J. N. and Harget, A. J. (1972), *Semi-Empirical Self-Consistent Field Molecular Orbital Theory of Molecules*, Wiley, New York.

Neely, W. B. (1965), *Molec. Pharmacol.*, **1**, 137.

Nogrady, T. (1988), *Medicinal Chemistry—A Biomedical Approach*, Oxford University Press, Oxford.

Olaru, N. and Simon, Z. (1981), *Revue Roumaine Biochim.*, **18**, 51.

Olsen, E. C. and Christofferson, R. E. (1979), *Computer-Assisted Drug Design*, American Chemical Society, Washington.

Osman, R., Namboodiri, K., Weinstein, H. and Rabinowitz, J. R. (1988), *J. Am. Chem. Soc.*, **110**, 1701.

Otto, P., Seel, M., Ladik, J. and Muller, R. (1979), *J. Theoret. Biol.*, **78**, 197.

Pariser, R. and Parr, R. G. (1953), *J. Chem. Phys.*, **21**, 466.

Parke, D. V. (1987), *Arch. Toxicol.*, **60**, 5.

Parke, D. V., Ioannides, C. and Lewis, D. F. V. (1986), in *Toxicology in Europe in the Year 2000, Federation of the European Societies of Toxicology*, Suppl. (C. M. Hodel, ed), p. 14, Elsevier, Amsterdam.

Parke, D. V., Lewis, D. F. V. and Ioannides, C. (1988), *Chemicals in the Environment* (M. R. Richardson, ed), p. 45, Royal Society of Chemistry, London.

Peradejordi, F. (1971), in *Aspects de la Chimie Quantique Contemporaine*, p. 261, CNRS, Paris.

Pople, J. A. (1953), *Trans. Faraday Soc.*, **49**, 1375.

Pople, J. A. and Beveridge, D. L. (1970), *Approximate Molecular Orbital Theory*, McGraw-Hill, New York.

Pople, J. A., Santry, D. P. and Segal, G. A. (1965), *J. Chem. Phys.*, **43**, Suppl. 129.

Pople, J. A., Beveridge, D. L. and Dobosh, P. A. (1967), *J. Chem. Phys.*, **47**, 2026.

Pullman, B. (1962), *Electronic Aspects of Biochemistry.*, Academic Press, New York.

Pullman, B. (1970), in *Molecular Orbital Studies in Chemical Pharmacology* (L. B. Kier, ed), p. 1, Springer-Verlag, Berlin.

Pullman, B. (1976), *Quantum Mechanics of Molecular Conformations*, Wiley, New York.
Pullman, B. (1979), *Int. J. Quantum Chem.*, **16**, 669.
Pullman, B. and Courriere, P. (1973), *Theoretica Chimica Acta.*, **31**, 19.
Pullman, B. and Pullman, A. (1960), *Rev. Mod. Physics*, **32**, 428.
Pullman, B. and Pullman, A. (1963), *Quantum Biochemistry*, Wiley, New York.
Pullman, B. and Pullman, A. (1969), *Prog. Nucleic Acid Res.*, **9**, 328.
Purcell, W. P. (1966), *J. Med. Chem.*, **9**, 294.
Purcell, W. P., Singer, J. A., Sundaram, K. and Parks, G. C. (1970), *Medicinal Chemistry* (A. Burger, ed), Ch. 10, Wiley, New York.
Recanatini, M., Klein, T., Young, C-Z., McClarin, J., Langridge, R. and Hansch, C. (1986), *Molec. Pharmacol.*, **29**, 436.
Rekker, R. F. (1977), *The Hydrophobic Fragmental Constant*, Elsevier, Amsterdam.
Richards, W. G. (1983), *Quantum Pharmacology*, Butterworths, London.
Richards, W. G. and Black, M. E. (1975), *Prog. Med. Chem.*, **11**, 67.
Roothaan, C. C. J. (1951), *Rev. Mod. Phys.*, **23**, 69.
Rusu, I., Medesan, A., Grigoras, S., Moldoveaunu, S. and Pausescu, E. (1979), *Revue Roumaine Biochimie*, **16**, 321.
Sankar, D. V. and Kumber, D. V. (1974), *Res. Commun. Chem. Path. Pharmacol.*, **7**, 259.
Saunders, M. R. (1986), Ph.D. Thesis, University of Surrey, England, UK.
Saxena, A. K. and Ram, S. (1979), *Prog. Drug Res.*, **23**, 199.
Schnaare, R. L. (1971), *Drug Design*, **1**, 405.
Schnaare, R. S. and Martin, A. N. (1965), *J. Pharmaceut. Sci.*, **54**, 1707.
Schrödinger, E. (1926), *Phys. Rev.*, **28**, 1049.
Schwalbe, C. H., King, M. E., Wong, K. P., Lambert, P. A., Bliss, A. and Stevens, M. F. G. (1987), *Anti-Cancer Drug Design.*, **2**, 289.
Segal, G. A. (1977), *Semi-Empirical Methods of Electronic Structure Calculation*, Plenum, New York.
Selassie, C. D., Fang, Z-X., Li, R., Hansch, C., Klain, T., Langridge, R. and Kaufman, B. R. (1986), *J. Med. Chem.*, **29**, 621.
Seydel, J. K. (1985), *QSAR and Strategies in the Design of Bioactive Compounds*, VCH, Weinham.
Seydel, J. K. and Schaper, K. J. (1982), *Pharmacol. Therapeut.*, **15**, 131.
Shorter, J. (1973), *Correlation Analysis in Organic Chemistry*, Clarenden, Oxford.
Simon, Z. (1976), *Quantum Biochemistry and Specific Interactions*, Abacus, London.
Sinclair, J., Cornell, N. W., Zaitlin, L. and Hansch, C. (1986), *Biochem. Pharmacol.*, **35**, 707.
Sklener, H. and Jaeger, J. (1979), *Int. J. Quantum Chem.*, **16**, 467.
Smith, G. J., Macrae, C. F. and King, P. M. (1986), *J. Molec. Graphics.*, **4**, 238.
Snyder, S. H. and Merril, C. R. (1965), *Proc. Nat. Acad. Sci. USA*, **54**, 285.
Stedman, N. J., Morris, G. M. and Atkinson, P. J. (1987), *J. Molec. Graphics*, **5**, 211.
Steward, E. G. and Clarke, G. R. (1975), *J. Theoret. Biol.*, **52**, 493.
Steward, E. G. and Lowe, R. H. (1978), in *Iontophoresis and Transmitter Mechanisms in the Mammalian CNS* (R. W. Ryan and J. S. Kelly, eds), p. 394, Elsevier, Amsterdam.
Streitwieser, A. (1961), *Molecular Orbital Theory for Organic Chemists*, Wiley, New York.
Stuper, A. J. and Jurs, P. C. (1975), *J. Am. Chem. Soc.*, **97**, 182.
Tanford, C. (1980), *The Hydrophobic Effect*, Wiley, New York.
Taft, R. W. (1956), in *Steric Effects in Organic Chemistry* (M. S. Newman, ed), p. 556, Wiley, New York.
Taylor, J. L. and Durant, J. C. (1985), *J. Molec. Graphics*, **3**, 158.
Testa, B. (1981), *Chem.-Biol. Interactions*, **34**, 287.

Testa, B., El Tayar, N., Carrupt, P. A., van de Waterbeemd, H., Kilpatrick, G. J., Jenner, P. and Marsden, C. D. (1987), *J. Pharmacy Pharmacol.*, **39**, 767.

Thornton, J. M., Barlow, D. J. and Sternberg, M. J. E. (1986), in *Neuropharmacology and Pesticide Action* (M. G. Ford, ed), p. 102, Ellis Horwood, Chichester.

Tichy, M. (1976), *Quantitative Structure—Activity Relationships*, Birkhauser-Verlag, Basel.

Tichy, M. (1985), *QSAR in Toxicology and Xenobiochemistry*, Elsevier, Amsterdam.

Timmermans, P. B. M. W. M. and Van Zwieten, P. A. (1977), *J. Med. Chem.*, **20**, 1636.

Topliss, J. G. (1972), *J. Med. Chem.*, **15**, 1006.

Topliss, J. G. and Costello, R. J. (1972), *J. Med. Chem.*, **15**, 1066.

Turner, L., Choplin, F , Dugard, P., Hermens, J., Jaeckh, R., Marsmann, M. and Roberts, D. (1987), *Toxicol. in Vitro*, **1**, 143.

Tute, M. S. (1971), *Adv. Drug Res.*, **6**, 1.

Upton, R. and Gasking, H. (1988), *Int. Lab.*, (Sept), 24..

van de Waterbeemd, H. and Testa, B. (1987), *Adv. Drug Res.*, **16**, 87.

Wald, R. W. and Feuer, G. (1971), *J. Med. Chem.*, **14**, 1081.

Wohl, A. J. (1970), *Molec. Pharmacol.*, **6**, 195.

Wohl, A. J. (1971), *Drug Design.*, **1**, 381.

Wold, S. (1976), *Experientia* (Suppl. 23), 87.

Yates, K. (1978), *Hückel Molecular Orbital Theory*, Academic Press, New York.

Young, R. C., Durant, G. J., Emmett, J. C., Ganellin, C. R., Graham, M. J., Mitchell, R. C., Prain, M. D. and Roantree, M. L. (1986), *J. Med. Chem.*, **29**, 44.

Xiao-Yuan F. and Shu-Jun, S. (1981), *Int. J. Quantum Chem.*, *Quantum Biol. Symp.*, **8**, 197.

CHAPTER 6

Enantiospecific analytical methodology : applications in drug metabolism and pharmacokinetics

A. J. Hutt

Department of Pharmacy, Brighton Polytechnic, Brighton, BN2 4GJ, , UK[1]

[1] Present address: Chelsea Department of Pharmacy, King's College London, University of London, London, SW3 6LX, UK

1. Introduction

Stereochemistry is that area of chemistry concerned with the three dimensional nature of molecules. The term stereochemistry was first used by Victor Meyer, in 1890, and was derived from the title of a booklet, *La Chimie dans l'Espace* (Chemistry in Space) published by van't Hoff in 1875 (Ramsay, 1981), the prefix stereo originating from the Greek *stereos* meaning solid or volume. Stereoisomers are compounds which differ only in the three-dimensional arrangement of their constituent atoms in space; such isomers may be further divided into two groups namely enantiomers and diastereoisomers.

Enantiomers are pairs of compounds which are non-superimposable mirror images of one another and, in terms of physicochemical properties, differ only in their ability to rotate the plane of plane polarized light. Such isomers are said to be chiral (Greek *chiros* meaning handed) and are variously referred to as optical isomers or enantiomorphs (Greek *enantios*—opposite, *morph*—form). The term diastereoisomers refers to all other stereoisometric compounds regardless of their ability to rotate plane polarized light and the definition, therefore, includes both optical isomers and geometrical or cis/trans isomers (Gunstone, 1975). A fundamental distinction between enantiomerism and diastereoisomerism is that in a pair of enantiomers the distances between non-bonded atoms are identical, whereas in diastereoisomers they are not. Thus, the energy content of enantiomers is identical, whereas diastereoisomers differ in energy content and hence in their physical and chemical properties. This fundamental difference in the properties of the two types of isomer has considerable significance as mixtures of enantiomers cannot be separated by standard chemical techniques, whereas diastereoisomers may be separated by, for example, distillation, recrystallization and most importantly in the present context, chromatography.

In terms of compounds of interest in medicinal chemistry and pharmacology, the most frequent cause of chirality is due to the presence of asymmetric centres in organic molecules, generally tetracoordinate centres to which four different atoms or groups are bonded. Examples of tetrahedral centres of importance are associated with carbon, nitrogen, sulphur and phosphorus atoms in organic molecules. A less frequently found situation is that of atropoisomerism (Greek *atropos*—inflexible), a term used to characterize stereoisomers which are chiral due to hindrance of rotation around a single bond, e.g. *ortho*-substituted biphenyl derivatives are chiral due to restricted rotation; examples of interest include methaqualone and gossypol (see below).

Enantiomers behave in an achiral environment, in an identical manner and to distinguish between a pair of enantiomers it is necessary to place the isomers in a chiral environment, a point that has considerable significance for both the biological properties and the analysis of a mixture of enantiomers. Biological environments are highly chiral environments being composed of chiral biopolymers, e.g. the right-handed helices of DNA, the backbone of which contains D-deoxyribose; the α helix of proteins comprised of L-amino acids and carbohydrates exclusively of the D-configuration. As nature has made a preference in terms of chirality it is not surprising that enzyme and receptor systems frequently exhibit a preference towards one of a pair of enantiomers. The interaction between the chiral biopolymer and the individual enantiomers results in the formation of a pair of diastereoisomeric complexes.

The differential pharmacodynamic properties of the enantiomers of chiral drugs has been known for a number of years (see, for example, Cushny, 1926). In contrast stereochemical considerations in drug metabolism and disposition developed much later and only relatively recently has become an 'issue' for both the pharmaceutical industry and the regulatory authorities (Smith and Caldwell, 1988). The late development of stereochemical considerations in drug metabolism arose due to the lack of appropriate methodology suitable for the determination of material in biological media and the complexity of enantiomeric differentiation. The recent resurgence of interest in both the pharmacodynamic and pharmacokinetic properties of the enantiomers of chiral drugs has been stimulated in part, by the rapid developments in methodology for both the analytical and preparative resolution of racemic drug mixtures, particularly in the area of chromatography.

Differences between enantiomers may occur during their absorption, distribution, metabolism and excretion and hence it is not surprising that following the administration of a racemic drug, the individual enantiomers do not reach their site of action in equal concentrations. These differences in metabolism and disposition have obvious consequences for the related disciplines of clinical pharmacology and toxicology. Over recent years a number of useful monographs and reviews concerned with the biological properties of chiral drugs and the problems associated with a lack of appreciation of this area have appeared and those interested are referred to these for further information (Ariens, 1984; Ariens *et al.*, 1983, 1988; Caldwell *et al.*, 1988 d; Drayer, 1986; Hutt and Caldwell, 1984; Simonyi, 1984; Testa and Mayer, 1988; Trager and Jones, 1987; Vermeulen, 1989; Wainer and Drayer, 1988; Williams and Lee, 1985).

Until relatively recently much of our knowledge concerning the fate of drug enantiomers resulted from their individual administration to an animal or man, the advantage of this approach being that non-stereoselective analytical methods could be used for the determination of drug-related material in biological fluids. This approach is now unacceptable as 1. the majority of chiral drugs are used as racemates and the effect of one enantiomer on the disposition of the other is unknown and 2. racemization, either chemically or enzymatically mediated, may occur and would go undetected. Also the formation and detection of chiral metabolites from either achiral or chiral drug molecules may yield valuable information concerning the nature of the substrate—enzyme interaction and the topology of the active site of the enzyme system. In addition, the use of stereochemical probe compounds may yield useful information concerning the composition of hepatic cytochrome P450 isozymes (Kaminsky *et al.*, 1984). It is, therefore, appropriate to consider the various approaches and analytical methodologies available to carry out such metabolic and pharmacokinetic studies.

Enantiospecific analysis generally requires the presence of a chiral environment or an interaction with a second chiral agent. This may involve the use of plane-polarized light, e. g. polarimetry or circular dichroism; derivatization with a chiral compound to yield a pair of diastereoisomeric derivatives followed by achiral chromatography or nuclear magnetic resonance spectroscopy (NMR); interaction with a chiral complex, solvent or surface, e.g. chiral shift reagents or solvents in NMR, a chiral mobile phase in high-performance liquid chromatography (HPLC), chiral stationary phases for HPLC, gas chromatography (GC) or thin-layer chromatography (TLC); or alternatively utilization of the inherent chirality of nature in enantioselective immunoassay or radioreceptor techniques.

All of these approaches offer advantages and limitations in terms of ease of sample manipulation or preparative work required to establish the methodology. Various aspects of these methods have been reviewed in recent years and the interested reader is referred to the general overviews of Testa and Jenner (1978), Cook (1983), Hutt and Caldwell (1988 a, 1989), reviews of chromatographic methods by Testa (1986) and Vermeulen and Testa (1988) and the monograph edited by Wainer and Drayer (1988). More general overviews not specifically related to bioanalytical chemistry have appeared, e.g. Morrison (1983), as have more specialized monographs on various aspects of chromatography, e.g. König (1987), Zief and Crane (1988) and Allenmark (1988).

The classical methods of distinguishing between a pair of enantiomers and determination of the enantiomeric composition of a non-racemic mixture of isomers, makes use of the unique property of chiral compounds of rotation of plane-polarized light. This may involve an examination of their specific rotation at a specific wavelength (polarimetry), over a range of wavelengths (optical rotatory dispersion) or by the difference in absorption of right and left circular polarized light (circular dichroism) (Schurig, 1985; Lyle and Lyle, 1983).

The determination of optical rotation is fraught with potential pitfalls and is dependent on temperature, sample concentration, solvent and wavelength of light used, as not only may the magnitude of the measured rotation vary but the direction of rotation may also alter with both concentration and solvent. Also the presence of trace achiral impurities or contaminants can influence the observed rotation and there are several reports of enhancement of observed rotation due to the presence of contaminants (Lyle and Lyle, 1983). Additional problems are associated with the magnitude of the rotation of the substance under investigation which may be quite low. This obviously limits the sensitivity of the determination, a situation compounded by the relatively small quantities of material generally isolated in metabolic experiments. It is also essential to know the specific rotation of the pure enantiomers of the material under investigation.

Whilst the optical methods have been largely superseded by the advances made in other areas of enantiomeric analysis, optical rotation determinations are frequently reported in the literature as an initial indication that stereoselective metabolism has taken place. However, the use of such measurements, other than as supportive/comparative data for quantitative determinations, is outdated. The major advance in this area involves the use of optical activity detectors as specific detector systems for HPLC (see below).

2. Enantioselective immunoassay

The potential of immunoassay methodology for the discrimination of enantiomers has been known since the late 1920s when Landsteiner and van der Scheer (1928, 1929) were able to prepare antibodies that could differentiate between the optical isomers of N-(p-aminobenzoyl)phenylglycine and the enantiomers and meso form of tartaric acid.

Similar studies by Karush (1956) resulted in the preparation of enantioselective antibodies to a series of chiral azo dyes related to N-(p-aminobenzoyl) phenylglycine. Since these initial observations, radioimmunoassay (RIA) methods have become relatively commonplace in clinical biochemistry, therapeutic drug monitoring and drug screening laboratories (Findlay, 1987). The area of chiral drug immunoassay has until relatively recently received little interest, both in terms of the development of enantioselective antibodies for drug enantiomer analysis and also in terms of the problems that may arise due to the production of antibodies using racemic molecules to prepare haptens and hence antigens. Examples of enantioselective immunoassays are presented in Table 1.

Drugs and drug enantiomers are not normally immunogenic, due to their small molecular size, and require the formation of a drug-carrier complex, generally a protein, before immunization of animals to elicit the production of antibodies. A 'bridging' group between the drug molecule and the carrier-protein is also frequently introduced to facilitate the coupling of the drug to the carrier. The preparation of a drug-carrier complex required for the production of enantioselective antibodies obviously requires the availability of enantiomerically pure compounds and may involve several chemical transformations before immunization may be carried out (Figure 1). Such chemical transformations must be carried out under mild conditions which will not result in partial racemization of the drug moiety, as the specificity of the antibodies produced is dependent on the enantiomeric purity of the material used. Small impurities in the antigen, due to lack of enantiomeric purity of the starting material, or partial racemization, may result in disproportionate quantities of a pair of antibodies, the use of which will produce data of limited value.

The size and position of substitution of the 'bridge' on the drug molecule may also be of significance as the immunogenic determinants will be specific for that area of the molecule which protrudes from the carrier and hence increasing the surface accessibility of the drug moiety may be advantageous. An additional problem associated with the above is that the position of substitution may influence the cross-reactivity of the antibody with the metabolic products of the drug. The production of two enantioselective antibodies produced to (R) and (S)-warfarin coupled through the 4'-position to the bridging group and ultimately to Bovine Serum Albumin (BSA) showed minimal cross-reactivity to each drug enantiomer, but both showed 50 per cent cross-reactivity with racemic 4'-hydroxywarfarin implying 100 per cent cross-reaction with each antiserum (Cook *et al.*, 1979 a).

Similar problems have been found on preparation of antibodies to the drug cyclazine (Figure 2). Using the racemate, a series of hapten-BSA conjugates were prepared in which the length and position of substitution of the bridging group were varied (Maeda and Tsuji, 1981). Of eleven antisera produced to the racemate, three were selected for further investigation. One was found to be highly specific for the leavorotatory isomer whilst the others yielded results indicative of a mixture of unequal quantities of two enantioselective antibodies and it is noteworthy that an antibody showing equal cross-reactivity to both isomers was not obtained (Figure 2). These antisera were used to examine the disposition of the racemic drug following administration to dogs. As expected, the serum concentration–time profiles obtained were totally dependent on the antisera used and illustrate the limitations of the use of material prepared in response to racemic drugs (Maeda and Tsuji, 1981).

Similar results have been found on the production of antisera to the drug atropine ((±)-hyoscyamine). Several groups have attempted to develop RIAs

Table 1. Enantioselective immunoassays for chiral drugs.

Drug enantiomer	Cross-reactivity (%)		Application	Reference
	Enantiomer	Metabolites and related compounds		
(S)-Amphetamine	4.5	—	—	Gross and Soares (1974)
(S)-Methamphetamine	3.9	(R,S)-Methamphetamine 52	Disposition in man following administration of both (S) and (R,S)-methamphetamine	Niwaguchi *et al.* (1982)
		(R,S)-Amphetamine <0.9		
		(±)-Methylephedrine 26		
		(±)-Ephedrine 0.8		
(S)-Methamphetamine	—	Data presented for 45 rigid and non rigid analogues	Disposition of (S)-amphetamine in dogs	Faraj *et al.* (1976)
(1S,2R)-Ephedrine	<2	(±)-Norephedrine 0	Disposition in man following administration of racemic ephedrine	Midha *et al.* (1983)
		(±)-*p*-hydroxyephedrine 0		
		(±)-pseudoephedrine <1		
(1R,2S)-Ephedrine	<2	(±)-Norephedrine <1		
		(±)-*p*-hydroxyephedrine 0		
		(±)-pseudoephedrine <1		
(1S,2S)-Pseudoephedrine	<0.05	(+)-norpseudoephedrine 5	Bioequivalence study in man	Findlay *et al.* (1981)
		(−)-ephedrine <0.44		
		(+)-ephedrine 0.35		
		(−)-norephedrine 0.02		
(S)-Propranolol	c. 7	Propranolol glycol c. 11	Drug disposition in rats following administration of the racemate	Kawashima *et al.* (1976)
		4-Hydroxypropranolol c. 2.9		
(R)-Pentobarbital	1.0	Racemate 50	Pharmacokinetics of enantiomers following administration of the racemate to rabbits and men	Cook *et al.* (1987)
		4'-Hydroxypentobarbital <0.1–0.6		
		5-Ethyl-5-(3-carboxy-2-propyl) barbituric acid 0.06–0.11		
		(R)-Secobarbital 180		
		(S)-Secobarbital 2.2		
		(R)-Thiopental 144		
		(S)-Thiopental 3.2		

(*continued*)

Progress in Drug Metabolism

Table 1. (*Continued*).

Drug enantiomer	Enantiomer	Cross-reactivity (%) Metabolites and related compounds		Application	Reference
(S)-Pentobarbital	1.4	Racemate	49	Disposition in man following administration of racemate	Cook *et al.* (1979 b)
		4'-Hydroxypentobarbital	0.1–0.32		
		5-Ethyl-5-(3-carboxy-2-propyl) barbituric acid	0.09		
		(R)-Secobarbital	1		
		(S)-Secobarbital	83		
		(R)-Thiopental	0.9		
		(S)-Thiopental	84		
(R)-Secobarbital	1–2	3'-Hydroxy metabolite	<1		Cook (1983)
(S)-Secobarbital	1–2	3'-Hydroxy metabolite	<1		
(R)-Hexobarbital	<0.0005	Norhexobarbital	6–19	—	
(S)-Hexobarbital	0.005	Other metabolites	0.1–4	—	
(−)-Pentazocine	0.08	Racemate	51.2	Disposition in man following administration of the racemate	Nambara *et al.* (1979)
		(±)-*trans* alcohol	0.63		
		(±)-*trans* acid	<0.01		
(S)-Methadone	<1	Racemate	56	—	McGilliard *et al.* (1979)
		α-(−)-methadol	93		
		α-(−)-acetylmethadol	204		
		α-(+)-methadol	<1		
		α-(+)-acetylmethadol	1		
(R)-Methadone	3	Racemate	57	—	
		α-(+)-methadol	89		
		α-(+)-acetylmethadol	154		
		α-(−)-methadol	<1		
		α-(−)-acetylmethadol	3		

			Description	Reference
α-(−)-(3S,6S)-Acetylmethadol	0.2			
		Racemate	50.6	Disposition of	McGilliard and Olsen
		α-(+)-(3S,6R)-Acetylmethadol	<0.1	α-(−)-Acetylmethadol	(1980)
		β-(+)-(3R,6S)-Acetylmethadol	25	in dogs	
		α-(−)-(3S,6S)-Methadol	2.6		
		β-(+)-(3R,6S)-Methadol	0.3		
		(3S,6R)-Methadol	<0.1		
		(3R,6R)-Methadol	<0.1		
		(S)-Methadone	6.6		
		(R)-Methadone	<0.1		
		α-(−)-ncracetylmethadol	12		
		α-(−)-dinoracetylmethadol	<0.1		
(R)-Warfarin	3.3				
		(R,S)-4-Hydroxywarfarin	55	Disposition of enantiomers	Cook *et al.* (1979 a)
		(R,S)-7-Hydroxywarfarin	0.14	following administration of	
		(R,S)-6-Hydroxywarfarin	0.32	the racemate to rats	
		Warfarin alcohol 1	0.24		
		Warfarin alcohol 2	0.87		
		4-Hydroxycoumarin	0.07		
(S)-Warfarin	0.33				
		(R,S)-4-Hydroxywarfarin	51		
		(R,S)-7-Hydroxywarfarin	3.8		
		(R,S)-6-Hydroxywarfarin	3.0		
		Warfarin alcohol 1	1.2		
		Warfarin alcohol 2	0.04		
		4-Hydroxycoumarin	0.004		
(S)-Nicotine	5.9				
		(S)-cotinine	0.0006	—	Matsukura *et al.*
		6-Hydroxynicotine	1.7		(1975)
		Nicotine-N'-oxide	0.04		
		Nornicotine	0.03		
(S)-Bioallethrin (1R,3R,4'S)	0.75				
		Diastereoisomers of configuration:		—	Wing and Hammock
		1R,3R,4'R	57		(1979)
		1S,3S,4'S	5		
		1R,3S,4'R	2.9		
		1S,3R,4'S	2.0		
		1R,3S,4'S	<0.12		
		1S,3R,4'R	≤0.12		

using the racemic drug coupled to BSA via either formation of a succinate ester or diazotized *p*-aminobenzoic acid derivative. Many of the early studies reported selectivity towards (+)-hyoscyamine (Fasth *et al.*, 1975; Wurzburger *et al*, 1977) whilst others reported cross-reactivity with 'equal efficiency' (Berghem *et al*. 1980) or 'identically to both' enantiomers (Virtanen *et al.*,

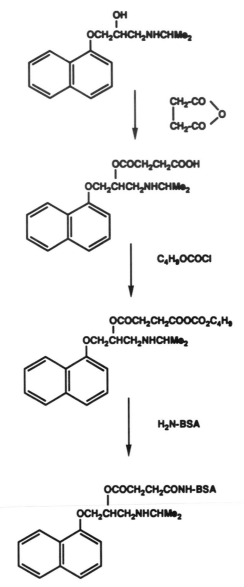

Figure 1. Propranolol immunogen synthesis by the method of Kawashima *et al.* (1976). BSA = bovine serum albumin.

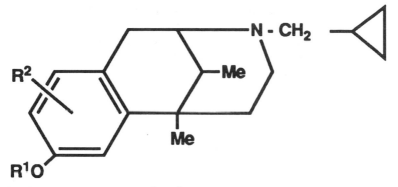

Figure 2. Structure of cyclazine ($R^1 = R^2 = H$) and two hapten-BSA conjugates: I ($R^1 = $ -CH$_2$CH$_2$CONH-BSA; $R^2 = H$) and II ($R^1 = H$; $R^2 = $ -CH$_2$NH-BSA). Immunization of rabbits using immunogens prepared from racemic cyclazine using conjugate I produced antibodies stereoselective for (−)-cyclazine, whilst II produced unequal amounts of two enantioselective antibodies (Maeda and Tsuji, 1981).

1980) even when the antigen was prepared using the (−)-isomer. Such a result may be due to the facile racemization of the pure enantiomer.

The possible problems that may arise using racemic drugs for the formation of haptens illustrates the importance of stereochemical considerations when preparing antisera to such compounds. This is not to say that antisera to racemic drugs may not be formed. For example, antibodies prepared to racemic methadone showed 50 per cent cross-reactivity to both enantiomers (Bartos *et al.*, 1977); however, the importance of an examination of the cross-reactivity to the individual isomers should be emphasized.

A solution to this problem has been proposed by Cook *et al.* (1982). During studies on the development of an RIA to a potential antimalarial agent, racemic 1-(1,3-dichloro-6-trifluoromethyl-9-phenanthryl)-3-dibutylaminopropan-l-ol, it was found that the antibodies prepared showed different selectivities for the individual isomers and the racemate. A solution to the problem was found by using a non-chiral analogue of the drug which produced essentially non-enantioselective antibodies (Figure 3; Cook *et al.*, 1982). Enantioselective antibodies could have arisen due to stereoselective formation of the hapten-carrier complex via the selective reaction of one of the chiral hapten molecules with the chiral protein. That this did not occur was shown by hydrolysis of the conjugate and determination of the optical rotation of the incorporated drug moiety which was found to be zero (Cook *et al.*, 1982).

The solution to the problem of enantioselective antibodies generated in response to racemic drugs outlined above has obvious limitations when dealing with compounds containing two or more chiral centres. This situation has been addressed by Rominger and Albert (1985) in their considerations of the drug fenoterol. Fenoterol contains two chiral centres and the marketed material is the racemate containing the enantiomers of the (RR) and (SS) configurations. Rominger and Albert (1985) have presented a theoretical analysis

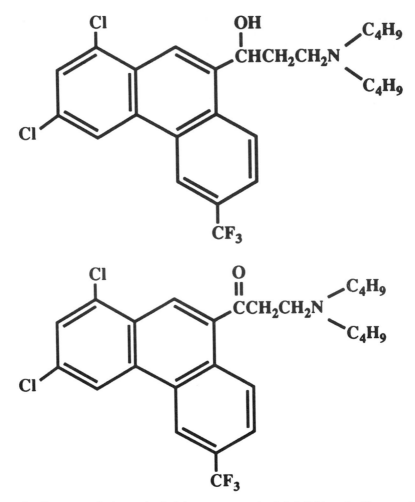

Figure 3. Structure of the antimalarial agent, racemic 1-(1,3-dichloro-6-trifluoromethyl-9-phenanthryl)-3-dibutylaminopropan-l-ol (top) and the achiral analogue (bottom) used for the preparation of a non-enantioselective RIA (Cook *et al.*, 1982).

of the situation assuming two stereospecific antibodies are produced in differing concentrations, with differing affinities and enantiomeric cross-reactivities. Assuming that one antibody has a low and the other a high cross-reactivity these authors generated a series of displacement curves for the individual isomers and the racemic drug, which are in fairly good agreement with the experimentally determined data of Cook *et al.* (1982).

The examples discussed so far and for which brief details are presented in Table 1, have involved the production of polyclonal antibodies and as yet there are few examples where monoclonal antibody production has been used for the production of enantioselective antisera. Monoclonal antibodies have been prepared and used to develop an enzyme linked immunosorbent assay (ELISA) to both (S)-nicotine and (S)-cotinine (Bjercke *et al.*, 1986). The cross-reactivity of the (S)-nicotine antibody with the (R)-enantiomer was around 4 per cent.

The above antibodies were prepared using optically active alkaloids; however, using hybridoma technology the production of enantioselective antibodies from a racemic immunogen is possible. Thus Wang *et al.*, (1986) have produced enantioselective antibodies using racemic propranolol. These authors isolated a number of hybridomas and selected two clones for further characterization, one of which showed a preference for the (S)-enantiomer, the other antibody was more specific for the (S)-enantiomer, the cross-reactivities to the racemic drug, the (S) and (R)-enantiomers being 100, 169 and 35 respectively. The hybridoma cells bearing these latter monoclonal antibodies were fixed by glutaraldehyde treatment to produce an artificial 'receptor', the specificity of which was almost identical to the soluble antibodies. The K_D of (S)-propranolol to this 'receptor' being of the same order of magnitude as that of the β-adrenergic receptor at 4.1 nM (Wang *et al.*, 1986).

A similar technique has also been used to produce antibodies to the cholinesterase inhibitor soman, a compound containing two chiral centres which exists as a mixture of four stereoisomers (Brimfield *et al.*, 1985). Two antibodies were produced following immunization of mice with a phenyldiazonium analogue of the drug conjugated to either keyhole limpet haemocyanin or BSA. One antibody-producing clone was obtained from each antigen and whilst both showed a preference for the more toxic isomers, (−)-phosphorus centres, the stereoselectivity was 'modest' for both. This was explained by the fact that the major sites for interaction with the antibodies was associated with the *t*-butyl group and the phosphonyl oxygen, i.e. a two-point interaction rather than a three-point interaction, which would be more likely to produce a stereoselective response (Brimfield *et al.*, 1985).

The further application of this technology to the problem of enantioselective immunoassays may be expected to increase over the next few years and may ultimately offer a relatively facile approach to enantiomeric analysis.

3. Radioreceptor assays

The stereoselectivity of biological systems is also utilized in the radioreceptor analysis technique. Radioreceptor analysis (RRA) is based on the competitive binding of an unlabelled ligand with a radiolabelled ligand for a specific receptor system. If a competitive ligand is added to a receptor preparation containing a fixed quantity of radiolabelled ligand the competing ligand will displace a certain amount of the radiolabel and at equilibrium the bound radioactivity remaining is a function of the quantity of the unlabelled ligand added. The quantity of unlabelled material present may be determined by reference to a standard curve prepared with the same concentration of radio-ligand and the receptor system in the presence of varying known concentrations of the unlabelled ligand (Barnett and Nahorski 1983; Crevat-Pisano *et al.*, 1986; Ferkany 1987).

RRAs have the advantages of being simple, rapid, sensitive and accurate provided that optimal conditions for ligand binding have been determined (Crevat-Pisano *et al.*, 1986). Such conditions include incubation buffer, temperature, reaction time, receptor preparation, separation of bound and free radioligand and assessment of both specific and non-specific binding (Barnett and Nahorski, 1983). Also of significance is the availability of the labelled ligand at an appropriate specific activity and also, in the present context, non-specific interference of constituents of the media under examination, e.g. plasma or serum (Barnett and Nahorski, 1983). The advantages and limitations of the technique have been discussed in detail elsewhere (Crevat-Pisano *et al.*, 1986; Barnett and Nahorski, 1983; Enna, 1985; Ferkany, 1987; Ensing and de Zeeuw, 1984).

As biological receptor systems are 'chiral' then it is not surprising that RRA may be used as an enantioselective analytical method. The enantioselectivity of such methods depends upon the relative binding affinities of the two enantiomers under examination and differences of about 100 are not uncommon. Receptor enantioselectivity is well known and it is therefore surprising that several authors have appeared to ignore this selectivity when reporting their methodology (Gould *et al.*, 1983).

Of the chiral drugs for which RRA have been developed, the β-blocking agent propranolol has received most attention; however, the reported assays vary considerably in the choice of the biological tissue used and to a lesser extent in the radioligand. Nahorski *et al.*, (1978) developed an RRA for propranolol using bovine lung membranes as the receptor system and $(-)$-$[^3H]$-dihydroalprenolol as the radioligand. The binding of the radiolabel to the tissue was found to be saturable and have a dissociation constant (K_D) of 0.95 nM. Under the conditions of the assay the K_i values, the equilibrium dissociation constant of the inhibitor, were 8×10^{-10} and 6×10^{-8} M for (S)-and (R)-propranolol respectively, the (R)-enantiomer having about 1.3 per cent of the competitive activity of the pharmacologically active (S)-enantiomer. Such K_i values facilitate the detection and quantification of drug enantiomer plasma concentrations of the order of 0.5–2 ng/ml.

One of the advantages of RRAs is that relatively crude biological samples may be used for analysis. For example, with the propranolol assay, addition of 20 μl of neat plasma, to a total assay volume of 250 μl, had no effect on the propranolol standard curve (Nahorski *et al.*, 1978). In addition the sensitivity of the assay was such that plasma samples required dilution, either 1 in 3 or 1 in 10, prior to drug determination.

RRAs are essentially bioassay systems, i.e. they are sensitive to all 'active' drug-related material present in crude samples of biological origin. This is of particular significance if pharmacologically active metabolites are likely to be present in a sample, their contribution to radioligand displacement being proportional to their affinity at the receptor system (Barnett and Nahorski, 1983). 4-Hydroxypropranolol is an active metabolite of propranolol known to contribute to the β-blocking activity of the drug. It is of interest to note that the RRA of Nahorski *et al.* (1978) yielded a K_i of 1.5×10^{-8} M for racemic 4-hydroxypropranolol, which is equivalent to about 5 per cent of the activity of the (S)-enantiomer of the drug. As this K_i value was obtained with the racemic metabolite it is likely that the majority of the activity resides in the enantiomer of the (S)-configuration. Such metabolite interactions require the results obtained from samples of pharmacokinetic or metabolic studies to be expressed in terms of 'drug enantiomer equivalents'.

The (S)-propranolol assay of Nahorski *et al.* (1978) has been modified, using a rat lung membrane tissue preparation with $(-)$-[^{3}H]-dihydroalprenolol by Barnett *et al.* (1980) and Jackman *et al.* (1981). Innis *et al.* (1978) used a calf cerebellum membrane preparation as a source of membrane bound β-receptors and $(-)$-[^{3}H]-dihydroalprenolol as the radioligand to develop an assay for propranolol. These workers found that human plasma (as little as 0.01 ml in a volume of 1.0 ml) reduced the binding of the ligand by between 25 and 40 per cent and routinely carried out their analysis using plasma dialysates. These authors were presumably measuring the (S)-enantiomer of propranolol but no statements are made in their report concerning the stereoselectivity of this method (Innis *et al.*, 1978).

A similar stereoselective RRA for (S)-propranolol using a turkey erythrocyte plasma membrane preparation and [^{125}I]iodohydroxybenzylpindolol has been described by Bilezikian *et al.* (1979). These authors also found that the presence of drug-free serum resulted in the inhibition of binding of the radioligand to the receptor. This interference necessitated extraction of the drug from serum prior to the RRA, which also had the additional advantage that two metabolites, 4-hydroxypropranolol and desisopropylpropranolol, which also interacted in the assay, were only poorly extracted into the solvent. The limit of detectability for (S)-propranolol was found to be between 0.25 and 0.50 ng/ml, which exceeds the normal therapeutic range of the drug. The analytical results obtained using this assay were compared with data generated from both HPLC and RIA methods, the correlation between the RRA and other techniques being 0.91 and 0.85 respectively. This agreement is surprising as neither of the two alternative techniques was stereospecific, and the results were interpreted by the authors as indicating that the major circulating material in plasma was (S)-propranolol (Bilezikian *et al.*, 1979).

Spahn *et al.* (1989 b) have recently developed an RRA to metoprolol using $(-)$-[^{3}H]-4-(3-*tert*-butylamino-2-hydroxypropoxybenzimidazole-2-one as the radioligand and rat salivary gland membranes and reticulocytes to determine drug activity to both β_1- and β_2-receptors respectively. The K_i values for racemic metoprolol to the β_1- and β_2-receptors were 67 and 1390 nM respectively and the β_1 preparation was examined with respect to the enantioselectivity of the assay. The K_i value for the (S)-enantiomer was found to be 85 nM compared to a value of 4 μM for the (R)-isomer, and the detection limit was found to be 1–2 ng/ml. The RRA was used to determine the plasma (S)-metoprolol concentrations following the administration of the racemic drug to extensive (EM) and poor metabolizers (PM) of sparteine. The results obtained from the RRA were compared with those obtained using a stereospecific HPLC method involving precolumn derivatization with (R)-phenylethylisocyanate to yield a pair of diastereoisomeric urea derivatives (see below). Good analytical agreement was found between the two methodologies and, in addition, the plasma concentrations of (S)-metoprolol were above the K_i value for a significantly longer period, up to 24 hours post drug administration, in the PM subject compared to the EM subject (Spahn *et al.*, 1989 b).

The problems associated with the development of an RIA to atropine have been referred to above. Aaltonen *et al.* (1984) have compared the results obtained from a pharmacokinetic study using the RIA method of Virtanen *et al.* (1980) with a radioreceptor assay. These workers used a rat brain tissue preparation and [^{3}H]-quinuclidinylbenzilate radioligand for the RRA. The binding of the radioligand was found to be saturable and of high affinity with a K_D of 0.48 nM, the K_i value for atropine being 1.21 nmol/l and (−)-hyoscyamine, the active enantiomer, was reported to be 'about twice as potent as atropine' (Aaltonen *et al.*, 1984). Using this method neat plasma or serum could be used in the assay, 25 μl of drug free plasma being found to decrease total radioligand binding by about 0.5–2 per cent.

Plasma samples, obtained from a pharmacokinetic study following administration of atropine, were analysed using both RIA and RRA. It was found that the area under the plasma concentration time curves were between two to three times greater using data from the RIA compared to the RRA and also the RRA data indicated a more complex model to describe the plasma pharmacokinetics of the drug than did the RIA data (Aaltonen *et al.*, 1984). As the RIA of Virtanen *et al.* (1980) is reputed to have equal cross-reactivity to both (−)-hyoscyamine and atropine, the RIA data may be interpreted as being due to the sum of the plasma (+)- and (−)-hyoscyamine concentrations whilst the RRA data is due solely to the (−) enantiomer. This would appear to be an example where the limitations of non-specific RIA lead to data which are of limited value, whereas the data from the RRA give a clearer indication of enantiomer disposition.

4. *Chromatographic methods of enantiomeric resolution*

The most significant advances in enantiomeric analysis over the last ten years have been made in the area of chiral chromatographic techniques and several useful monographs and reviews have appeared in this area describing the applicability of the wide variety of systems presently available (Konig, 1987; Zief and Crane, 1988; Allenmark, 1988; Gal, 1987; Testa, 1986; Vermeulen and Testa, 1988). The object of this section is to briefly examine the available methodologies and to illustrate the applications of these systems and the potential problems associated with their use in the bioanalytical area.

Two main approaches to enantiomeric analysis are available to the bioanalyst:

1. formation of stable diastereoisomeric derivatives, the so-called indirect resolution approach, by reaction of the analyte(s) under examination with an optically pure chiral derivatizing agent (CDA) involving a precolumn derivatization step during sample 'work up';
2. formation of unstable diastereoisomeric complexes or direct resolution approach, involving formation of labile diastereoisomeric complexes between the analyte(s) and a chiral environment arising from either a chiral stationary phase (CSP) in HPLC or GC or a chiral mobile phase additive (CMPA) in HPLC.

A chiral environment may also be provided by the detector system, both polarimetric and circular dichroic detectors having been described for HPLC analysis. Also it should not be forgotten that many metabolic processes yield diastereoisomeric derivatives which may be readily separated by chromatographic procedures (see below).

Chromatographic separation of compounds may be assessed by two parameters, the separation factor (α) and the resolution factor (R) (see Figure 4).

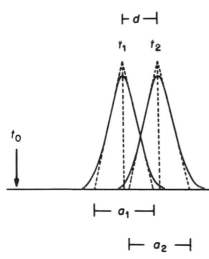

retention time : t_1

capacity factor: $k_1' = (t_1 - t_0)/t_0$

separation factor: $\alpha = k_2'/k_1'$

resolution factor: $R = 2d/(a_1 + a_2)$

peak separation	α	R
no	1	0
yes, useless		0 – 0·5
yes, fair	>1	0·5 – 1
yes, good		>1

Figure 4. Idealized chromatogram illustrating chromatographic definitions, where t_0, t_1 and t_2 are the retention times of a non-retained compound and the first and second eluting peaks, respectively, and a_1 and a_2 are the baseline peak widths of the first and second eluting peaks. Reproduced from Testa (1986) with permission of the author and *Xenobiotica*.

The separation factor is defined thus:

$$\alpha = \frac{k_2^1}{k_1^1}$$

where k_1^1 and k_2^1 are the capacity ratios of the first and second eluting peaks respectively, the capacity ratio being defined as the ratio of the difference between the retention volume of an analyte and a non-retained solute (i.e. the void volume of the system) to the void volume. The capacity ratio is directly related to the equilibrium distribution constant (K) of the analyte between the chromatographic mobile phase and stationary phase. This may be related to the free energy of adsorption of the process by:

$$\Delta G = - RT \ln K$$

and the difference in free energies (ΔG) for a pair of enantiomers may be related to the separation factor (α) by:

$$\Delta(\Delta G) = - RT \ln \alpha$$

The separation factor is a measure of relative peak separation and is independent of the column size, particle size, flow rate or how well the column is packed and is a constant under a given set of conditions, e.g. stationary phase, mobile phase and temperature. From a practical viewpoint α is of limited value, as values greater than 1 indicate that peak separation has occurred but yield no information on how good the resolution is in terms of peak separation or utility of the system for analytical or preparative separation of enantiomers. A more practically useful parameter is the *resolution factor* (R) which is given by:

$$R = \frac{2d}{(a_1 + a_2)}$$

where d is the difference between the retention times of the two peaks and a_1 and a_2 are the baseline peak widths of the first and second eluting peaks respectively. Resolution is a measure of the completeness of the separation and depends on the magnitude of α and also on the column efficiency and hence particle size, column size, column packing and flow rate, etc. An R value $\geqslant 1$ indicates effectively complete band separation.

Indirect methods of separation

The indirect method of chromatographic resolution has been known for a number of years and is the most common approach applied in drug metabolism studies. However, until relatively recently such separations were carried out in an empirical manner; only recently have systematic studies been carried out and the mechanisms of the resolution examined and it is presently appreciated that broad classes of diastereoisomeric derivatives exhibit chromatographic separability.

Covalent diastereoisomeric derivatives may be readily prepared using a variety of chiral reagents, however, several problems may arise from the use of such reagents all of which may affect the conclusions drawn from the analysis. These include:

1. The enantiomeric purity of CDA. Ideally the CDA should be 100 per cent enantiomerically pure and also be both chemically and stereochemically stable to storage. If the CDA is not 100 per cent enantiomerically pure, then the stereochemical purity of the material should be known so that the analytical results obtained may be 'corrected' for the enantiomeric contamination. It may be possible to obtain useful data using CDAs which contain low concentrations of contaminating enantiomers; however, analysis of the results obtained will be necessarily complex. If this methodology is used to determine the enantiomeric purity of an 'optically pure' analyte, i.e. detect trace quantities of an enantiomeric impurity, then it is essential that the CDA be 100 per cent pure if useful data is to be obtained. It should be noted that several CDAs are now available resulting from chemical modification of natural products, e.g. carbohydrates, hence they are likely to be of very high or total optically purity.

2. The CDA should react quantitatively with the analyte. If quantitative derivatization does not occur then care must be taken to ensure that stereoselective derivatization or kinetic resolution has not taken place, i.e. is the measured ratio of diastereoisomers equal to that of the starting enantiomeric ratio. It is, therefore, essential to examine the time course of the derivatization reaction.

Published accounts of derivatization methods frequently do not state the overall reaction yield and data are presented as 'final values' or as derivative recovery on a percentage basis. Such data is of limited value and is potentially highly misleading in an analysis of the derivatization step. Our studies on the resolution of the 2-arylpropionic acid derivative pirprofen, using (S)-1-(naphthen-1-yl)ethylamine as a CDA were greatly eased as the availability of the individual enantiomers of the acid enabled us to prepare synthetic samples of the required diastereoisomeric amide derivatives prior to an examination of the derivatization step. Using these derivatives it was possible to determine the optimal conditions for the derivatization reaction, to show that product yields were in excess of 90 per cent and that the reaction was not stereoselective (Hutt *et al.*, 1986; Hutt and Caldwell, 1988 b). We have since used the same technique for the determination of the enantiomeric composition of both 2-phenylpropionic acid and ibuprofen in animal and human samples (Fournel and Caldwell, 1986; Avgerinos and Hutt, 1987).

Care is also required when transferring what may be regarded as a general derivatization method to related compounds. We have recently used the above technique to derivatize the enantiomers of tiaprofenic acid and found on resolution by HPLC that the yields of the two products were different, hence kinetic resolution may be taking place with this 2-arylpropionic acid analogue.

3. The derivatization reaction should take place under conditions such that racemization of either the analyte or the CDA does not occur. Some CDAs, particularly those based on derivatives of L-proline, have attained notoriety due to their stereochemical instability, enantiomeric impurity and unpredictable racemization. Silber and Riegelman (1980), in the first report of a chromatographic method for the determination of the enantiomers of propranolol, found that commercially available N-trifluoroacetyl-L-prolyl chloride (TPC) was contaminated with its optical antipode to the extent of between 4 and 15 per cent and rapidly underwent racemization on storage. Using a sample which they prepared themselves, of greater than 98 per cent enantiomeric purity, these authors found that the extent of racemization of the reagent during derivatization of the drug varied considerably with temperature, up to 25 per cent at $60°$ C and hence the derivatization reaction was carried out at $-78°$ C where less than 2 per cent racemization was observed (Silber and Riegelman, 1980). Similarly, problems were also found by Adams *et al.* (1982) who attempted to resolve the enantiomers of ketamine using (S,S)-N-trifluoroacetylproline anhydride as a CDA. It was found that the reaction proceeded stereoselectively, in poor yield and with racemization of the acylating agent.

4. Detection. Ideally both diastereoisomers will respond identically to the detector system. If this does not occur then appropriate analytical corrections must be made. There are relatively few reports in which the differential detector response of diastereoisomeric derivatives has been addressed. A recently published example will serve to illustrate the point. Lindner *et al.* (1984) systematically examined a range of O-diacyl and O-dialkyl derivatives of (R,R)-tartaric acid anhydride for their suitability as CDAs for a range of fifteen β-blocking drugs. The advantage of these agents as CDAs is that the secondary hydroxyl group of the alkanolamines react to yield a monoester with the anhydride and the free carboxyl group so formed appears to form an internal salt with the basic secondary amino functions, (Figure 5) resulting in chromatographic resolution values of between 4 and 6 (Lindner *et al.*, 1984). On adaptation of this method for the quantitative determination of the enantiomers of propranolol in human plasma using (R,R)-O,O-diacetyltartaric acid as the CDA, the ratio of the peak areas of the two derivatives, determined by UV, differed by a factor of 1.08. This could be accounted for by differences in the yield of the diastereoisomers; however, that selective derivatization was not the cause was shown by the quantitative yield of the derivatives. Examination of the diastereoisomers by fluorescence indicated greater differences, the (S)-propranolol derivative being 20 per cent less fluorescence active than the (R)-enantiomer derivative. Similar results were also

observed with the internal standard, the racemate of the t-butyl analogue of propranolol (Lindner *et al.*, 1989).

Careful choice of the CDA may well facilitate analysis by, for example, increasing the sensitivity of detection, e.g. fluorinated derivatives for use with GC electron capture detectors or fluorescent derivatives for HPLC.

For reaction with a CDA it is obviously essential for the analyte under investigation to contain a functional group which may be readily derivatized. An additional complication may arise if the analyte contains two potentially reactive functional groups. For example, reaction of either (R) or (S)-1-phenylethylisocyanate with the aryloxypropanolamine β-blocking agents, e.g. propranolol, may potentially yield either urea or carbamate derivatives depending on the site of reaction with the secondary amine or alcohol functions respectively (Thompson *et al.*, 1982). It is, therefore, of considerable importance to characterize the product of such derivatizations. Additionally, the diastereoisomeric derivatives formed may also contain functional groups which interfere with the chromatography, resulting in either poor peak shape and/or incomplete resolution of the derivatives. Such groups may need to be masked by derivatization with an achiral reagent.

The chromatographic separation of a pair of diastereoisomeric derivatives is enhanced by such factors as the close proximity of the chiral centres (ideally these should be three to four atoms apart), and conformational rigidity of groups in the region of the chiral centre. For example, resolution may be enhanced if one of the chiral centres is part of a ring system or if the groups surrounding the chiral centres are bulky and hence conformationally inflexible, and also if either polar or polarizable groups are in relatively close proximity to the chiral centres (Helmchen *et al.*, 1979; Helmchen and Nill, 1979; Pirkle and Finn, 1983; Feitsma and Drenth, 1988). The final choice of CDA will obviously depend on the specific application. For example, if preparative resolution of diastereoisomers is required in order to obtain the original compound in an enantiomerically pure form then the formation of either amide or ester derivatives is preferable as there are several methods, e.g. diazotization or mild hydrolysis, which allow cleavage of the derivatives under mild conditions which will not result in racemization. Under such circumstances, the cost of the CDA may also be of some significance. Isolation of the diastereoisomeric derivatives as such may be required for determination of analyte absolute configuration by, for example, NMR. Many of the synthetic CDAs are available as both enantiomeric forms which is of significance as the elution order of the analyte(s) may be reversed by reversing the chirality of the CDA so that the minor component present in a non-racemic mixture of enantiomers may be eluted from the column first resulting in an increase in analytical sensitivity.

An additional problem that is of particular relevance is the incorrect configurational designation of some CDAs found in some companies' catalogues. For example, the two enantiomers of 1-phenylethylisocyanate have been incorrectly assigned absolute configurations and sign of optical rotation (Thompson *et al.*, 1982). It is also of interest to note that Mosher's acid, α-methoxy-α-trifluoromethylphenylacetic acid, changes configurational designation on formation of the acid chloride, i.e. the acid enantiomer of the (S)-absolute configuration becomes the (R)-acylchloride for the same three-dimensional spatial arrangement about the chiral centre (Dale and Mosher, 1973), a point which appears to be lost on some manufacturers. As this reagent is frequently used for determination of absolute configuration of alcohols and amines by NMR it is of some significance that the spatial arrangement about the chiral centre is known with certainty (Davis *et al.*, 1985; Drummond *et al.*, 1989).

The most commonly used CDAs are those which involve formation of either amide or ester bonds; relatively few examples yielding alkylated or other derivatives are known.

Chiral acylating agents

A wide variety of reagents have been used as acylating agents, e.g. acid chlorides, acyl imidazole derivatives and acid anhydrides.

In spite of the potential problems associated with the use of CDAs based on L-proline, referred to previously, these reagents remain useful, provided appropriate precautions are taken and also as the stereochemical instability does not extend to all such derivatives. Examples of reagents based on L-proline are given in Figure 6.

An enantiospecific GC assay for fenfluramine, and its dealkylated metabolite norfenfluramine, has been developed using heptafluorobutyryl-(S)-prolyl chloride (Srinivas *et al.*, 1988). The use of the heptafluorobutyryl derivative in combination with an electron-capture detector facilitated analysis of the drug and metabolite enantiomers in plasma for 96 and 168 hours respectively post drug administration. The same reagent has been used by Roy and Lim (1988) for the derivatization of methoxyphenamine and its metabolites (Figure 7). Resolution of the diastereoisomeric derivatives was carried out using capillary GC. The two amines methoxyphenamine and 2-methoxyamphetamine, on derivatization yield a pair of monoderivatized diastereoisomers whereas the two phenolic metabolites yielded mixtures of the mono and di-derivatized diastereoisomers, and in addition, stereoselective derivatization was observed for 2-hydroxymethamphetamine (Roy and Lim, 1988). This example serves to illustrate the difficulties which may arise when two reactive groups are present in an analyte.

A GC method for the determination of the enantiomeric composition of 3,4-methylenedioxymethamphetamine and 3,4-methylenedioxyamphetamine in micro samples (200µl) of whole blood has been reported by Fitzgerald *et al.*, (1989). The method involves liquid–liquid extraction of the drugs from blood followed by on-column derivatization using N-trifluoroacetyl-L-prolyl chloride. The derivatization was carried out by injecting a chloroform

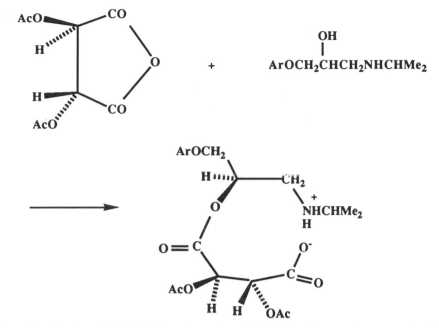

Figure 5. Reaction of (R,R)-0,0-diacetyltartaric acid anhydride with an aryloxypropanolamine to yield intramolecularly ion-paired diastereoisomeric esters.

solution (3 μl) of the drugs together with 1 μl of a 0.1 M solution of the derivatizing agent in CHCl₃, rapidly into the gas chromatograph which was equipped with a split liner packed with 5 mm of OV-101 on 80–100 mesh supelcoport held in place with silanized glass wool. Under the conditions used, no racemization of the reagent was observed (Fitzgerald *et al.*, 1989).

A new CDA based on L-proline, (S)-N-1-(2-naphthylsulphonyl)-2-pyrrolidine carbonyl chloride (Figure 6) has been prepared by Shimizu *et al.* (1986). This reagent has been used to resolve the enantiomers of the drug diltiazem (Figure 8) by HPLC. The drug contains two chiral centres and therefore exists as four isomeric forms, i.e. two enantiomeric pairs. Interestingly the compound does not possess a functional group suitable for derivatization and the first step in the derivatization procedure was the base catalysed hydrolysis of the acetate ester to yield the corresponding alcohol which subsequently undergoes derivatization with the acyl chloride (Shimizu *et al.*, 1986).

Banfield and Rowland (1983) have used carbobenzyloxy-L-proline to prepare diastereoisomeric ester derivatives of the enantiomers of warfarin (Figure 9). The coupling of the CDA and the analyte(s) was achieved using dicyclohexylcarbodiimide in the presence of imidazole as a catalyst; other diimides, e.g. 1-cyclohexyl-3-(2-morpholinoethyl)carbodiimide metho-*p*-cleaving, following resolution by HPLC, which was achieved by mixing the failed to react or gave incomplete derivatization. Resolution of the esters was

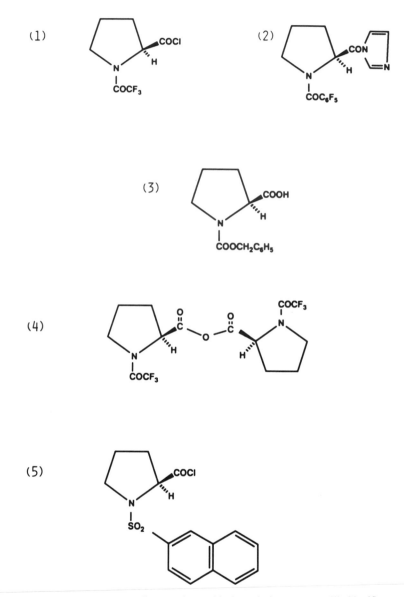

Figure 6. Derivatives of L-proline used as chiral acylating agents: (1) N-trifluoroacetyl-L-prolylchloride; (2) N-pentafluorobenzoyl-L-prolylimidazolide; (3) carbobenzyloxy-L-proline; (4) (S,S)-N-trifluoroacetylproline anhydride; (5) (S)-N-1-(2-naphthylsulphonyl)-2-pyrrolidine carbonyl chloride.

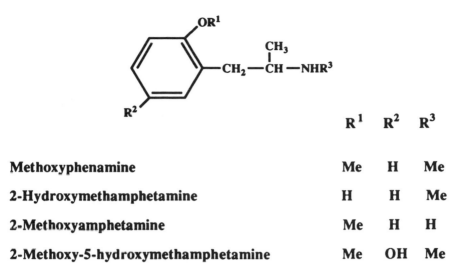

	R^1	R^2	R^3
Methoxyphenamine	Me	H	Me
2-Hydroxymethamphetamine	H	H	Me
2-Methoxyamphetamine	Me	H	H
2-Methoxy-5-hydroxymethamphetamine	Me	OH	Me

Figure 7. Methoxyphenamine and three dealkylated and hydroxylated metabolites.

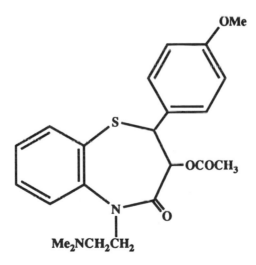

Figure 8. Structure of diltiazem.

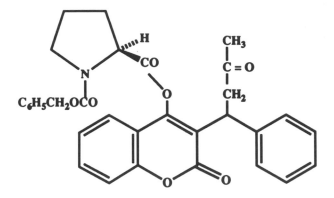

Figure 9. Structure of warfarin carbobenzyloxy-L-prolyl diastereoisomeric esters.

achieved using a silica HPLC column, an ethylacetate-hexane-methanol-acetic acid mobile phase and detection was carried out using a UV detector. The method was found to be suitable for the determination of the enantiomers in plasma following either administration of large single oral doses of the racemate or for subjects on chronic warfarin therapy. These workers later extended their method to enable analysis of the major metabolites of the drug to be carried out and also increased the analytical sensitivity by use of a fluorescence detector (Banfield and Rowland, 1984). The enantiomers of the drug and metabolites were derivatized as described above and resolved using the same HPLC system. The derivatized esters were not fluorescent and required cleaving, following resolution by HPLC, which was achieved by mixing the HPLC eluent with a post column reagent containing *n*-butylamine and methanol (1 : 1) and passing the whole through a bed reactor packed with glass beads. The residence time in the bed reactor was about 1.5 min, which did not result in any significant band broadening; aminolysis of the ester derivatives occurred and produced fluorescent species. The analytical method allowed determination of both enantiomers of the unchanged drug and the 6- and 7-hydroxylated metabolites, together with two of the diastereoisomeric alcohol reduction products, and yielded good correlations when compared to a GC-mass spectrometry assay method using stable isotopes (Banfield and Rowland, 1984).

Other useful acylating agents include the enantiomers of O-methylmandelic acid and α-methoxy-α-trifluoromethylphenylacetic acid (MTPA). (R)-O-methylmandelic acid, activated by formation of the acylchloride, has been used to derivatize the enantiomers of tocainide which were resolved by normal phase HPLC (Hoffman *et al.*, 1984). MTPA is of particular interest as a CDA as, lacking a hydrogen on the carbon α to the carboxyl group, it is

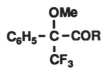

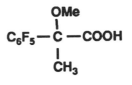

R = OH

R = Cl

Figure 10. Derivatives of phenylacetic acid used as acylating CDAs. Left: α-methoxy-α-trifluoromethylphenylacetic acid (R = OH) and the corresponding acylchloride (R = Cl) and right, α-methyl-α-methoxypentafluorophenylacetic acid.

stereochemically stable (Figure 10). As a result of this stability several authors have compared results obtained with this reagent to those obtained with N-trifluoroacetyl-L-prolyl-chloride (Nichols *et al.*, 1983; Gal, 1977). Davis *et al.* (1985) have developed a reverse phase HPLC method for the determination of the enantiomeric composition of the alcohols produced by the ketone reduction of pentoxifylline, following the formation of diastereoisomeric esters using (R)-MTPA.

A similar reagent to the above is (+)-α-methyl-α-methoxypentafluoro-phenylacetic acid (MMPA, Figure 10) a reagent originally reported by Pohl and Trager (1973) for the acylation of a variety of amphetamines. The derivatization reaction being carried out using 1,1′-carbonyldiimidazole, to yield an activated imidazolide, which subsequently reacts with the amine. This reagent has recently been utilized for the GC resolution of the enantiomers of the antiviral drug rimantadine (Miwa *et al.*, 1988). The derivatization reaction was carried out using dicyclohexylcarbodiimide as the coupling agent, in the presence of 1-hydroxybenzotriazole (1-HOBT). The two diastereoisomers were resolved by capillary GC and quantified by selective ion monitoring negative-ion-chemical-ionization mass-spectrometry and stable isotope dilution using the tetradeutero racemic drug as internal standard (Miwa *et al.*, 1988). It was noted that the peak heights of the two diastereoisomeric derivatives varied from 1:2 to about 1:1 for a given set of samples; however, the use of the tetradeuterated internal standard enabled quantification to be carried out.

Spahn and co-workers have utilized the fluorescent properties of some of the chiral 2-arylpropionic acid non-steroidal anti-inflammatory drugs, namely benoxaprofen, flunoxaprofen and naproxen (Figure 11), for the analysis of the enantiomers of a variety of chiral amines and alcohols by both TLC and HPLC (Spahn *et al.*, 1984; Weber *et al.* 1984; Spahn, 1988 a,b). Both naproxen and flunoxaprofen are marketed as the (S)-(+)-enantiomers and hence offer advantages over benoxaprofen which was available as a racemate and hence required resolution before use as a CDA. Some care is required

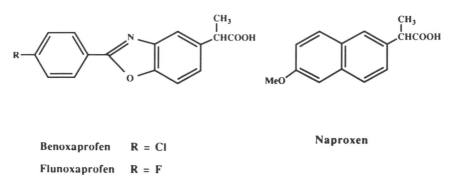

Benoxaprofen　R = Cl

Flunoxaprofen　R = F

Naproxen

Figure 11.　2-Arylpropionic acids used as CDAs due to their fluorescent properties.

when using naproxen as a CDA as Singh *et al.* (1986) have found (S)-naproxen to be contaminated with small quantities of the (R)-enantiomer. Büyüktimkin *et al.* (1988) have used (S)-naproxen as a CDA for the determination of the enantiomeric composition of a variety of amino acid methyl esters by GC. The use of these reagents has been reported for the determination of the enantiomeric composition of β-blocking drugs in urine (Pflugmann *et al.*, 1987 a) and for the determination of baclofen and its fluoro analogue, in both urine and plasma (Spahn *et al.*, 1988 a).

Reid *et al.* (1989) have recently reported a similar approach for the analysis of the enantiomers of cyclophosphamide in human plasma (Figure 12). The initial step in the derivatization reaction involves amidoalkylation of cyclophosphamide using anhydrous chloral. This reaction proved to be problematical due to the formation of several by-products thought to be associated with the instability of the aldehyde, which was solved by the addition of dimethylformamide (1 per cent) to the chloral. The initial reaction results in the formation of a carbinolamine derivative which may be relatively easily acylated. Also a second chiral centre is introduced into the molecule which could give rise to a series of diastereoisomeric products. On analysis of the products formed on reaction of racemic and the individual enantiomers of cyclophosphamide, by both normal and reverse phase chromatography, only one peak was observed and the authors concluded that either the reaction takes place in a highly stereospecific manner or that the possible diastereoisomers could not be resolved using their systems (Reid *et al.*, 1989). The final step in the derivatization involved reaction of the carbinolamine with (S)-naproxen acylchloride in the presence of a catalyst, 4-dimethylaminopyridine. Under these conditions, the reaction was found to go to completion within 20 min at room temperature. The diastereoisomers produced were easily resolved by both normal and reverse phase HPLC and examination of plasma samples indicated that drug concentrations at 100 ng/ml could be detected (Reid *et al.*, 1989).

Other recently reported applications using acylating agents as CDAs include

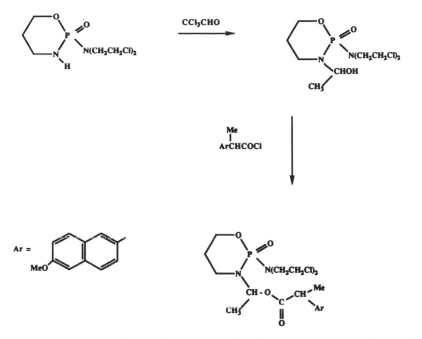

Figure 12. Derivatization of cyclophosphamide using (S)-naproxen acyl chloride as a CDA (Reid *et al.*, 1989).

the resolution of the enantiomers of the bronchodilator proxyphylline using camphanoyl chloride (Ruud-Christensen and Salvesen, 1984) and (+)-endo-1,4,5,6,7,7-hexachlorobicyclo[2.2.1]hept-5-ene-2-carboxylic acid (HCA; Figure 13) for the resolution of the enantiomers of hydroxylated aza-aromatic hydrocarbons (Duke and Holder, 1988). This latter report is of particular interest as a comparison of the utility of (+)-HCA, (+)-MTPA and (−)-menthoxyacetic acid as CDAs is presented.

Chiral amines and alcohols

Compared to amines there are relatively few examples of alcohols being used for the formation of diastereoisomeric derivatives. This is probably due to the relative instability of esters (Testa, 1986) and also the resolution of esters, on silica and alumina columns, is generally not as good as that of the corresponding amides (Pirkle and Finn, 1983). This may be due to the lack of the amide hydrogen which is capable of hydrogen bonding interactions with the adsorbent.

Examples of the use of alcohols as derivatizing agents include (S)-2-octanol for the resolution of the NSAIDs ibuprofen (Lee *et al.*, 1984) and naproxen (Johnson *et al.*, 1979), and Ballard *et al.* (1983) have describe the synthesis of 0-menthyl-N,N'-diisopropylisourea from (−)-menthol (Figure 14). This

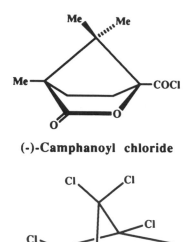

(-)-Camphanoyl chloride

endo-1,4,5,6,7,7-hexachlorobicyclo[2.2.1]hept-5-ene-2-carboxylic acid

Figure 13.   Structures of alternative acylation agents used as CDAs.

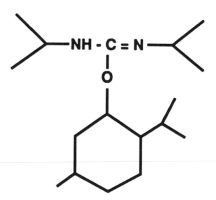

Figure 14.   O-((−)-menthyl)-N,N′-diisopropylisourea CDA used for the preparation of diastereoisomeric esters.

Table 2. Chiral amines used for the chromatographic resolution of the enantiomers of some 2-arylpropionic acid and related chiral acidic NSAIDs.

Amine CDA	Derivatization method†	Acid	Chromatography	Reference
(S)-2-Aminobutane	1	2-[3-(2-Chlorophenoxyphenyl)] propionic acid	Normal phase HPLC	Tamegai et al. (1979)
(R) or (S)-1-Phenylethylamine	1	Ibuprofen	GC	Brooks and Gilbert (1974)
	1	Indoprofen	GC	Tosolini et al. (1974)
	3	Ibuprofen	GC	Van Giessen and Kaiser (1975)
		2-[4-(2-Hydroxy-2-methylpropyl) phenyl]propionic acid	GC	Kaiser et al. (1976)
		2-[4-(2-carboxypropyl)phenyl] propionic acid	Capillary GC	Young et al. (1986)
	3	Benoxaprofen	GC	Bopp et al. (1979)
	3	Benoxaprofen	Normal phase HPLC	McKay et al. (1979)
		Ketoprofen		
		Fenoprofen		
	1	Benoxaprofen	TLC	Simmonds et al. (1980)
	4	Clidanac	TLC	Tamura et al. (1981)
	3	Carprofen	Normal phase HPLC	Kemmerer et al. (1979)
			Normal phase HPLC	Stoltenborg et al. (1981)
	3	2-Phenylpropionic acid	Normal phase HPLC	Maitre et al. (1984)
		Ibuprofen		
		Naproxen		
		2-(2-Naphthyl)propionic acid		
		2-(4-Biphenyl)propionic acid		
		Flurbiprofen		
		Cicloprofen		
		Carprofen		
		Suprofen		
	3	Fenoprofen	GC	Rubin et al. (1985)
	3	2-Phenylpropionic acid	GC	Yamaguchi and Nakamura (1985)
	1	2-Phenylpropionic acid	Normal phase HPLC	Sallustio et al. (1986)
		Ketoprofen		
		Fenoprofen		
	3	Flunoxaprofen	Reverse phase HPLC	Pedrazzini et al. (1987)
	2	Etodolac	Normal phase HPLC	Jamali et al. (1988)

(continued)

Table 2. (*Continued*).

Amine CDA	Derivatization method†	Acid	Chromatography	Reference
(R) or (S)-l-(Naphthen-1-yl) ethylamine	4	2-Phenylpropionic acid Ibuprofen Carprofen Pirprofen Pirprofen 'pyrrole'	Normal phase HPLC	Fournel and Caldwell (1986) Hutt *et al.* (1986)
(S)-1-(4-Dimethylaminonaphthen -l-yl) ethylamine	4 2	Ibuprofen Ibuprofen	Normal phase HPLC Reverse phase HPLC	Avgerinos and Hutt (1987) Mehvar *et al.* (1988 b)
	4	Ibuprofen Indoprofen Naproxen	Normal phase HPLC	Goto *et al.* (1980)
	4 4	Naproxen Loxoprofen *cis* and *trans* mono hydroxylated metabolites	Normal phase HPLC Normal phase HPLC	Goto *et al.* (1982) Nagashima *et al.* (1985)
(−) or (+)-1-(1-Anthryl) ethylamine and (−) or (+)- 1-(2-anthryl)ethylamine	4	Naproxen	Normal phase HPLC	Goto *et al.* (1986)

Chiral reagent	No.	Compound	Method	Reference
(R) or (S)-Amphetamine	3	Ibuprofen Ketoprofen Naproxen Fenoprofen Flurbiprofen Pirprofen Cicloprofen Tiaprofenic acid Etodolac	Capillary GC	Singh *et al.* (1986)
L-Leucinamide	2 2	Indoprofen Ketoprofen	Reverse phase HPLC Reverse phase HPLC	Bjorkman (1985) Bjorkman (1987) Foster and Jamali (1987)
	2	Benoxaprofen Carprofen Cicloprofen Fluncaprofen Flurbiprofen Indoprofen Naproxen Pirprofen	Reverse phase HPLC	Spahn (1987)
	2 2 2 2	Flurbiprofen Fenoprofen Tiaprofenic acid‡ Carprofen	Reverse phase HPLC Reverse phase HPLC Reverse phase HPLC Reverse phase HPLC	Berry and Jamali (1988) Mehvar and Jamali (1988 a) Mehvar *et al.* (1988 a) Spahn *et al.* (1988 b)

† Derivatization method used to activate the carboxylic acid prior to reaction with the chiral amine CDA (see Figure 16)
‡ Ethylchloroformate replaced by trichloroethylchloroformate

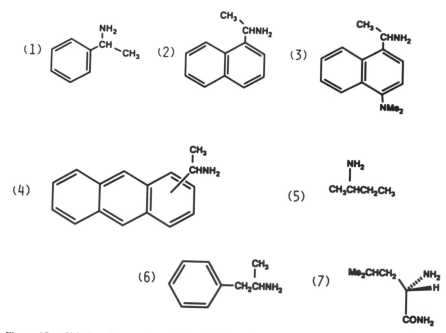

Figure 15. Chiral amines used as CDAs: (1) (R)-and (S)-1-phenylethylamine; (2) (R)-and (S)-1-(naphthen-l-yl) ethylamine; (3) (R)-and (S)-1-(4-dimethylaminonaphthen-l-yl)ethylamine; (4) (−)-1-(1-anthryl)ethylamine and (−)-1-(2-anthryl)ethylamine; (5) (S)-2-aminobutane; (6) (R)-and (S)-amphetamine; (7) L-leucinamide.

reagent has been used to prepare diastereoisomeric esters of mandelic acid and naphthoxylactic acid, a metabolite of propranolol. The menthol esters obtained were resolved by capillary GC and their structures confirmed by mass spectrometry (Ballard *et al.*, 1983).

In contrast to the above a wide variety of chiral amines have been used as CDAs (Figure 15). The variety of techniques used for the resolution of chiral carboxylic acids using amine CDAs may be illustrated using the 2-aryl-propionic acid NSAIDs as examples. This class of compounds has been the subject of some interest in recent years due to their metabolic chiral inversion in both animals and man (Hutt and Caldwell, 1983; Caldwell *et al.* 1988 c). A summary of the various amine CDAs and techniques applied to their analysis is presented in Table 2.

The derivatization reaction requires prior chemical activation of the carboxyl group and this may be achieved in one of four ways (Figure 16). Amongst the favoured methods one of the most commonly used is formation of an imidazolide via reaction of the acid with 1,1′-carbonyldiimidazole (Maitre *et al.*, 1984; Van Giessen and Kaiser, 1975; Singh *et al.*, 1986; Pedraz-zini *et al.*, 1987). There are several disadvantages associated with this method, e. g. formation of N,N′-disubstituted urea derivatives unless acetic acid is added to the reaction mixture before the chiral amine (Van Giessen and

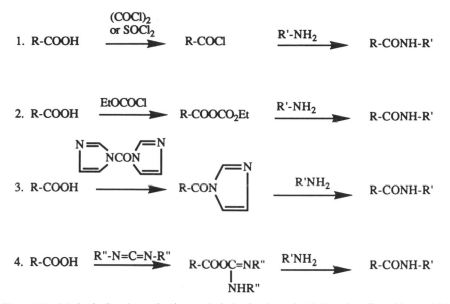

Figure 16. Methods for the activation and derivatization of chiral carboxylic acids to yield diastereoisomeric amides: (1) formation of acylchlorides using thionyl and oxalyl chlorides; (2) formation of mixed anhydrides using ethylchloroformate; (3) reaction with 1,1'-carbonyldiimidazole to yield an imidazolide; (4) reaction with a carbodiimide to yield an O-acyldialkylisourea derivative.

Kaiser, 1975). In addition, for the derivatization to take place the conditions seem to vary considerably. Some workers, for example, find the reaction to proceed relatively easily at room temperature in about 30 min (Maitre *et al.*, 1984; Rubin *et al.*, 1985; Pedrazzini *et al.*, 1987) whilst others indicate that a reaction time of 2 hours at 85° C is required (Singh *et al.*, 1986). These differences in conditions are presumably associated with the concentrations of the activating agent used as the optimal concentration remains the subject of some debate (Maitre *et al.*, 1984; Singh *et al.*, 1986). Singh *et al.*(1986) have observed additional chromatographic peaks when the concentration of the carbonyldiimidazole reagent is increased to the milligram range used by other workers, their own studies using very low quantities of the activating agent (low microgram range).

An alternative method of amine bond formation involves the use of a carbodiimide (Figure 16). During studies on the derivatization of pirprofen (Hutt *et al.*, 1986; Hutt and Caldwell, 1988 b), we investigated the application of two such reagents, namely dicyclohexylcarbodiimide (DCC) and 1-(3-dimethylaminopropyl)-3-ethylcarbodiimide. Using DCC to derivatize the enantiomers of pirprofen using (S)-1-(naphthen-1-yl) ethylamine, the chromatograms produced showed additional peaks which were not due to either the amine, the acid or the required diastereoisomeric amides. Isolation of the major contaminant and examination by direct insertion mass spectrometry indicated the material to be due to the intermediate adduct (Figure 16, equation 4) formed between the diimide and the carboxylic acid. Changing to the alternative diimide resulted in a more efficient reaction and no additional peaks (Hutt and Caldwell, 1988 b). This example, together with that cited previously of Banfield and Rowland (1983), indicates the importance of examining several compounds within a chemical group rather than dismissing a class of activating agent if one does not react satisfactorily. One disadvantage of the diimide reaction is the time course of the derivatization, which may be up to 2 hours to attain a yield in excess of 90 per cent (Avgerinos and Hutt, 1987; Hutt *et al.*, 1986).

A more rapid derivatization procedure for these compounds has been developed by Björkman (1985; 1987). This method involves reaction of the acid with ethylchloroformate in the presence of triethylamine (Figure 16, equation 2), followed by addition of L-leucinamide. The reaction is complete within 2 to 3 min and may be used with other chiral amines, e.g. (S)-1-(naphthen-l-yl) ethylamine (Mehvar *et al.*, 1988 b). This technique appears to be widely applicable, Spahn (1987) having derivatized and resolved eight 'profen' NSAIDs using this method; Jamali and co-workers (see Table 2 for references) have also developed analytical methods for four 2-arylpropionic acids using L-leucinamide as the CDA. The application of this method whilst being of general utility does indicate that within a series of compounds some variation in conditions may be required. Thus, derivatization of tiaprofenic acid required the use of an alternative, more reactive activating agent 2,2,2,-trichloroethylchloroformate (Mehvar *et al.*, 1988 a) and alternative amine CDAs were found to be required for resolution and analysis of the acids following isolation from biological fluids (Mehvar *et al.*, 1988 b; Jamali *et al.*, 1988; Mehvar and Jamali, 1988 b). The general principle of the activation step does however appear to be widely applicable (Spahn, 1988 c) and the choice of amine CDA will depend on both the chromatographic resolution and spectroscopic properties of the diastereoisomeric amides produced.

A similar rapid activation step has recently been described for the derivatization of the bactericidal drug ofloxacin (Lehr and Damm, 1988). The activation step involves reaction of the acid with diphenylphosphinylchloride, in the presence of triethylamine, to yield a mixed anhydride prior to reaction with L-leucinamide. The total reaction time is about 10 min. The diastereoisomers were resolved by reverse-phase HPLC and detected by fluorometry allowing plasma and urine concentrations of the drug to be determined down to about 0.03 and 0.3 $\mu g/ml$ respectively (Lehr and Damm, 1988).

Chiral isocyanates and isothiocyanates

Isocyanates react readily with alcohols and amines to yield urethane and urea derivatives respectively, whilst the reaction of isothiocyanates with amines yields the corresponding thiourea derivatives (Figure 17). Over the last few years, several chiral derivatives of these agents have become commercially

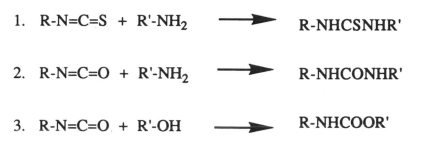

1. R-N=C=S + R'-NH₂ ⟶ R-NHCSNHR'

2. R-N=C=O + R'-NH₂ ⟶ R-NHCONHR'

3. R-N=C=O + R'-OH ⟶ R-NHCOOR'

Figure 17. Reactions of isothiocyanates and isocyanates with alcohols and amines to yield thiourea (1), urea (2) and urethane (3) derivatives.

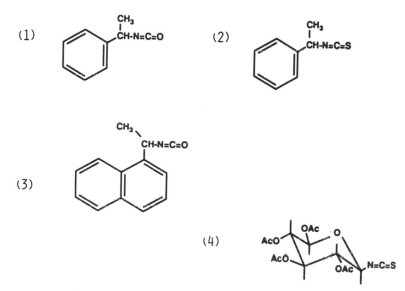

Figure 18. Chiral isocyanates and isothiocyanates used as CDAs: (1) 1-phenylethylisocyanate; (2) 1-phenylethylisothiocyanate; (3) 1-(naphthen-1-yl)ethylisocyanate; (4) tetra-O-acetyl-β-glucosylisothiocyanate.

available and many of these are related to the chiral amines referred to previously, e.g. 1-phenylethylisocyanate and isothiocyanate and 1-(naphthen-l-yl) ethylisocyanate (Figure 18). However, in addition to these derivatives, two compounds based on carbohydrates have also been used namely 2,3,4,6-tetra-O-acetyl-β-D-glucopyranosylisothiocyanate (GITC) and 2,3,4-tri-O-acetyl-α-D-arabinopyranosyl isothiocyanate (AITC).

These reagents are particularly useful in the resolution of aminoalcohol derivatives which may be associated with intramolecular hydrogen bonding involving the hydroxyl group. Hydrogen bond formation in the diastereoisomers would be expected to result in a reduction in the conformational flexibility of the molecules and hence alter their physicochemical properties which contributes to their degree of chromatographic resolution (Pirkle and Finn, 1983).

These compounds have been widely used for the enantiomeric resolution of a variety of medicinal amines and aminoalcohols, e.g. amphetamines, ephedrines and β-blocking agents by TLC and HPLC (Thompson *et al.*, 1982; Sedman and Gal, 1983; Dieterle and Faigle, 1983; Miller *et al.* 1984; Wilson and Walle, 1984; Pflugmann *et al.*, 1987 b; Schuster *et al.*, 1988; Gietl *et al.*, 1988). The papers of Sedman and Gal (1983) and Miller *et al.* (1984) are of particular interest as in both these reports several CDAs are compared.

Thus, Sedman and Gal (1983) examined the resolution of the enantiomers of nine β-blocking drugs following their derivatization with either GITC or AITC, using a reverse-phase (C-18) HPLC system. The GITC derivatives all gave baseline resolution with relatively minor changes in the separation factor (α) over the range of compounds examined. In contrast, the resolution of the AITC derivatives was somewhat poorer. An additional noteworthy observation was that the elution order of the GITC diastereoisomers was the reverse of that obtained for the AITC derivatives. This reversal of elution is thought to be associated with conformational differences between the carbohydrate residues particularly at the anomeric carbon atom (Sedman and Gal, 1983). A similar reversal of elution order using the same two reagents was observed for a series of diastereoisomers produced by reaction with amphetamine and some ring substituted amphetamine derivatives (Miller *et al.*, 1984).

The resolution of the enantiomers of metoprolol and α-hydroxymetoprolol by HPLC has been recently reported using GITC as a CDA (Schuster *et al.*, 1988). The solvent system employed in this case was an acetonitrile-water (48 : 52 by volume) mixture containing 0.1 per cent v/v triethylamine. The high water content enabled the simultaneous determination of both the drug and the metabolite.

The mild reaction conditions and the rapid derivatization using GITC has been utilized by Walle *et al.* (1985) for the chiral derivatization of the intact sulphate conjugates of 4-hydroxypropranolol and prenalterol. Using a reverse-phase (C-18) column and a mobile phase consisting of a mixture of acetonitrile-methanol-water-acetic acid (35 : 5 : 59 : 1 by volume), the two diastereoisomeric derivatives of 4-hydroxypropranolol sulphate showed complete baseline resolution with R = 2.1. Using their method, these workers were able to determine the enantiomeric composition of the conjugate in plasma obtained from a patient undergoing chronic drug treatment (Walle *et al.*, 1985). The major disadvantage of the method was the sample clean up, by ion-pair solvent extraction and HPLC prior to the derivatization being carried out. The same derivatization technique has recently been applied for the analysis of terbutaline sulphate conjugates by HPLC in an examination of the *in vitro* metabolic conjugation of the drug by rat liver cytosol (Walle and Walle, 1989).

GITC has also been used for the determination of the enantiomeric composition of some chiral epoxides or oxiranes (Gal, 1985). Mono-substituted epoxides were reacted with a variety of alkylamines resulting in the formation of ring opened amino alcohols. The nucleophilic attack of the amine took place at the least hindered carbon atom of the oxirane; the amino alcohols produced, therefore, retain the configuration of the oxirane. The amino alcohols were then derivatized with GITC and the diastereoisomeric derivatives resolved by reverse phase HPLC.

Chiral alkylating and arylating agents

There are presently few reports of the use of alkylating agents as CDAs for the analysis of chiral drugs; much of the work in this area is associated with the determination of the enantiomeric composition of amino acid mixtures.

Pre- or post-column derivatization with *ortho*-phthaldialdehyde and 2-mercaptoethanol is a commonly used method for the HPLC determination of amino acids (Figure 19; Alvarez-Coque *et al.*, 1989). The advantages of this method are that the reaction conditions are simple and the products obtained exhibit intense fluorescence and may also be detected electrochemically. Buck and Krummen (1984) have modified this method for the determination of the enantiomeric composition of amino acids by replacing the 2-mercaptoethanol in the derivatization step by a chiral thio compound, e.g. N-acetyl-L-cysteine

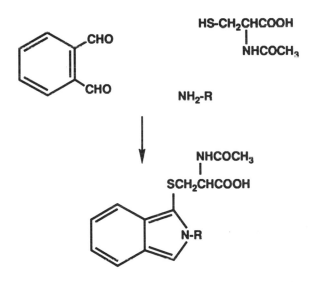

Figure 19.   Reaction of *ortho*-phthaldialdehyde with N-acetylcysteine and primary amines to yield fluorescent isoindole derivatives.

or N-*tert*-butyloxycarbonyl-L-cysteine. These authors were also able to auto-
mate the pre-column derivatization step and hence integrate the derivatization
into the HPLC system. Using this technique the resolution of twenty-one
amino acid enantiomers was achieved (Buck and Krummen, 1984).

Alternative chiral thio compounds which have been successfully used for
the derivatization of amino acid enantiomers include 1-thio-β-D-glucose and
its tetra acetyl derivative (Figure 20; Einarsson *et al.*, 1987; Jegorov *et al.*,
1988). Euerby *et al.* (1988) have recently reported the application of this
method for the determination of the enantiomeric composition of lombricine,
a serine-containing compound, found in earthworms. The HPLC resolution
of the enantiomers of noradrenaline, dopa and baclofen has been achieved by
reaction with *ortho*-phthaldialdehyde using N-acetyl-L-cysteine as a CDA
(Nimura *et al.*, 1987; Wuis *et al.*, 1987)

An alternative reagent which has been used for the determination of the
enantiomeric composition of β-leucine is Marfey's reagent (Figure 21; N-(5-
fluoro-2,4-dinitrophenyl)-L-alaninamide). This reagent reacts with primary
amino groups via an aromatic nucleophilic substitution reaction to yield a pair
of diastereoisomeric products which may be resolved by reverse phase HPLC
(Aberhart and Cotting, 1988).

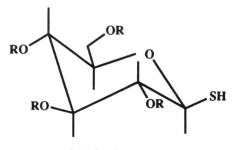

1-thio-ß-D-glucose   **R = H**

2,3,4,6-tetra-O-acetyl-1-thio-ß-D-glucose   **R = CH₃C O**

Figure 20.   Thioglucose derivatives used as CDAs with *ortho*-phthaldialdehyde.

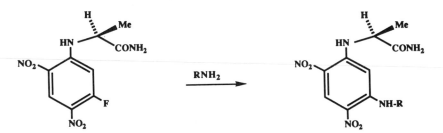

Figure 21.   Reaction of Marfey's Reagent (N-(5-fluoro-2,4-dinitrophenyl)-L-alaninamide) with a
primary amine to yield a chiral derivative.

One of the few reports on the use of alkylating CDAs for the determination of drug molecules is that of Knorr *et al.* (1984). These workers used (+)-(R)-tetrahydrofurfuryl-(1S)-camphor-10-sulphonate to derivatize the enantiomers of the adrenergic drug etilefin, the chiral tetrahydrofurfuryl moiety alkylating the nucleophilic nitrogen of the drug molecule (Knorr *et al.*, 1984).

Other chiral derivatizing agents

Gossypol is a male antifertility agent which has antitumour activity and in addition may be potentially useful in the treatment of some gynaecological disorders. This compound, a polyphenolic binaphthyl derivative, is chiral due to restricted rotation about the carbon–carbon bond linking the two aromatic rings (Figure 22), and may be resolved into (−) and (+) forms and represents an example of atropisomerism. The resolution of the enantiomers of gossypol has been achieved by Schiffs base formation on reaction with the CDA (R)-2-aminopropanol. The derivatization resulted in reaction of both aldehyde groups in the molecule to yield the corresponding diimine derivatives (Wu *et al.*, 1988). The diastereoisomeric imines produced could be resolved by reverse-phase (C-18) HPLC and using an electrochemical detector, the plasma concentrations of the individual enantiomers could be determined in samples obtained from both two dogs and two patients following chronic administration of the racemic drug (Wu *et al.*, 1988).

The genetically determined oxidation of debrisoquine to 4-hydroxydebrisoquine (Figure 23) results in the formation of a chiral metabolite from an achiral substrate. The stereochemistry of this oxidation has been recently determined by Meese *et al.* (1988). The 4-hydroxy compound was initially converted to a pyrimidinyl derivative by reaction with 1,1,1,5,5,5,-hexafluoro-2,4-pentandione and this was further derivatized by reaction with a CDA. Using three CDAs namely (R)-(−)-menthylchloroformate, (S)-(−)-1-camphanyl chloride and (S)-1-phenylethylisocyanate the 4-hydroxy pyrimidinyl derivative of the metabolite was converted into diastereoisomeric carbonate, ester and carbamate derivatives respectively. Analysis of these was

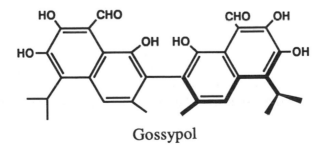

Gossypol

Figure 22. Structure of gossypol.

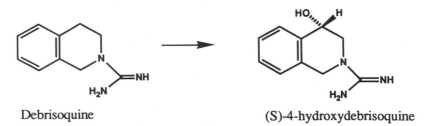

Debrisoquine   (S)-4-hydroxydebrisoquine

Figure 23.   Metabolic oxidation of debrisoquine to yield (S)-4-hydroxydebrisoquine.

carried out using a chemically bonded SE-30 capillary GC column with negative-ion-chemical-ionization mass-spectrometry detection using deuterated
internal standards. All three diastereoisomeric derivatives of the metabolite
were resolved using this system and the metabolic product, in extensive metabolizers of the drug, was shown to be mainly of the (S)-absolute configuration
with an enantiomeric excess of $\geqslant 90$ per cent (Meese *et al.*, 1988). An
additional point of note from these studies is that the 4-hydroxy metabolite
undergoes partial racemization to the extent of 2–7 per cent after 1 hour and
30 per cent after 17 hours at 110° C, during derivatization with the diketone,
a reaction that was found to be of less importance using samples of biological
origin (Meese *et al.*, 1988). Hence if a non-chiral derivatization of a chiral
analyte is required, careful examination of the possible stereochemical consequences of such a reaction should be taken into account.

(–)-Menthylchloroformate has also been used recently for derivatization
and resolution of the β-blocking drugs propranolol and flavodilol by reverse
phase (C-8) HPLC (Schmitthenner *et al.*, 1989).

Direct methods of separation

Chiral high-performance liquid chromatography

Since the introduction of the first HPLC-chiral stationary phase (CSP), in
1981, the number of commercially available columns has increased considerably, around forty being marketed at the present time. These CSPs may be
divided into two groups:

1. the designed CSPs where the mechanisms involved in the resolution
   process are fairly well understood and the elution order of a pair of enantiomers may be predicted, e.g. the 'brush type' or Pirkle CSPs;
2. the empirical CSPs which are dependent on a more trial-and-error
   approach for the resolution of enantiomers, e.g. the protein based chiral
   affinity phases.

Many of the designed CSPs are available in both enantiomeric forms so that
the elution order of a pair of enantiomers may be reversed and hence the

isomer present in excess may be eluted last. Such peak reversal is not possible on CSPs derived from natural products, such as the protein-based CSPs.

Many of the constraints discussed above, using CDAs for the formation of stable diastereoisomers, are of less importance with the application of CSPs. For example useful resolutions may be obtained using CSPs which are not 100 per cent enantiomerically pure. Under these conditions the resolving power of the system is obviously not optimal but the resolution may be useful. Also, should derivatization of the analyte(s) be necessary for optimal resolution, the derivatization reagent need not be chiral and hence the considerations of kinetic resolution, enantiomeric purity and possible racemization of the reagent and differential detector responses of derivatives are eliminated.

The mechanism of enantiomeric resolution using CSPs is generally attributed to the '3-point' fit model of Dalgliesh (1952). For chiral recognition and hence enantiomeric resolution to occur on a CSP the functional groups of one of the enantiomers of the analyte must be involved in three simultaneous interactions with the CSP, with at least one of these interactions being stereochemically dependent, whilst its antipode may only interact at two sites (Figure 24; Pirkle and Pochapsky, 1989). The diastereoisomeric complexes thus formed will have different energies of interaction and the enantiomer forming the most stable complex will be retained longer by the CSP (Pirkle and Pochapsky, 1987). The types of interaction involved in the resolution process vary depending on the system used, however; they may be due to hydrogen bonding, dipole–dipole interactions, charge transfer complexes, hydrophobic interactions and steric repulsion. Optimal conditions for resolution occur when three different types of interaction take place as this

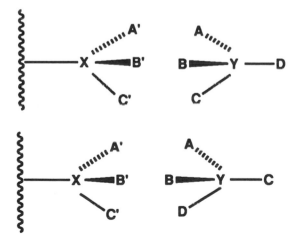

Figure 24. Interaction model for the chromatographic resolution of enantiomers using chiral stationary phases. The upper analyte enantiomer has the correct configuration for three simultaneous interactions (A-A′; B-B′; C-C′) with complimentary sites on the CSP whilst its antipode (lower) has two interactive sites (A-A′; B-B′).

prevents interchange between recognition sites (Pirkle and Finn, 1983). The three interactions do not necessarily have to result in stabilization of the diastereoisomeric complex, i.e. result in bonding interactions; one of the interactions may result in destabilization of the complex, e.g. repulsive steric interactions, and in this case the enantiomer interacting at three sites would be eluted from the column first.

There has in recent years been considerable interest in this area and the interested reader is referred to the monographs by Allenmark (1988), Souter (1985) and Wainer (1988), together with the edited work of Zief and Crane (1988) and the reviews of Armstrong (1984; 1987), Dappen *et al.* (1986), Feitsma and Drenth (1988), Mehta (1988) and Pirkle and Pochapsky (1987; 1989).

Wainer (1988) has classified the commercially available CSPs into five groups depending on the separation principles involved and the remainder of this section will be divided according to this classification.

a. TYPE I: DONOR–ACCEPTOR OR PIRKLE CSPs. The first commercially available CSP, (R)-N-(3,5-dinitrobenzoyl) phenylglycine ionically bonded to γ-aminopropylsilica (Figure 25, number 2) is of this group (Pirkle *et al.*, 1981). These systems have the advantage that the CSP–analyte interactions are fairly well understood and as a result they are the most readily adaptable CSPs to the design approach, reports of new phases frequently appearing in the literature (Salvadori *et al.*, 1989). Some eighteen different CSPs of this type are available (Wainer, 1989) examples of which are presented in Figure 25. The types of interaction involved in the formation of the diastereoisomeric complexes include hydrogen bonding, π-donor/acceptor, dipole-stacking and steric interactions (Figure 25) (Pirkle and Pochapsky, 1989), and considerable effort has been devoted to computational studies of the CSP–analyte interactions in order to rationalize the resolution process (Lipkowitz *et al*,, 1987; 1988; Topiol *et al*,, 1988). The elution order of a pair of enantiomers, or their derivatives, on a given CSP is related to their absolute configuration, and chiral recognition models have been developed, which have the added advantage that absolute configuration as well as enantiomeric purity may be determined using nanogram quantities of material (Pirkle and Finn, 1981). Some care is required, however, as reversals in elution order are occasionally observed, and such reversals may be indicative of two or more mechanisms associated with chiral recognition (Pirkle *et al*,, 1984).

Many of the analytes resolved on CSPs of this type require precolumn derivatization to extend the π-system and also to introduce groups which are capable of taking part in either dipole–dipole or hydrogen bonding interactions. The type of derivative formed will depend on both the nature of the CSP and the analyte, e.g. carboxylic acids and amines, are generally converted into amide derivatives using an aromatic amine or acid, the formation of the amide bond increasing the possible dipole–dipole and hydrogen bonding interactions. The choice of the derivatizing agent depends on the π-donor/acceptor properties of the CSP e.g. π-acceptor derivatives commonly include 3,5-dinitrobenzoyl or 3,5-dinitroanilide derivatives, whilst π-donor derivatives include phenyl, substituted phenyl and naphthyl systems (Figure 26).

Mobile phases used with CSPs of this type are frequently non-polar, e.g. hexane or hexane–dichloromethane mixtures containing low concentrations of alcohols, e.g. propan-2-ol or ethanol, or acetonitrile as modifiers. Mobile phases of polarity greater than 20 per cent propanol in hexane should not be used with the ionically bonded phases. However, more polar phases may be used with the covalently bonded CSPs and there are examples of highly polar aqueous buffer-methanol systems giving useful resolutions (Lin and Hsieh, 1988). The effect of mobile phase composition, temperature, interstrand distance on the CSP, and analyte structure, with particular reference to the steric and electronic properties of derivatizing agents, on the resolutions produced using these CSPs have been the subject of a number of investigations (see, for example, Pescher *et al.*, 1986; Wainer and Alembik, 1986 a; Pirkle and Hyun, 1985; Pirkle and Pochapsky, 1988; Zief, 1988).

A wide variety of analytes have been resolved using these systems including: α and β-amino acids (Griffith *et al.*, 1986; Pirkle *et al.*, 1985), monoalkyl and acylglycerols (Takagi and Itabashi, 1986; Itabashi and Takagi, 1986), phosphine oxides (Pescher *et al.*, 1986), pyrethroid insecticides (Cayley and Simpson, 1986), sulphoxides (Light *et al.*, 1982), alcohols (Pirkle and McCune, 1988), dipeptides (Hyun *et al.*, 1988), amides (Wainer and Alembik, 1986 a,b; Pirkle and Welch, 1984), barbiturates and succinimides (Yang *et al.*, 1985), hydroxyeicosatetraenoate derivatives (Kuhn *et al.*, 1987; Hawkins *et al.*, 1988; Turk *et al.*, 1988), amphetamines (Lee *et al.*, 1986; Alembik and Wainer, 1988), ephedrine (Wainer *et al.*, 1983), propranolol (Wainer *et al.*, 1984), 2-tetradecyglycidic acid (Weaner and Hoerr, 1987), the 4,6-dimethyl-2-pyrimidinyl derivative of 4-hydroxydebrisoquine (Meese *et al.*, 1987) and 2-arylpropionic acid NSAIDs (Wainer and Doyle, 1984; McDaniel and Snider, 1987; Nicoll-Griffith, 1987; Nicoll-Griffith *et al.*, 1988).

Bioanalytical applications of these CSPs are widespread, particularly in the area of alcohol derivatives of the polycyclic aromatic hydrocarbons (Yang and Weems, 1984; Yang *et al.*, 1986; McMillan *et al.*, 1987; Yang, 1988 and references therein).

The report of Yang and Weems (1984) is of interest from an analytical viewpoint. These authors examined the elution order of a number of dihydrodiol derivatives using both covalently and ionically bonded (R)-N-(3,5-dinitrobenzoyl) phenylglycine CSPs and observed a reversal of elution order between the two CSPs for the enantiomers of *trans*-5,6-dihydrodiol-7,12-dimethylbenz[a]anthracene.

Metabolic transformations frequently result in minor alterations in drug structure, which in the present context may have a small effect on the properties of the molecule. This is the case for the chemical and metabolic oxidation product of the NSAID pirprofen, a reaction which results in the

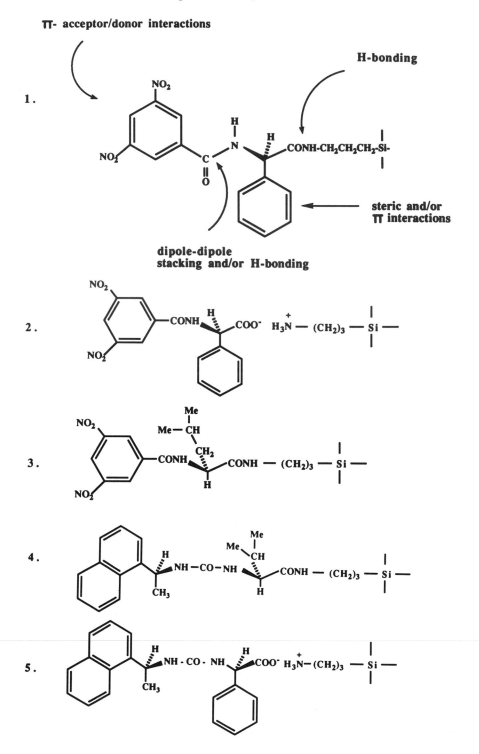

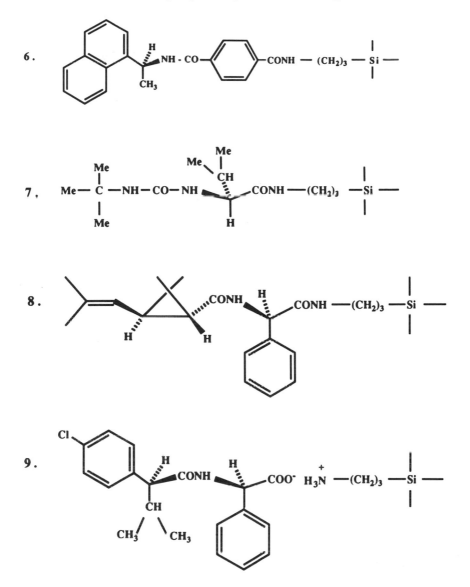

Figure 25. Examples of Type I CSPs which are commercially available and CSP–analyte inter-actions which may contribute to the resolution process. (1) (R)-N-(3,5-dinitrobenzoyl)phenyl-glycine (covalently bonded to silica); (2) (R)-N-(3,5-dinitrobenzoyl)phenylglycine (ionically bonded to silica) also available in the (S)-absolute configuration; (3) (S)-N-(3,5-dinitrobenzoyl) leucine (covalently bonded, also available ionically bonded); (4) (S)-N-1-(α-naphthyl)-ethylaminocarbonyl-(S)-valine (covalently bonded) also available with the 1-(α-naphthyl)ethyl-amino moiety in the (R)-absolute configuration; (5) (S)-N-1-(α-naphthyl)ethylaminocarbonyl-(R)-phenylglycine (ionically bonded) also available with the 1-(α-naphthyl)ethylamino moiety in the (R)-absolute configuration; (6) (S)-N-1-(α-naphthyl)ethylaminoterephthalic acid (covalently bonded); (7) N-*tert*-butylaminocarbonyl-(S)-valine (covalently bonded); (8) (1R,3R)-N-chrysan-themoyl-(R)-phenylglycine (covalently bonded); (9) (S)-2-(4-chlorophenyl)isovaleroyl-(R)-phenyl-glycine (ionically bonded).

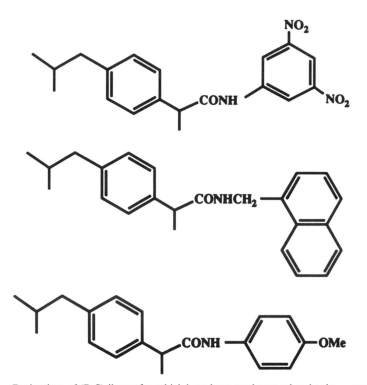

Figure 26. Derivatives of (R,S)-ibuprofen which have been used to resolve the drug enantiomers using Type I CSPs. From the top (derivative; CSP; elution order; reference): (1) 3,5-dinitroanilide; (S)-N-(2-naphthoyl)alanine; not reported; Pirkle *et al.* (1986); (2) 1-naphthalenemethylamide; (R)-N-(3,5-dinitrobenzoyl)phenylglycine (covalent); (S) before (R); Wainer and Doyle (1984); (3) 4-methoxyanilide; (R)-N-(3,5-dinitrobenzoyl)phenylglycine (covalent); (S) before (R); Nicoll-Griffith (1987).

aromatization of the heterocyclic ring system (Figure 27). Using a CDA, (S)-1-(naphthen-1-yl) ethylamine, we were unable to separate the diastereoisomeric amides of the drug from those of the oxidation product (Hutt *et al.*, 1986). Similar difficulties were also observed by Sioufi *et al.*, (1987) who attempted to resolve the enantiomers of the drug using a (R)-N-(3,5-dinitrobenzoyl) phenylglycine CSP. The resolved drug enantiomers could not be separated from those of the metabolite. The similarity in structure of the drug and the metabolite required the combined use of both a CDA, (R)-1-phenylethylamine, and the CSP for both resolution of the drug enantiomers and their separation from those of the metabolite (Sioufi *et al.*, 1987).

b. TYPE II: CELLULOSE DERIVATIVES AS CSPs. A number of synthetic ester, ether and carbamate derivatives of cellulose adsorbed on macroporous silica are presently available as HPLC–CSPs (Figure 28) (Okamoto *et al.*, 1984 b; Ichida *et al.*, 1984; Ichida and Shibata, 1988). The mechanism of resolution

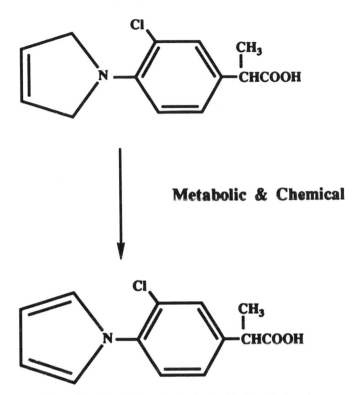

Figure 27. Metabolic and chemical oxidation of pirprofen.

of these systems involves hydrogen bonding, dipole–dipole stacking, π-donor/acceptor interactions together with partial inclusion complex formation between the analyte and the CSP (Wainer and Alembik, 1986 b). Mobile phases commonly employed include hexane-propan-2-ol mixtures and occasionally more polar alcohols, e.g. methanol or ethanol and also aqueous–alcohol mixtures (Dappen *et al.*, 1986; Ichida and Shibata, 1988).

A variety of chiral drugs have been resolved using these systems, e.g. barbiturates, glutethimide and aryloxypropanolamine β-blocking agents, together with molecules containing chiral sulphur and phosphorus centres (Wainer *et al.*, 1986; Ichida and Shibata, 1988; Wainer, 1988). Compounds containing amino or carboxyl functions bonded to the chiral centre may be resolved following derivatization to yield arylamide derivatives (Wainer and Alembik, 1986 b). The cellulose tricinnamate coated CSP has been used recently to determine the enantiomeric composition of the flavouring agent 2-(4-methoxyphenoxy)propanoic acid in roasted coffee beans (Rathbone *et al.*, 1989). Adequate resolution of the free acid enantiomers could not be obtained using this CSP and derivatization to yield the corresponding methyl esters was required.

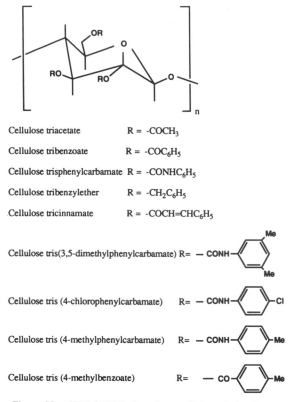

Cellulose triacetate	R = -COCH₃

Cellulose triacetate $R = -COCH_3$

Cellulose tribenzoate $R = -COC_6H_5$

Cellulose trisphenylcarbamate $R = -CONHC_6H_5$

Cellulose tribenzylether $R = -CH_2C_6H_5$

Cellulose tricinnamate $R = -COCH=CHC_6H_5$

Cellulose tris(3,5-dimethylphenylcarbamate) $R = -CONH-$

Cellulose tris (4-chlorophenylcarbamate) $R = -CONH-$

Cellulose tris (4-methylphenylcarbamate) $R = -CONH-$

Cellulose tris (4-methylbenzoate) $R = -CO-$

Figure 28. HPLC CSPs based on cellulose derivatives.

Two analytical methods for the resolution of the enantiomers of pro-pranolol using the tris(3,5-dimethylphenylcarbamate) CSP have been reported (see Table 3; Straka *et al.*, 1988; Takahashi *et al.*, 1988). These assays have been used to monitor the plasma pharmacokinetics of the enantiomers fol-lowing the oral administration of the racemic drug to man (Straka *et al.*, 1988) and their tissue distribution following i.v. administration to rats (Taka-hashi *et al.*, 1988).

The preparation of silica bonded cellulose and amylose tris(substituted phenylcarbamate) CSPs have been reported (Okamoto *et al.*, 1987). The resolution of a number of chiral drugs has been investigated, including β-blockers, antihistamines and calcium antagonists (Okamoto *et al.*, 1988); however, no bioanalytical applications of these columns have appeared.

c. TYPE III: CHIRAL INCLUSION COMPLEX CSPs

i. *Cyclodextrins.* The cyclodextrins (CDs) are cyclic, non-reducing oligo-saccharides composed of D-glucose units bonded via α-(1, 4)-linkages (Figure

Table 3. Analysis of propranolol enantiomers in plasma using a cellulose tris(3,5-dimethyl-phenylcarbamate) CSP.

Parameter	Straka *et al.* (1988)	Takahashi *et al.* (1988)
Extraction solvent	Diethylether	Chloroform
Recovery (%)	85–89	85–97
Internal standard	(±)-Verapamil	(−)-Penbutolol
Mobile phase	Hexane : propan-2-ol: N,N-dimethyloctylamine (92 : 8 : 0.1 by vol)	Hexane : propan-2-ol: diethylamine (90 : 10 : 0.1 by vol)
Flow rate (ml/min)	1.0	1.4
Resolution factor	3.7	3.75
Elution order	R before S	
Detection	Fluorescence	
Limit of detection (ng/ml)	7.5	3.0

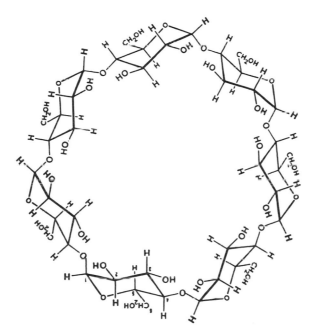

Figure 29. Structure of β-cyclodextrin. Reproduced from Däppen *et al.* (1986) with permission of the authors and Elsevier Science Publishers BV.

29). The shape of these molecules is like a hollow truncated cone, the inner surface of which is relatively hydrophobic. In contrast, the mouth of the cavity is hydrophilic, the larger opening being encircled by a ring of relatively rigidly held secondary hydroxyl groups, whilst the narrow opening is surrounded by a rim of more polar primary hydroxyl groups which may rotate and hence partially block the cavity (Ward and Armstrong, 1988). Three CSPs are available containing either α-, β- or γ-CD, bonded to silica via a 6–10 atom spacer unit. The letters used designate the size of the ring system in terms of the number of D-glucose units, α, β and γ corresponding to 6, 7 and 8 units respectively. The internal diameter of the cavity therefore also varies being α, 5.7 Å; β, 7.8 Å and γ, 9.5 Å (Ward and Armstrong, 1988). As the resolution process involves the formation of an analyte–CD inclusion complex (Figure 30) the size of the cavity is of some significance for successful resolution to take place. One of the major advantages of the CD-CSPs is that aqueous-based mobile phases may be used, e.g. water–methanol or water–acetonitrile mixtures.

A variety of chiral compounds have been resolved using the β-CD-CSP including amino acid derivatives, carboxylic acids (Hinze *et al.*, 1985; Feitsma *et al.*, 1985), barbiturates, β-blocking drugs (Armstrong, 1984; Armstrong *et al.*, 1986), the tropane derivatives scopolamine, cocaine, atropine and homatropine (Armstrong *et al.*, 1987 a) and nomifensine (Aboul-Enein *et al.*, 1988). In contrast, there are relatively few reports of the resolution of enantiomers using α-CD or γ-CD phases. The resolution of some amino acids, and their derivatives on a α-CD-CSP has been reported (Armstrong *et al.*, 1987 b) and the resolution of (±)-norgestrel has been reported using γ-CD as a mobile phase additive (Gazdag *et al.*, 1986).

A bioanalytical application of the β-CD-CSP has been reported by Krstulovic *et al.* (1988) for the resolution of *trans*-6, 6a, 7, 10, 10a, 11-hexahydro-8,9-dimethyl-11-oxodibenz[b,e]oxepin-3-acetic acid, a potential anti-inflammatory agent (Figure 31). The two enantiomers were resolved using a mobile phase of potassium dihydrogen phosphate (0.05 M): methanol (35 : 65 v/v). The analytical method was sufficiently sensitive to determine the

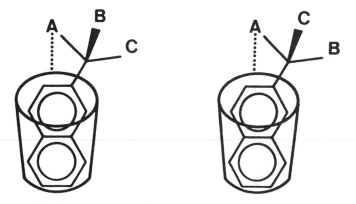

Figure 30. Model of the chiral inclusion complex formed between the cyclodextrins and the enantiomers of a chiral analyte. Reproduced from Däppen *et al.* (1986) with permission of the authors and Elsevier Science Publishers BV.

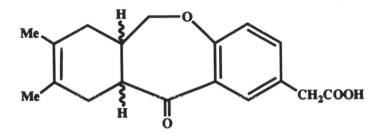

Figure 31. Structure of (±)-*trans*-6,6a,7,10,10a,11-hexahydro-8,9-dimethyl-11-oxodibenz [b,e]oxepin-3-acetic acid a potential anti-inflammatory agent.

enantiomeric composition of the drug in rat plasma samples for up to 24 hours post drug administration (Figure 32).

Other bioanalytical applications of β-CD include: the resolution of the enantiomers of 5-(4-hydroxyphenyl)-5-phenylhydantoin, a metabolite of phenytoin (McClanahan and Maguire, 1986), following isolation of the compound from urine by reverse phase HPLC prior to determination of enantiomeric composition, and also the disposition of hexabarbitone enantiomers in rat blood (Huang-Chandler *et al.*, 1987).

ii. *Synthetic polymer phases.* Polymerization of triphenylmethyl methyl-acrylate, in the presence of a chiral anionic initiator, results in the formation of an optically active synthetic polymer which is chiral as a result of helicity (Okamoto and Hatada, 1988). Two polymers are produced as a result of this process, a highly crystalline high molecular weight polymer which is insoluble in common organic solvents and a soluble low molecular weight polymer. The low molecular weight polymer is used as a CSP following adsorption onto macroporous silanized silica, which, as a result of its solubility, limits the choice of mobile phases which may be used (Okamoto and Hatada, 1988).

Two columns are commercially available, one based on (+)-poly(triphenyl-methyl methacrylate) and the other poly(2-pyridyldiphenylmethyl meth-acrylate) (Dappen *et al.*, 1986). These columns are useful for the resolution of chiral molecules which possess rigid non-planar structures, are hydrophobic and/or lack functional groups which in the majority of cases cannot be resolved using other CSPs. The resolution of a variety of compounds containing chiral sulphur and phosphorus centres has been reported (Okamoto *et al.*, 1984 a) and these CSPs are particularly applicable for the resolution of atropisomers (Okamoto and Hatada, 1988).

The resolution of the enantiomers of the dihydropyridine calcium antagonist, nilvadipine, using (+)-poly(triphenylmethyl methacrylate) and a mobile phase of methanol : water (95 : 5) has been reported by Tokuma *et al.*, (1987). The analytical method was not sensitive enough to determine the drug enantiomers in biological fluids following administration of the racemate to man. The problem of sensitivity was solved by the addition of deuterated racemic nilvadipine as internal standard and collection of the appropriate eluent fractions following resolution of the enantiomers by the CSP. The samples were then analysed by negative-ion-chemical-ionization GC-MS. Using this method it was possible to show that the plasma half-lives of the two enantiomers were similar but that the area under the plasma concentration time curves of the (+)-isomer was about three times greater than that of the

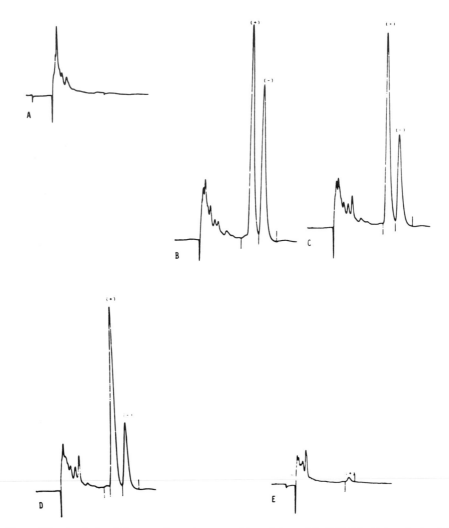

Figure 32. Analysis of the enantiomeric composition of *trans*-6,6a,7,10,10a,11-hexahydro-8,9-dimethyl-11-oxodibenz [b,e] oxepin-3-acetic acid in rat plasma using a β-cyclodextrin bonded CSP. Samples taken predosing (A) and postoral administration of the racemate, 1 h (B); 3 h (C); 6 h (D) and 24 h (E). (+) and (−) indicate the respective isomers. Reproduced from Krstulovic *et al*. (1988) with permission of the authors and Elsevier Science Publishers BV.

(−)-enantiomer (Tokuma *et al.*, 1987). This analytical method was found to be labour intensive, twenty-five assays taking four days.

Similar synthetic polymers, based on polyacrylamide and polymethacrylamide have been prepared by reaction of the anhydrides or acid chlorides of either acrylic acid or methacrylic acid with chiral amines [(S)-phenylalanine, (S)-1-phenylethylamine or (S)-1-cyclohexylethylamine] followed by polymerization (Blaschke, 1988). Polyamide gels have been shown to be useful for the low-pressure preparative resolution of a variety of drugs (Blaschke, 1986, 1988) and for the determination of the enantiomeric composition of thalidomide following administration of the drug to mice (Blaschke, 1988).

iii. *Microcrystalline cellulose triacetate.* Microcrystalline cellulose triacetate (MCTA) may be used as a CSP in low pressure LC. The properties of MCTA as a chiral sorbent are due to the formation of inclusion complexes of the analyte within cavities in the chiral matrix, the crystallinity of the sorbent having a considerable influence on the resolving power of the material (Francotte *et al.*, 1985). Mobile phases consisting of anhydrous ethanol or up to 5 per cent aqueous ethanol being commonly used with this CSP (Wainer, 1988).

The CSP has been extensively used for the preparative resolution of a number of chiral drugs including atropisomers, e.g. methaqualone (Figure 33) (Allenmark and Thompson, 1987; Blaschke, 1986; Mannschreck *et al.*, 1984; Shibata *et al.*, 1986; Ichida and Shibata, 1988). Problems due to reversal of elution order with analyte concentration have been reported using MCTA (Roussel *et al.*, 1989). To date there are no reports of bioanalytical applications of this CSP.

d. TYPE IV: CHIRAL LIGAND-EXCHANGE CHROMATOGRAPHY. Chiral ligand-exchange chromatography (CLEC) involves the reversible formation of complexes between metal ions and chiral complexing agents. The chiral complexing agents for the commercially available columns are amino acids, e.g. proline, hydroxyproline and valine, bonded to silica via a 3-glycidoxypropyl spacer group (Dappen *et al.*, 1986; Wainer, 1988; Allenmark, 1988). The most common mobile phases used with these CSPs are aqueous solutions of the metal ion, e.g. copper sulphate solution, to prevent loss of the ion from the stationary phase (Dappen *et al.*, 1986: Allenmark, 1988). Increased operating temperatures have been reported to improve both the enantiomer separation factor and column efficiency indicating that the resolution is entropy controlled.

The enantiomeric resolution is based on the formation of an enantioselective ternary complex between the fixed ligand, i.e. the bonded amino acid, a metal ion, e.g. Cu^{2+}, and the mobile ligand, the analyte. The differences in stability between the two diasteroisomeric complexes result in resolution. For resolution to take place, the analyte must have two functional

Progress in Drug Metabolism

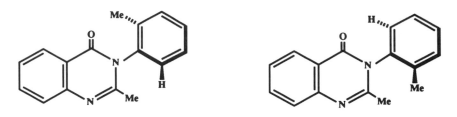

Methaqualone

Figure 33. Methaqualone atropisomers.

groups, appropriately spaced, such that they may simultaneously act as ligands for the metal ion. This latter requirement obviously limits the type of compounds which may be examined using this technique.

This approach has been successfully used for the resolution of a variety of amino acids and their derivatives, hydroxy acids, amino alcohols and derivatives of dopa (Allenmark, 1988; Grierson and Adam, 1985; Takeuchi *et al.*, 1986). In some cases derivatization of the analyte may be required prior to HPLC resolution; for example, for the determination of penicillamine, the compound was first reacted with formaldehyde to yield 5,5-dimethylthiazolidine-4-carboxylic acid, the enantiomers of which were resolved on a reverse phase (C-8) column coated with a copper II complex of (2S,4R,2′R,S)-4-hydroxy-1-(2^1-hydroxydodecyl)proline (Busker *et al.*, 1985).

There are a few examples of CLEC being used in bioanalytical chemistry. One recent report involves the determination of the enantiomeric composition of 5-(4-hydroxyphenyl)-5-phenylhydantion (HPPH) in human urine following administration of the prochiral drug phenytoin to subjects of known oxidation status (Fritz *et al.*, 1987). The metabolite was isolated from urine and purified by TLC prior to the determination of enantiomeric composition by CLEC. The HPLC system consisted of a reverse phase (C-18) column and a mobile phase containing L-proline-n-octylaminde (1.5 mM) and nickel (II) acetate (1.5 mM) together with ammonium acetate (0.1 M) in a methanol : water mixture (45 : 55 v/v) at pH 9. Under these conditions baseline resolution of the enantiomers of HPPH was obtained together with resolution of the related compounds 5-phenyl-5-ethylhydantoin and 5-(4-hydroxyphenyl)-5-ethylhydantoin (Figure 34). A model for the chiral complex involving interaction of the carbonyl (position 2) and the nitrogen (position 3) of the hydantoin ring with the chiral metal complex was proposed (Figure 35). This model is supported by the fact that methylation at position 3, i.e. mephenytoin and 4-hydroxymephenytoin, resulted in a loss of resolution (Fritz *et al.*, 1987).

In the case of the above example it is not entirely clear whether the L-proline-n-octylamide is acting as a CSP coating the reverse phase column or as a chiral mobile phase additive (see below).

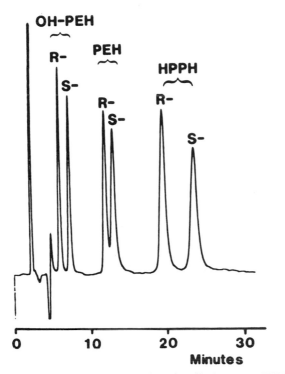

Figure 34. Resolution of 5-(4-hydroxyphenyl)-5-phenylhydantoin (HPPH), 5-phenyl-5-ethylhydantoin, (PEH) and 5-(4-hydroxyphenyl)-5-ethylhydantoin (OH-PEH) by CLEC. R- and S- represent the respective isomers. Reproduced from Fritz *et al.* (1987) with permission of the authors and the American Society for Pharmacology and Experimental Therapeutics.

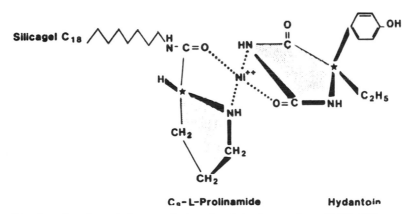

Figure 35. Complex formed between hydantoin derivatives and a CLEC–CSP, octyl-L-prolinamide and nickel (II) ions. Reproduced from Fritz *et al.* (1987) with permission of the authors and the American Society for Pharmacology and Experimental Therapeutics.

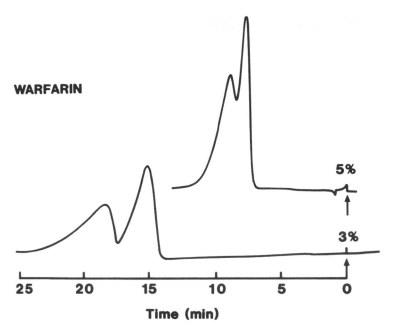

Figure 36. Effect of organic modifier concentration on the resolution of racemic warfarin using a BSA bonded-CSP. (Solvent: phosphate buffer, 0.1 M, pH 7.8 containing either 3 or 5 per cent v/v propan-1-ol, flow rate 2 ml/min). Reproduced from Hutt and Caldwell (1989) with the permission of Taylor & Francis.

e. TYPE V: AFFINITY OR PROTEIN CSPs. The enantiodifferentiating properties of proteins have been utilized as CSPs by bonding these macromolecules to silica. Two CSPs are presently available, namely bovine serum albumin (BSA; Resolvosil® ; Allenmark *et al.*, 1983) and α_1-acid glycoprotein (α_1-AGP, orosomucoid; EnantioPac® ; Hermansson, 1983). The mechanism of chiral recognition of these protein phases is complex and not clearly understood; however, factors such as hydrophobic, polar and steric interactions are known to be of importance (Allenmark, 1986; 1988; Dappen *et al.*, 1986).

Mobile phases used with these CSPs are generally phosphate buffers of varying composition, in terms of pH (5–9), ionic strength (0–500 mM), and may contain low concentrations of organic modifiers, e.g. 1- or 2-propanol (up to 5 per cent v/v) or N,N-dimethyloctylamine, *tert*-butylammonium bromide or octanoic acid (0–10 mM). The efficiency of the phases is also influenced by temperature. The efficiency and stereoselectivity of the CSPs are extremely sensitive to these parameters and it is difficult to predict their effect on the required resolution (Dappen *et al.*, 1986; Wainer, 1988). The effect of propan-1-ol concentration on the resolution of the enantiomers of warfarin using a BSA-CSP is shown in Figure 36 (Hutt and Caldwell, 1989). Allenmark (1988) has presented a logical approach, based on manipulation of mobile

MANDELIC ACID

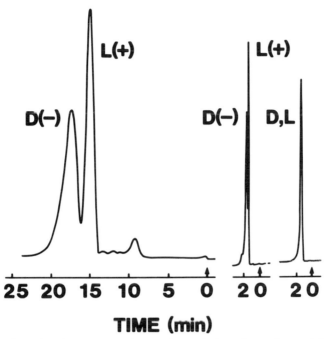

Figure 37. Effect of analyte concentration on the resolution of racemic mandelic acid using a BSA bonded-CSP. Chromatograms, right to left: 25 μg on column, abs 0.1, flow rate 2.0 ml/min; 2.5 μg on column, abs 0.01, flow rate 2.0 ml/min; as before, flow rate 0.2 ml/min. (Solvent phosphate buffer, 0.1 M, pH 7.0). Reproduced from Hutt and Caldwell (1988 a) with the permission of Taylor & Francis.

phase pH and addition of propan-1-ol, for the optimization of both retention and resolution using the BSA-CSP.

Additional problems associated with these phases include low sample capacities as the protein load on the column is low indicating a limited number of binding sites. The effect of analyte concentration on the resolution of the enantiomers of mandelic acid using a BSA-CSP is illustrated in Figure 37 (Hutt and Caldwell, 1988 a). Also, as the chiral recognition process may involve a variety of binding sites, the enantioselectivity of each may differ and hence rational prediction of enantiomer elution order is generally difficult (Pirkle and Pochapsky, 1989).

The major advantage of these phases is that they are useful for a wide range of analytes, which do not require derivatization prior to resolution, and they are compatible with aqueous mobile phases and hence may be used in combination with reverse phase HPLC systems for coupled column chromatography (see below).

The resolution of a large number of pharmaceuticals, including cationic and anionic compounds and the effects of mobile phase additives and pH on resolution have been reported using α_1-AGP phases (Schill *et al.*, 1986 a,b; Hermansson and Eriksson, 1986; Hermansson and Schill, 1988). Lee *et al.* (1987) reported the resolution and analysis of the enantiomers of bupivacaine in serum, using α_1-AGP following the intrapleural administration of the racemic drug. The enantiomeric composition of salbutamol in human urine has been reported by Tan and Soldin (1987). These authors used an α_1-AGP phase and a mobile phase consisting of triethylamine (0.1 per cent) in 5.3 mM citrate buffer (pH 7.2) in combination with an electrochemical detector. Using this assay, the urinary disposition of the drug enantiomers were investigated following i.v. and oral administration of the racemate to volunteers. The results indicated the stereoselective sulphate conjugation of the $(-)$-enantiomer in man (Tan and Soldin, 1987).

The resolution of the enantiomers of diisopyramide using α_1-AGP has been reported by Hermansson and Eriksson (1984), using a mobile phase of phosphate buffer (pH 6.2) containing both propan-2-ol and N,N-dimethyl-octylamine (1.95 mM). A problem arose due to the incomplete separation of the enantiomers of the drug from those of the monodesisopropyl metabolite. This was solved by the use of a precolumn (reverse phase, C-2) which separated the drug from the metabolite such that the enantiomers of both compounds were resolved by the CSP.

α_1-AGP has also recently been used to resolve the enantiomers of the N-oxide metabolite of the monoamine oxidase inhibitor pargyline (Lindeke *et al.*, 1987). Incubation of the drug with a rat liver microsomal preparation produced one of the possible chiral N-oxides and this compound represents one of the few examples of metabolic formation of a chiral nitrogen centre from a prochiral substrate. The stereochemistry of the metabolite has not yet been elucidated but the CSP used was shown to resolve the enantiomers of a synthetic racemic sample of the compound.

Leucovorin (5-formyltetrahydrofolate) contains two chiral centres, in the glutamic acid residue and the pteroic acid moiety; the commercially available material is a 1:1 mixture of the diastereoisomers of the (6R) and (6S) configurations as L-glutamic acid is used in the synthetic process. The (6S)-isomer is more biologically active than the (6R)-compound and these two also differ in their pharmacokinetic behaviour; the (6S)-isomer is selectively absorbed from the gastrointestinal tract and has a short plasma half-life (Choi and Schilsky, 1988). The resolution of these two diastereoisomers, and their major metabolite, the 5-methyl derivative, has been achieved using a BSA-CSP with a mobile phase of sodium phosphate buffer (pH 7.4:5 and 25 mM) (Choi and Schilsky, 1988). Using this system the elution order of leucovorin isomers was (6S) before the (6R)-isomer but this was reversed (6R) before the (6S) for the metabolite, indicating the difficulty of prediction of elution order using these phases. For bioanalytical work these authors suggested quantification and isolation of the drug and the metabolite, using a reverse phase (C-18) system, prior to the determination of enantiomeric composition using the CSP (Choi and Schilsky, 1988).

Other protein based CSPs have been reported. Miwa *et al.* (1987) used ovomucoid, a stable protein present in egg white, bonded to silica for the resolution of chlorpheniramine, chlorprenaline and phenylpropanolamine. Wainer and co-workers have immobilized active α-chymotrypsin (ACHT) on a silica support (Wainer *et al.*, 1988; Jadaud *et al.*, 1989). Whilst this CSP has not yet been used in bioanalytical chemistry it is of interest as the mechanism of resolution involves both hydrophobic interactions and also hydrolytic activity at the enzyme active site. The resolution of a variety of N-,O- and N,O-derivatized amino acids has been investigated in the presence and absence of compounds which either block the hydrolytic site or a hydrophobic pocket near to the active site. It would appear from these studies that chiral recognition for most of the compounds examined takes place at one of these sites and that if the compound is a substrate for the enzyme then the stereoselectivity of the phase is a function of enzyme activity (Jadaud *et al.* 1989).

Coupled column liquid chromatography

Many of the chromatographic systems described above are not directly applicable for the analysis of drug enantiomers in biological fluids due to problems associated with structurally similar metabolites and the presence of contaminants either from the biological matrix or from the components of the extraction media. The presence of these substances may interfere with the analytical resolution by either coelution or by alteration of the mobile phase composition. In the case of the CSPs the resolution and retention behaviour of an analyte may be highly sensitive to mobile phase composition and adversely affected by the presence or absence of low concentrations of organic solvents or water present in samples. It may also be difficult to separate the analytes of interest from those of a structurally similar metabolite, e.g. pirprofen (Sioufi *et al.*, 1987), and the diastereoisomeric glutathione conjugates of the enantiomers of 5,6-benz[a]anthracene-5,6-oxide (Dostal *et al.*, 1986). Several authors have overcome this problem in bioanalytical work by incorporation of an achiral TLC or HPLC isolation step prior to chiral analysis by either a CSP or CDA (see for example Crowther *et al.*, 1984).

An alternative approach is to use two chromatographic columns connected via a column-switching technique. This method is referred to as either coupled column chromatography or two-dimensional chromatography. Using this technique the major problem is the choice of systems such that the mobile phases are compatible with one another. The most common approach is to use an achiral phase initially for separation of the analytes of interest from the contaminants of the biological media or drug metabolites, followed by transfer of an appropriate volume of eluate to the CSP for enantiomeric analysis.

The problem of solvent compatibility is reduced to some extent with the designed CSPs; for example the N-(3,5-dinitrobenzoyl)phenylglycine phase is available in both the (R), (S) and racemic forms. In such cases the 'racemic' column yields identical separations to the chiral phases with the exception of the chiral resolution (Dappen *et al.*, 1986). Masurel and Wainer (1989) have used this technique for the enantiomeric analysis of ifosfamide and cyclophosphamide in plasma. A number of achiral systems were examined but mobile-phase compatibility and selectivity proved to be a problem (Wainer, 1989). Use of the 'racemic' form of a naphthylalanine column as the achiral system and cellulose tris(3,5-dimethylphenylcarbamate) as the CSP resulted in a useful analytical system and the mobile phases for both columns was identical, hexane : propan-2-ol mixtures (Masurel and Wainer, 1989).

This approach cannot be applied for the majority of CSPs as few are available in racemic forms. In these cases an achiral phase must be chosen such that the solvent used is compatible with the CSP. Using this approach Roston and Wijayaratne (1988) have resolved the isomers of the antiulcer drug misoprostol (methyl (11α, 13 E)-($\pm$)-11,16-dihydroxy-16-methyl-9-oxoprost-13-en-1-oate) which contains two chiral centres, 11 and 16, and samples consist of two pairs of enantiomers, the pharmacologically active isomer being the (11 R,16 S)-enantiomer. The individual pairs of enantiomers may be resolved using an α_1-AGP-CSP; however, coelution of the diastereoisomers rendered this system useless for analysis (Roston and Wijayaratne, 1988). The problem was solved by partial resolution of the diastereoisomeric pairs by conventional reverse phase chromatography followed by column switching of the fraction containing the active isomer to the CSP. The 'cut' size of the eluate from the achiral system was found to be crucial for the performance of the CSP; the solvent system consisting of a methanol : water (3 : 2) mixture (achiral chromatography) was found to deactivate the CSP, after two or three injections, if volumes $<250\,\mu$l were transferred (Roston and Wijayaratne, 1988).

There have been several reports of coupled column chromatography being used in bioanalytical studies. Edholm *et al.* (1988) used a β-cyclodextrin CSP linked to a phenyl achiral phase for the analysis of terbutaline enantiomers. The mobile phase for the achiral step consisted of ammonium acetate (0.01 M) at pH 4.6, whilst that for the CSP was methanol : ammonium acetate (0.05 M) (10 : 90) at pH 6.0. The use of the second stronger eluent resulted in peak compression and a reduction of band broadening which may be a problem in some instances as a reduction in sensitivity may result.

The resolution and bioanalysis of the enantiomers of warfarin has been achieved by coupled column chromatography using a Pinkerton internal-surface reverse phase column linked to a BSA-CSP (Chu and Wainer, 1988). The mobile phase for the achiral system consisted of phosphate buffer (0.2 M, pH 6.5) : propan-1-ol (99 : 1) whilst for chiral chromatography the composition was slightly altered to phosphate buffer (0.2 M, pH 7.5) : propan-1-ol (97 : 3) containing trichloroacetic acid (3 mM). The advantage of using this approach is the minimal sample preparation required before analysis is carried out. The achiral process was also used for the determination of the total drug content present in plasma, whilst the enantiomeric composition of the warfarin was determined by relative peak area following resolution by the CSP. Thus the problems associated with the selection of a suitable internal standard for the chiral analysis are circumvented (Chu and Wainer, 1988).

Wainer and Stiffin (1988) have also used this approach for the analysis of leucovorin isomers using a phenyl column for the separation of the drug from the methyl metabolite, followed by resolution of the (6R)- and (6S)-leucovorin isomers using a BSA-CSP.

Coupled-column chromatography obviously has a number of advantages, particularly in terms of preliminary sample 'work-up' and also in increasing the life of expensive CSPs which may be particularly sensitive to the type of trace contaminants found in samples of biological origin. In some instances the achiral-chiral arrangement of the system may not be very useful due to the low efficiency of the CSP, band broadening reducing the sensitivity of the method. A reversal of the columns may overcome this problem and thus increase the sensitivity of the system by compression of the peaks obtained using the CSP on the achiral phase (Edholm, cited in Wainer, 1989).

Chiral mobile phases for HPLC

The advantage of the addition of chiral additives to an HPLC mobile phase is that conventional highly efficient columns, either reverse or normal phase, may be used for analysis. Several approaches have been adopted in this area each of which will be briefly examined.

CHIRAL COUNTER IONS

Ion-pair chromatography is a commonly used technique in HPLC, a charged analyte forming a neutral ion pair with a counter ion of opposite charge as a component of the mobile phase, the neutral ion-pair being retained by the stationary phase. Enantiomeric resolution may be achieved by the use of chiral counter ions, as enantiomeric analytes may be expected to form diastereoisomeric ion pairs which will have different distribution properties between the stationary phase and the mobile phase (Pettersson and Schill, 1986). This technique has been applied mainly for the resolution and analysis of chiral amines and acids. Important properties of the reagents are relatively strong acid-base characteristics, low polarity, optical purity and commercial availability (Szepesi and Gazdag, 1988). Commonly used agents include (+)-10-camphorsulphonic acid and quinine (Pettersson and Schill, 1981; Pettersson, 1984).

If electrostatic interactions only occur between the analyte and the chiral counter ion then chromatographic selectivity would not be expected and additional interactions, e.g. hydrogen bonding, or hydrophobic interactions, between the two ions are also thought to be of significance (Pettersson and

Schill, 1981). For example, the resolution of some β-aminoalcohol, β-blocking agents, using (+)-10-camphorsulphonic acid has been investigated by Pettersson and Schill (1981). The interactions between the analyte and the chiral counter ion involves electrostatic forces between the protonated amino function of the analyte and the sulphonic acid group and also a hydrogen bonding interaction between the keto carbonyl on the camphor moiety and the hydroxy group of the analyte, which is thought to be responsible for the enantiomeric resolutions observed. This view is supported by the fact that resolution is not observed if the hydroxyl function is absent or greater than two carbon atoms distant from the protonated amino group (Pettersson and Schill, 1988). Similarly, the resolution of a series of carboxylic acids has been investigated using quinine as a chiral counter ion. Again a two-point interaction was required for resolution, analytes containing hydrogen bonding functions in addition to the electrostatic interaction being resolved (Pettersson and Schill, 1986).

Enantiomeric resolution is influenced by the concentration of the chiral counter ion, the addition of solvent modifiers to the mobile phase, e.g. pentan-1-ol *ca* 1 per cent in dichloromethane and the water content of the solvent, e.g. of the order of 80–90 ppm (Pettersson and Schill, 1986). The nature of the stationary phase is also of considerable importance. Modified silica surfaces such as Lichrosorb DIOL are generally preferred, and different stereoselectivity may be observed using different phases. For example the enantiomers of naproxen may be resolved on a silica surface using quinine as a chiral counter ion and not on the DIOL phase, whereas the situation is reversed with α-methoxy-α-trifluoromethylphenylacetic acid (Pettersson, 1984). This difference is indicative of alternative interactions between the polar functions in the analyte ion-pair and the stationary phase.

Alternative chiral counter ions include derivatives of amino acids, e.g. N-benzoxycarbonylglycyl-L-proline which has been used to resolve a series of aryloxypropanolamine β-blocking agents (Pettersson and Schill, 1988) and has been used for the determination of the enantiomeric composition of propranolol in human plasma (Pettersson and Josefsson, 1986).

CHIRAL METAL COMPLEXATION ADDITIVES

Metal complexation mobile phase additives involving L-amino acids and metal ions, e.g. Cu (II) and Ni (II), have been used for enantiomeric resolution on reverse phase (C-8, C-18) columns (see, for example, Wernicke, 1985; Keller and Dick, 1986). This technique involves the formation of diastereoisomeric complexes in a similar manner to that for CLEC and these systems are particularly useful for the resolution of amino acid enantiomers (Wernicke, 1985). Similarly, the enantiomers of structurally related drugs, e.g. dopa, methyldopa and carbidopa, have also been resolved using this technique (Gelber and Neumeyer, 1983; Wernicke, 1985).

Bewick (1986) has used this approach for the analysis of the enantiomeric composition of the chiral herbicide fluazifop (R, S-2-[4-(5-trifluoromethyl-2-

pyridyloxy)phenoxy] propionate) following isolation of the compound from soil samples. The enantiomers of fluazifop were resolved using a mobile phase containing a L-proline-n-octylamide nickel (II) complex (3.4 mM) in a methanol–acetonitrile–water–acetic acid mixture at pH 7.8. Using this method, it was possible to demonstrate that chiral inversion of the (S)-enantiomer had taken place to yield residues of the (R)-isomer in high optical purity (Bewick, 1986).

CYCLODEXTRINS

The cyclodextrins (CD) and their derivatives, have the advantage that they may be used in aqueous-based solvent systems and with reverse phase columns (Zukowski *et al.*, 1986; Szepesi and Gazdag, 1988). The mechanism of resolution is inclusion complex formation, as for the CD–CSPs; enantiomer differentiation is due to either differences in the analyte–CD complex stability constants and/or differences in the adsorption of the complexes, i.e. retention by the stationary phase (Zukowski *et al.*, 1986). The resolution of mandelic acid and some derivatives, and some chiral barbiturates and hydantoin derivatives including mephenytoin, has been reported using β-CD and heptakis (2,6-di-0-methyl)-β-CD as mobile phase additives (Debowski *et al.*, 1983; Zukowski *et al.*, 1986).

That the formation of an analyte–CD complex alone is not sufficient for chromatographic resolution has been shown by Mularz *et al.* (1988). These latter authors attempted to resolve the isomers of both ephedrine and pseudoephedrine using β-CD as a mobile phase additive. It was found, by NMR that all four isomers formed inclusion complexes; however, only the enantiomers of pseudoephedrine could be resolved by HPLC. This was surprising as the formation constants for all four analyte–β-CD complexes were similar. Following NMR analysis of the inclusion complexes it was concluded that both the hydroxyl and protonated nitrogen of the analytes interact with the β-CD. The dual interactions are strongest with (+)-(S,S)-pseudoephedrine and weakest with (−)-(R,R)-pseudoephedrine, approximately equal intermediate values being obtained for the enantiomers of ephedrine. It was concluded that the chromatographic resolution of these agents was dependent on the dual interaction of the two functionalities with the β-CD (Mularz *et al.*, 1988).

Szepesi and Gazdaz (1988) have suggested that a mixture of α, β and γ-CDs should be used as an additive to the mobile phase. The analyte under these conditions will only form an inclusion complex with that CD with which it forms the strongest bond, the other CDs present having no significant effects on chromatographic retention. These same authors have also examined the combined use of both chiral ion-pairing agents and β-CD as mobile phase additives particularly for those compounds which cannot be resolved satisfactorily by the individual use of either technique (Szepesi and Gazdaz, 1988).

OTHER CHIRAL MOBILE PHASE ADDITIVES

Addition of proteins, e.g. human serum albumin (HSA) and α_1-acid glycoprotein, to mobile phases as chiral selectors has also been reported (Hermansson, 1984; Pettersson and Schill, 1986). The resolution of the enantiomers of tryptophan and a number of chiral carboxylic acid derivatives using HSA and reverse phase columns has been reported (Pettersson and Schill, 1986).

The resolution of the enantiomers of ephedrine, and related β-aminoalcohols, has been achieved using (+)-di-n-butyltartrate as a chiral complexing agent (Pettersson and Stuurman, 1984).

Optical activity detectors for HPLC

Both polarimetric and circular dichroic detectors have been described for HPLC instruments and combinations of achiral chromatography followed by a chiral detection system in series with a UV detector is a relatively facile method for enantiomer quantitation (see, for example, Scott and Dunn, 1985; Meinard *et al.*, 1985; Reitsma and Yeung, 1986). In addition these detectors in combination with a CSP allow the direct determination of enantiomer elution order (Salvadori *et al.*, 1984; Bertucci *et al.*, 1987). The utility of these detectors is due to their optical selectivity, i.e. only chiral compounds will be detected, and that the recorded responses are both positive and negative (Salvadori *et al.*, 1984).

Due to the constraints of small elution volumes and signal size, the sensitivity of these systems may be a problem; for example, polarimeter signals require amplification so that low optical rotations may be observed reproducibly. Because of this problem laser-based systems are the most suitable light sources for these detectors (Yeung, 1988; Purdie and Swallows, 1989) and Yeung *et al.* (1980) have described the construction of a micropolarimeter based on an argon ion laser for use as an HPLC detector. Bobbitt and Yeung (1984) have used microbore HPLC, in combination with an optical activity detector, which, due to the decreased analyte dilution, results in a decrease in the limit of detection. The construction of a polarimeter, with microdegree sensitivity, based on a semiconductor diode laser, has recently been described, its utility as an HPLC detector has been examined with the use of small volume flow cells (Lloyd *et al.*, 1989).

A laser-based polarimeter for use as an HPLC detector is presently commercially available in the UK (ACS ChiraMonitor®); however, sensitivity continues to be a problem, the limit of detection for glucose being quoted as 1 μg on column (ACS literature) and the sensitivity is not presently great enough for routine monitoring of drug plasma concentrations. To date there are no reports of the application of these detectors in bioanalysis, however, this is an area of obvious potential for these systems (Purdie and Swallows, 1989).

Chiral gas chromatography

Direct enantiomeric resolution by gas chromatography (GC) was first achieved by Gil-Av *et al.* (1966) using the lauryl ester of N-trifluoroacetyl-L-isoleucine as a chiral phase for the resolution of a series of N-trifluoro-acetylamino acid esters. Since this early success there has been considerable progress in the design and development of chiral phases for GC analysis (Liu and Ku, 1983; Schurig, 1984; König, 1987).

The mechanism of resolution on these early phases was assumed to be due to hydrogen bond formation between amide groups in the analyte and the CSP. Additional phases using esters of both di- and tripeptides have been examined and developments from these early peptide phases resulted in the preparation of diamide phases containing the functional grouping:

$$-NH-CO-CH(R)-NH-CO-$$

and the ureide or carbonyl bis(amino acid ester) phases:

$$R^1-O-CO-CH(R)-NII-CO-NII-CH(R)-COOR^1$$

Many of the early GC-CSPs were limited by their relatively low thermal stability; for example, many of these phases have operating temperatures below $150°$ C (Liu and Ku, 1983). The thermal stability problems of these columns are two-fold, involving phase breakdown and hence high column bleed and more importantly, racemization of the CSP with a loss in enantioselectivity.

The major advance with these systems occurred in the mid-1970s by the covalent bonding of the chiral selector L-valine-t-butylamide to a copolymer of dimethylsiloxane and carboxyalkylmethylsiloxane (Frank *et al.*, 1978). This diamide phase was wall coated on capillary columns and is commercially available as Chirasil-Val® (Figure 38). This column has the advantages of both high thermal stability, temperature range (70–240° C), and low volatility. The chiral selectors in the Chiralsil-Val® phase are separated from each

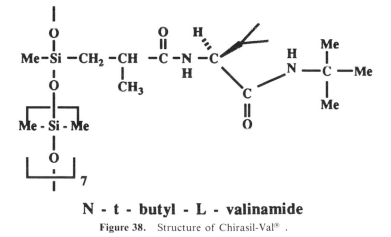

N - t - butyl - L - valinamide

Figure 38. Structure of Chirasil-Val® .

other by about seven dimethylsiloxane units (Figure 38) which appears to be of considerable importance for both thermal stability and useful analyte resolution, presumably by avoidance of interactions between adjacent selector residues. The presence of an additional chiral centre in the carboxyalkyl-methylsiloxane residue may also aid the resolution process (Figure 38).

An alternative commercially available diamide phase is XE-60-(S)-valine-(R) or (S)-α-phenylethylamide (Figure 39). Similar to the above, these phases have relatively high operating temperatures.

An alternative approach to GC-CSPs involves the use of chiral metal chelates coated onto capillary columns. The chiral selector is an optically active β-diketone of the type used as chiral shift reagents in NMR, e.g. 3-heptafluorobutyryl-(1R)-camphorate, complexed with a transition metal ion, e.g. nickel, europium or manganese (Schurig and Weber, 1984). The analyte(s) undergo enantioselective interactions with the chiral chelate complexes resulting in the formation of diastereoisomeric complexes. Chiral complexation GC is particularly useful for those compounds which cannot be derivatized or lack suitable functional groups for interaction with amide phases, e.g. chiral alkenes, epoxides, bicyclic spiroacetals, ketones and diol-acetonides (Schurig, 1986).

The application of GC-CSPs for the resolution of a number of chiral drugs has been reported. König and co-workers have examined the resolution of a variety of aminoalcohol sympathomimetic agents and the related β-blocking drugs using the XE-60-L-valine-(R)-α-phenylethylamide phase (König and Ernst, 1983; König *et al.*, 1984; Gyllenhaal *et al.*, 1985; König *et al.*, 1986; König, 1988). The initial studies involved formation of N,O-heptafluoro-butyryl derivatives. Whilst this approach resulted in the resolution of a number of compounds, it was found that ephedrine underwent partial racemization (König, 1988) and in addition the β-blocking agents containing a N-t-butyl group as opposed to an N-isopropyl function, could not be

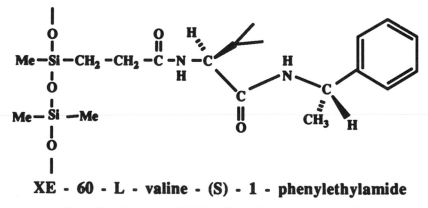

XE - 60 - L - valine - (S) - 1 - phenylethylamide

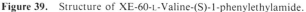

Figure 39.   Structure of XE-60-L-Valine-(S)-1-phenylethylamide.

resolved using this CSP even though diderivatization was confirmed by mass spectrometry (König and Ernst, 1983). This lack of resolution was explained by the steric bulk of the t-butyl group inhibiting formation of the required association complex with the CSP. An alternative approach was adopted involving reaction of the β-aminoalcohols with phosgene to yield oxazolidin-2-ones (Figure 40). Under the conditions of the derivatization, racemization of ephedrine was not observed and GC resolution of both isopropyl and t-butyl derivatives of the β-blockers was obtained (König *et al.*, 1986; König, 1988).

This method has also been used for the resolution of metoprolol, several analogues and two major metabolites α-hydroxymetoprolol and 4-(3-iso-propylamino-2-hydroxypropoxy)phenylacetic acid (Gyllenhaal *et al.*, 1985). The two metabolites required additional derivatization of the alcohol to the corresponding TMS derivative and the acid to the methyl ester. In the case of the alcohol, even though a new chiral centre is introduced, two peaks were observed with a separation factor similar to that of the drug. For the acid derivative, the resolution of a synthetic sample and material isolated from human urine indicated that stereoselective metabolism had not taken place (Gyllenhaal *et al.*, 1985).

Chirasil-Val® has been used for the resolution and analysis in plasma of the enantiomers of tocainide as their heptafluorobutyryl derivatives using an electron capture detector (Antonsson *et al.*, 1984).

The use of the same column for the analysis of the enantiomers of mephenytoin and its dealkylated metabolite 5-phenyl-5-ethylhydantoin in both plasma and blood has been reported by Wedlund *et al.* (1984). The technique involves the use of two internal standards 3-methyl-5-phenyl-5-isopropylhydantoin and 5-phenyl-5-propylhydantoin and the resolution of

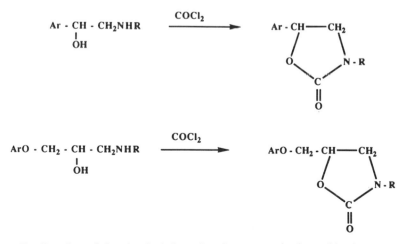

Figure 40. Reaction of β-aminoalcohols and aryloxypropanolamines with phosgene to yield oxazolidin-2-one derivatives prior to resolution using a GC–CSP.

both analytes and both internal standards is achieved in one chromatographic run. The assay relies on the selective 3-propylation of both the metabolite 5-phenyl-5-ethylhydantoin and the internal standard 5-phenyl-5-propyl-hydantoin using 1-iodopropane during the sample work up. Problems with this methodology occurred due to trace contaminants of iodomethane in the derivatizing agent resulting in the methylation of the dealkylated metabolite to yield the drug mephenytoin (Akrawi and Wedlund, 1986). The problem was partially solved by distillation of l-iodopropane prior to use, some 0.7 per cent of the total metabolite converted to mephenytoin being reduced to 0.1 per cent following distillation. Whilst these quantities appear to be low it should be noted that the metabolite levels may be 50 to 100 fold greater than that of the drug (Akrawi and Wedlund, 1986) and hence this example illustrates the importance of derivatizing agent purity.

The application of a combination of GC-CSPs for the separation of optical isomers may be illustrated using the organophosphorus anticholinesterase agents soman, sarin and tabun as examples. These agents all contain a chiral phosphorus atom and in the case of soman, a chiral carbon centre is also present, the drug consisting of a mixture of four stereoisomers (Figure 41; Benschop and De Jong, 1988). The absolute configuration of the chiral phosphorus centre in these agents has not yet been established and their stereochemistry is indicated by the sign of the enantiomer optical rotation. In the case of soman the four isomers are distinguished as C(+)-P(+), C(+)-P(−), C(−)-P(−) and C(−)-P(+), where C(+)/(−) refers to the chirality of the carbon centre in the 1,2,2-trimethylpropyl group which during synthesis arises from the sign of optical rotation of the pinacolylalcohol used (Benschop *et al.*, 1984). The enantiomeric alcohols are used to prepare two pairs of diastereoisomeric soman isomers, i.e. C(+)-P(+)/C(+)-P(−) and C(−)-P(−)/C(−)-P(+). The pairs of diastereoisomers may then be resolved by selective enzymic hydrolysis, e.g. those compounds designated P(−) selec-

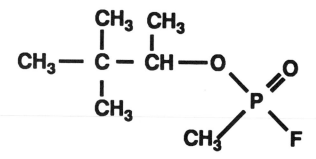

Figure 41. Structure of soman.

tively phosphoralylate α-chymotrypsin leaving those isomers designated P($+$). Alternatively, incubation with rabbit plasma shows the opposite stereoselectivity for hydrolysis leaving a residue of those isomers designated P($-$) (Benschop *et al.*, 1984; Benschop and DeJong, 1988). Synthetic soman consists of a mixture of the enantiomeric pairs C($+$)-P($+$) : C($-$)-P($-$) and C($+$)-P($-$) : C($-$)-P($+$) in a ratio of 45 : 55.

An enantiospecific analytical technique to determine the optical purity of the individual isomers of soman following selective hydrolysis was obviously required. Initially an examination of the four isomers by Chirasil-Val® was carried out. Using this system a total of three peaks were observed, the two outer peaks corresponding to the C($-$) isomers whilst the middle peak contained both C($+$) isomers (Benschop *et al.*, 1981). This result would indicate the resolution of the enantiomeric pairs but not the C($+$)diastereoisomers. As these diastereoisomers could be resolved by achiral capillary GC, a 30 m carbowax 20 M column was directly coupled to the Chirasil-Val® column (25 m). Using this system resolution of all four isomers was obtained (Benschop *et al.*, 1981).

These latter authors extended their studies and synthesized a sample of Chirasil-Val®, which, using a 50 m widebore column, resolved all four isomers directly. The elution order of the two peaks due to the C($+$) isomers was, however, reversed compared to the previous coupled achiral–chiral system (Benschop *et al.*, 1985). An additional advantage of this latter column was the separation and resolution of d_{13}-standards of C($\pm$)P($+$)-soman, prepared from complete deuteration of the 1,2,2-trimethylpropyl moiety, from those of the four hydrogen isomers, thus providing an internal standard without the requirement for GC-MS analysis (Benschop *et al.*, 1985). Using this assay, the authors developed an analytical method for the determination of the isomers in blood following administration of the compound to rats (Benschop *et al.*, 1985; 1987).

Chirasil-Val® columns were found not to resolve completely the isomers of the related compounds tabun and sarin. All three compounds could be resolved using lanthanide shift reagents in NMR. It therefore seemed reasonable that chiral complexation GC would be a possible solution to the problem. Using a column coated with bis[(1R)-3-((heptafluorobutyryl)camphorato)] nickel (II) in OV-101 on either a 2 m glass column or a 11 m wide bore column, both isomers of tabun and sarin could be resolved as could all four isomers of soman (Degenhardt *et al.*, 1986; Benschop and De Jong, 1988).

Several new GC-CSPs based on the cyclodextrins have recently become commercially available (Lipodex® columns, Macherey-Nagel). The hydrophobicity of the cyclodextrin is increased by alkylation and these derivatives have been used as liquid phases for capillary gas chromatography. The thermal stability of these columns appears to be high, no loss of column performance being observed after use at 200° C. The mechanism of resolution is not understood; however, it would appear that inclusion complex formation is unlikely and diastereoisomer association complexes via dipole–dipole interactions are more likely to be the mechanism of resolution (König *et al.*, 1988 a,c). These phases have been used for the resolution of carbohydrate derivatives, aminoalcohols, amino acid esters, acetylated amines and alkenes (König *et al.*, 1988 a,b,c; Ehlers *et al.*, 1988).

Chiral thin-layer chromatography

Many of the techniques applied for the HPLC and GC resolution of enantiomers have been examined for their application for resolution by thin-layer chromatography (TLC). Thus Gubitz and Mihellyes (1984) reported the TLC resolution of several β-blocking drugs using (R)-1-(naphthen-l-yl)ethyl isocyanate as a CDA and Maitre *et al.* (1986) have used centrifugal TLC for the preparative resolution of the diastereoisomeric amides of some 2-arylpropionic acid NSAIDs. Slégel *et al.* (1987) have described the TLC resolution of a number of chiral carboxylic acids as the diastereoisomeric carboxamide derivatives of the novel amine CDAs (−) and (+)-1-(4-nitrophenyl)-2-amino-1,3-propanediol.

Several of the techniques used for HPLC CSPs have been applied to TLC. Wainer *et al.* (1983) reported the resolution of the enantiomers of 2,2,2-trifluoro-1-(9-anthryl)ethanol using the CSP (R)-N-(3,5-dinitrobenzoyl) phenylglycine ionically bonded to γ-aminopropyl silanized silica TLC plates. Using a similar technique Wilson (1986) found that the plates rapidly discolour and no useful resolutions were obtained.

Commercially available TLC plates based on CLEC using ODS plates treated with (2S, 4R, 2′R,S)-4-hydroxy-1-(2-hydroxydodecyl)proline and copper (II) acetate have been used to resolve amino acid enantiomers (Brinkman and Kamminga, 1985). The resolution of the enantiomers of dopa, methyldopa and penicillamine has also been reported using the CLEC plates (Gunther *et al.*, 1985; Martens *et al.*, 1986 a,b). In the case of penicillamine, derivatization with formaldehyde to yield the corresponding 5,5-dimethylthiazolidine was required to effect resolution (Martens *et al.*, 1986 b).

Wilson (1986) attempted to resolve the enantiomers of propranolol, mandelic acid and a propionic acid NSAID using TLC plates coated with a solution of 1 per cent β-cyclodextrin in a mixture of ethanol : dimethylsulphoxide (80 : 20). Partial resolution of the enantiomers of mandelic acid was achieved using this system. The preparation of β-CD bonded TLC plates has been reported by Alak and Armstrong (1986). These plates were found to be useful for the resolution of dansyl and naphthylamide derivatives of amino acids.

There are no reports of TLC CSPs being used in bioanalytical chemistry; however, the development of suitable systems may be of considerable use in analysis and more importantly allow rapid screening of a number of CSPs for a resolution of interest and hence optimize the preparation of derivatives and choice of CSP for HPLC.

Resolution of diastereoisomeric drug conjugates by HPLC

Many metabolic transformations of racemic drugs result in the formation of diastereoisomeric metabolites. This is particularly the case for the conjugation reactions where the conjugating agent may be chiral, e.g. the carbohydrates D-glucuronic acid and D-glucose, the amino acid glutamine and the tripeptide glutathione. Hence racemic drugs which undergo conjugation with these agents may yield a pair of diastereoisomeric metabolites and achiral compounds may yield chiral conjugates. That such conjugates may be resolved by achiral chromatography is not surprising as derivatives of both amino acids and carbohydrates are frequently used as CDAs. The formation of such products may give rise to problems associated with the analysis of the material obtained, as the analysis of glucuronide conjugates for example frequently involves enzymatic hydrolysis, with β-glucuronidase, followed by analysis of the liberated aglycone. An approach of this type may result in misleading data due to the stereoselectivity of the enzymatic step.

The major metabolite(s) of the racemic antidepressant drug oxaprotiline in man are two diastereoisomeric glucuronide conjugates which can be resolved using micronized XAD-2 (Dieterle *et al.*, 1984 a). The hydrolysis of these two glucuronides requires different conditions. The more polar isomer, formed from (S)-oxaprotiline, is readily susceptible to enzyme hydrolysis whereas the less polar compound, from (R)-oxaprotiline could be cleaved by treatment with acid (Dieterle *et al.*, 1984 a,b).

A similar situation occurs with oxazepam, which also yields a pair of diastereoisomeric glucuronides which may be readily resolved by achiral HPLC (Sisenwine *et al.*, 1982). The enzymatic hydrolysis of these two glucuronides has been investigated under a variety of conditions and found to be dependent on both the stereochemistry of the compound and the enzyme preparation used (Ruelius *et al.*, 1979). The hydrolysis of (S)-oxazepam glucuronide is more rapid than that of the (R)-isomer, the ratio of the rates of hydrolysis (S/R) varying from 446, using β-glucuronidase from *Escherichia coli*, to 1.3 using an enzyme obtained from a marine mollusc (Ruelius *et al.*, 1979).

The glucuronidation of oxazepam is of particular interest as the drug rapidly undergoes racemization in aqueous media and in contact with glass surfaces and it is of interest to note that following hydrolysis of either of the isolated diastereoisomeric glucuronides the oxazepam obtained was racemic (Ruelius *et al.*, 1979). The formation of the diastereoisomeric glucuronides and their analysis by HPLC (see Table 4) thus facilitates an examination of the disposition of the drug. The species variability of metabolic conjugation has been reported (Sisenwine *et al.*, 1982) and oxazepam has also been used as a probe for induction of UDP-glucuronyltransferases in rabbits (Yost and Finley, 1985).

Glucuronidation of carboxylic acids is problematical and continues to be of interest due to the facile rearrangement of the conjugates produced, by intra-

Table 4. HPLC systems for the analytical resolution of diastereoisomeric glucuronide conjugates.

Compound	Column	Mobile phase	Detection	Elution	Reference
Benoxaprofen	ODS (250 × 4.6 mm, 5 µM)	0.01 M phosphate buffer, pH 6.3 in CH_3CN (gradient 30–35% in 3 min, isocratic at 35% for 12 min) flow-rate 1.0 ml/min	UV 254 nm	S,D before R,D (R_T 7.8 and 8.4 min)	El-Mouelhi *et al.* (1987)
Ibuprofen		0.1 M $NH_4^+ AcO^-$: $CH_3 CN$ (gradient 35 to 80% over 10 min) flow-rate 1.0 ml/min		S,D before R,D (R_T 5.4 and 6.0 min)	
Naproxen		0.05 M $NH_4^+ AcO^-$: $CH_3 CN$ (80:20) at pH 6.0 flow-rate 1.2 ml/min		S,D before R,D (R_T 14.3 and 15.2 min)	
2-Phenylpropionic acid	Lichrosorb-Hibar RT (250 × 4 mm, 7 µm)	CH_3CN : CF_3CO_2H : H_2O (38.0 : 0.08 : 162) flow-rate 1.0 ml/min	UV 254 nm	R,D before S,D (capacity values k^1 18.14, k^1 19.73 respectively R_s = 3.54)	Fournel-Gigleux *et al.* (1988)
2-Arylpropionic acids (9 compounds)	ODS (250 × 4.6 mm, 5 µm)	CH_3CN : Tetrabutylammonium hydrogen sulphate (10 mM) pH 2.5 (28:72) flow-rate 1.5 ml/min	Fluorescence or UV depending on compound	S,D before R,D (α values 1.03–1.14, R_s values 0.3–2.27)	Spahn (1988 d)
Indoprofen	As above	CH_3CN : Tetrabutylammonium hydrogen sulphate (8 mM) pH 2.5 (23:77)	Fluorescence (ex 275, em 433 nm)	SD before RD (α = 1.05, R = 1.54)	Spahn (1988 d)
Benoxaprofen	Ultrasphere (250 × 4.6 mm, 5 µm)	CH_3CN : Tetrabutylammonium hydroxide buffer (10 mM) pH 2.5 (28:72) flow-rate 1.8 ml/min	Fluorescence (ex 313 nm, em 365 nm)	SD before RD (α = 1.10, R = 2.39)	Spahn *et al.* (1989 a)
Propranolol	ODS (250 × 4.6 mm, 10 µm)	MeOH : 0.1 M $NH_4H_2PO_4$ (56:44) flow rate 1.0 ml/min	UV 225 nm	RD before SD (run time < 10 min)	Thompson *et al.* (1981)

Compound	Column	Mobile phase	Detection	Result	Reference
4-Hydroxy-propranolol	As above	As above composition 13:87, flow-rate 1.2 ml/min	As above	S,D before R,D (run time > 20 min)	
E-10-Hydroxy-nortriptyline	ODS (250 × 10 mm)	MeOH:Phosphate buffer 0.01 M, pH 2.6 (45:55) flow-rate 2.5 ml/min	UV 254 nm	(+) before (−) (R_T 10 and 11 min respectively)	Dumont *et al.* (1987)
Oxazepam	ODS (300 × 4.6 mm, 10 μm)	MeOH, 40%, in 0.025 M NaH_2PO_4 flow-rate 2 ml/min	UV 254 nm	R,D R_T 9.4 min S,D R_T 11.5 min	Ruelius *et al.* (1979)
	ODS (150 × 4.6 mm, 10 μm)	MeOH, 40% in phosphate buffer (0.1 M) pH6, flow rate 1.0 ml/min	UV 234 nm	(−) before (+) (run time c. 12 min)	Seideman *et al.* (1981)
	ODS (250 × 4.6 mm)	CH_3CN (14–25%) in $NH_4^+AcO^-$ (0.1 M) or MeOH (30%) in $NH_4^+AcO^-$ (0.1 M) flow-rates 1.4–2.5 ml/min depending on the sample	UV 254 nm	R,D before S,D	Sisenwine *et al.* (1982)
	Ultrasphere–RP (250 mm, 5 μm)	MeOH (40%) in 25 mM KH_2PO_4 at pH6 flow-rate 1 ml/min	UV 254 nm	R,D before S,D	Yost and Finley (1985)
5-(4-Hydroxy-phenyl)-5-phenyl-hydantoin (metabolite of phenytoin)	ODS (250 × 4.5 mm, 5 μm)	CH_3CN (8%) in phosphate buffer ($\mu = 0.1$) pH 7.5 flow-rate 1.0 ml/min	UV 225 nm	R,D before S,E $\alpha = 1.06$ run time c. 30 min	Hermansson *et al.* (1982)
2-(N-Propyl-N-2-thienylethylamine)-5-hydroxy-tetralin	ODS (150 × 4.6 mm, 3 μm)	CH_3CN (12%) in 0.01 M phosphate buffer pH 6.8 flow rate 1.5 ml/min	UV 225 nm	(−) before (+) $\alpha = 1.13$, R_S 3.6 (run time c. 70 min)	Gerding *et al.* (1989)
Amobarbital*	ODS (250 × 4.6 mm, 5 μm)	CH_3CN (20%) in 0.025 M sodium phosphate buffer pH 6.5 flow rate 1.4 ml/min	UV 198 nm	Conjugates A and B R_T 14.2 and 15.9 min respectively	Soine and Soine (1987)

* N-glucose conjugate

molecular acyl transfer to yield β-glucuronidase-resistant isomers and their reactivity toward nucleophilic centres (Faed, 1984; Caldwell and Hutt, 1986; Caldwell *et al.*, 1988 b). The metabolism and disposition of the 2-arylpropionic acid NSAIDs is of particular interest due to their metabolic chiral inversion and evidence is also available which would indicate that enantioselectivity in glucuronidation also occurs (Caldwell *et al.*, 1988 c). Several groups have resolved the diastereoisomeric glucuronides (Figure 42) of these agents by achiral chromatography and the methods are summarized in Table 4.

Spahn *et al.* (1989 a) have investigated the analysis of benoxaprofen glucuronides in some detail. Using an achiral chromatographic system, which gave baseline resolution of the two diastereoisomers, the conjugate derived from (R)-benoxaprofen was found to be less stable under physiological conditions of pH and temperature, than that derived from (S)-benoxaprofen. The rate of decomposition of these conjugates, in microsomal incubation media, was similar for both isomeric forms provided that inhibitors of hydrolytic enzymes were added; in the absence of inhibitors the (R)-benoxaprofen conjugate decomposed more rapidly than the (S)-isomeric form (Spahn *et al.*, 1989 a). Conjugates present in urine samples could be stabilized by dilution of the sample 1 : 10 and by reduction of pH to between 2.5 and 3.0. Freezing and thawing samples which were not pH-adjusted resulted in almost complete loss of β-glucuronidase hydrolyzable material and the appearance of chroma-

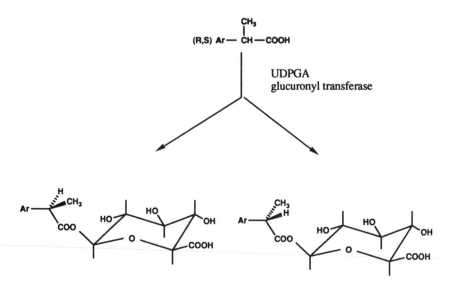

(R,D) - diastereoisomer   (S,D) - diastereoisomer

Figure 42. Conjugation of racemic 2-arylpropionic acids to yield diastereoisomeric glucuronide conjugates.

tographic peaks resistant to enzyme cleavage which could be hydrolyzed with alkali (Spahn *et al.*, 1989 a). Such data has obvious implications for the determination of these diastereoisomeric conjugates in samples of biological origin as the final analytical values obtained may not reflect their formation and/or renal clearance but their relative stability in the biological media.

It is common practice when using β-glucuronidase for conjugate hydrolysis to carry out control incubations containing saccharo-1,4-lactone as a specific enzyme inhibitor to confirm the formation of a glucuronide (Caldwell and Hutt, 1986). El-Mouelhi *et al.* (1987) have recently reported observations concerning the importance of enzyme and inhibitor concentration on the stereoselectivity of inhibition. Incubation of the diastereoisomeric glucuronides of (R)- and (S)-naproxen with β-glucuronidase obtained from bovine liver, resulted in the total hydrolysis of both conjugates. In the presence of saccharo-1,4-lactone, in a ratio of enzyme to inhibitor of 83 units : 5 mM only slight hydrolysis of both conjugates was observed; however, a ratio of 276 units : 2.5 mM resulted in total hydrolysis of the (R)-naproxen conjugate with some 73 per cent of the (S)-isomeric form remaining. Intermediate ratios of enzyme to inhibitor resulted in partial hydrolysis of both conjugates but to different extents (El-Mouelhi *et al.*, 1987).

The chromatographic resolution of glucuronide conjugates has recently resulted in the use of glucuronic acid as a 'biological' CDA for the resolution of the dopamine agonist 2-(N-propyl-N-2-thienylethylamino)-5-hydroxytetralin (Table 4; Gerding *et al.*, 1989). Using a bovine liver microsomal preparation, fortified by the addition of a twenty-fold excess of uridine 5′-diphosphoglucuronic acid (UDPGA) and a reaction time of 120 min, the total yield of the two glucuronides was found to be >99 per cent. Examination of the kinetic constants for the reaction indicated a $(+)/(-)$ ratio of 2.8 in Vmax, whereas the affinity of the $(-)$ enantiomer was about four times greater than that of the $(+)$-isomer (Gerding *et al.*, 1989). However, under the conditions of the reaction, both isomers are quantitatively converted to their respective conjugates. Using this system the authors were able to detect 1 per cent of the $(-)$-isomer as a contaminant in the $(+)$-enantiomer (Gerding *et al.*, 1989).

Resolutions of diastereoisomeric glucuronides may not always be possible using achiral chromatographic systems; for example the resolution of the glucuronide conjugates of the 2-arylbutanoic acid indobufen requires the use of a β-cyclodextrin CSP (Nicholls *et al.* cited in Hutt and Caldwell, 1989).

The formation of N-glucose conjugates of amobarbital has been known for some time (Tang *et al.*, 1978). Amobarbital is prochiral; formation of the N-glucose conjugate, however, confers asymmetry at carbon 5 of the barbiturate ring (Figure 43), the conjugate may therefore exist as a pair of diastereoisomers (Soine *et al.*, 1986). Soine and Soine (1987) have developed a chromatographic method based on a reverse phase (C-18) column for the analysis of these conjugates in human urine. Using a synthetic sample, both diastereoisomers could be readily resolved. On examination of material

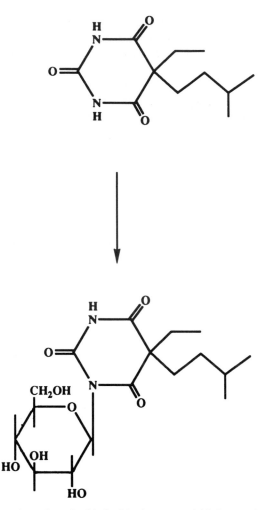

Figure 43. Conjugation of amobarbital with glucose to yield diastereoisomeric glucosides.

obtained from human urine, the metabolite formed was essentially stereochemically pure and corresponded to the less polar, longer eluting isomer (Soine and Soine, 1987). This stereoselectivity is of particular interest as the formation of this conjugate is under genetic control.

The formation and further metabolism of glutathione conjugates has been the subject of continued interest due to the importance of this tripeptide as a biological defence mechanism. As glutathione is composed of two chiral and one achiral amino acids, then the products of reaction with chiral substrates are diastereoisomers, as are the corresponding mercapturic acids.

The regioselectivity and stereoselectivity of conjugation of a variety of chiral epoxides of both polycyclic aromatic hydrocarbons, e.g. benze[a]pyrene-4,5-oxide, benz[a]anthracene-5,6-oxide and pyrene-4,5-oxide, cyclohexene oxide and styrene oxide have been reported (Dostal *et al.*, 1986; Delbressine *et al.*, 1981; van Bladeren *et al.*, 1981) as has the conjugation of chiral alkylhalides (Mangold and Abdel-Monem, 1983; Ridgewell and Abdel-Monem, 1987). These diastereoisomeric conjugates are readily amenable to chromatographic resolution, both normal and reverse phase HPLC systems being employed (Delbressine *et al.*, 1981; Dostal *et al.*, 1986). However, it may be necessary to utilize more than one system to analyse all possible conjugates (see, for example, Dostal *et al.*, 1986 who used two reverse phase systems for the total analysis of the conjugates formed from reaction of glutathione with a racemic mixture of benz[a]anthracene-5,6-oxide).

An example of particular interest is the conjugation of α-bromo-isovalerylurea, which appears to be a potentially useful substrate for the examination of glutathione conjugation *in vivo* (Te Koppele *et al.*, 1986 a,b). Metabolism involves nucleophilic substitution of the bromine, bonded to a chiral carbon atom, by the sulphur of glutathione and could therefore yield a pair of diastereoisomeric glutathione conjugates (Figure 44). *In vivo* in the rat, the major metabolites found in bile are glutathione conjugates and, in urine, mercapturic acids (Te Koppele *et al.*, 1986 b).

An examination of the stereochemistry of metabolism necessitated the development of an HPLC assay which would resolve the possible diastereoisomeric conjugates. The resolution of the two glutathione and mercapturic acid conjugates was achieved using a reverse phase column (C-18), a mobile phase based on aqueous buffer (pH 2.5) methanol mixtures and the presence or absence of sodium 1-decanesulphonate together with sodium nitrate, citric acid and potassium bromide (for the generation of bromine as an electrochemical amperometric detector was used). All four conjugates could be resolved using a concentration of 0.1 mM sodium 1-decane-sulphonate; however, the resolution of the two pairs of conjugates was affected differently by alteration in concentration, resolution of the glutathione conjugates being greater at high concentrations whilst that of the mercapturic acids was greater at low concentrations. Increasing both pH and methanol content of the mobile phase resulted in a decrease in the capacity factors of the analytes (Te Koppele *et al.*, 1988 a). The main advantage of this system involved the minimal sample preparation before analysis could be carried out, e.g. dilution of the bile or urine ten-fold with an appropriate buffer followed by direct injection into the HPLC system (Te Koppele *et al.*, 1988 a).

This analytical method has been used to examine the stereoselectivity of glutathione conjugation of α-bromoisovalerylurea both *in vivo* and *in vitro* and also to examine the stereoselectivity of purified rat glutathione transferase enzymes (Te Koppele *et al.*, 1986 b; 1988 a,b).

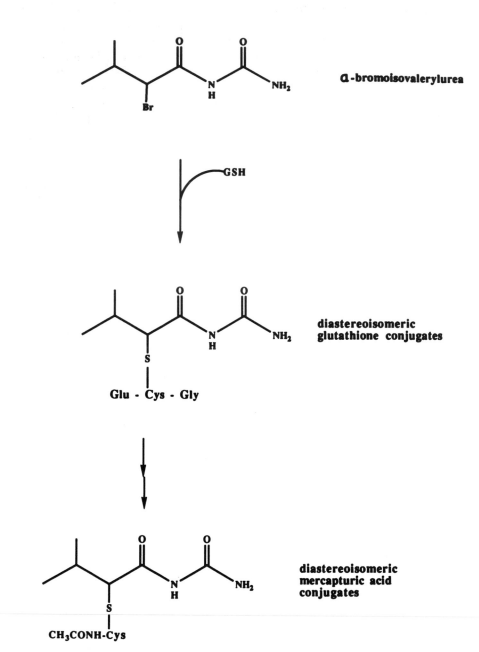

α-bromoisovalerylurea

diastereoisomeric
glutathione conjugates

diastereoisomeric
mercapturic acid
conjugates

Figure 44.   Conjugation of α-bromoisovalerylurea to yield diastereoisomeric glutathione and
mercapturic acid conjugates.

5. *Pseudoracemic mixtures*

As pointed out previously, determination of enantiomeric composition generally requires the interaction of the material under examination with a second chiral agent. One approach available to the bioanalyst which does not require an interaction between the analyte and a second chiral agent is the use of 'pseudoracemic' mixtures. A pseudoracemate is a 1 : 1 mixture of the enantiomers of a chiral compound in which the individual isomers are differentially isotopically labelled. The two components of the mixture are therefore no longer truly enantiomeric with one another. Following the administration of the pseudoracemic mixture to an animal, the drug and metabolites present in biological fluids and tissue may be examined in a conventional manner, e.g. solvent extraction followed by achiral chromatography etc., and the enantiomeric composition of the material determined by a suitable isotopic specific analytical method.

The choice of isotope utilized in the method will obviously be dependent upon the available facilities. Both stable and radioisotopes have been used, commonly used ones being carbon-13 or -14 and either deuterium or tritium; the enantiomeric composition of the material of interest is determined by mass spectrometry or liquid scintillation counting. The technique also enables an investigator to examine the differential disposition of enantiomers under conditions of chronic drug administration, or of the enantiomers of an endogenous chemical, together with the normal material, provided that both enantiomers are differentially isotopically labelled. For example, Iversen *et al.* (1971), examined the stereochemical aspects of noradrenaline uptake and metabolism in rat brain using a pseudoracemate prepared from carbon-14 and tritium-labelled neurotransmitter. Similarly, Nakamura *et al.* (1982), using differentially deuterated methadone, the (R)- and (S)-enantiomers being labelled in one of the aromatic rings $[d_5]$ and the terminal methyl group $[d_3]$ respectively, were able to examine the plasma and urinary disposition of the drug enantiomers in two subjects undergoing methadone maintenance therapy. A similar technique has been used by Küpfer *et al.*, (1982) in studies concerned with the chronic disposition of racemic mephenytoin. Four normal subjects received mephenytoin for fourteen days, with the radiolabelled pseudoracemate administered on days one and eleven of the study. The results obtained indicated that chronic drug treatment could result in autoinduction for the demethylation of (R)-mephenytoin to (R)-5-phenyl-5-ethylhydantoin (nirvanol).

Obviously preparation and possibly enantiomeric resolution and stereochemical analysis of the starting materials for the preparation of the pseudoracemic mixture is required prior to a metabolic experiment. The position of the label within the molecule is also a primary consideration and must obviously be in a metabolically stable position. Use of the isotopes of carbon is potentially the best solution to this problem as the relatively small change in mass would not be expected to result in kinetic isotope effects if metabolism does takes place at the site of the label. The use of deuterium and tritium labels may give rise to problems. Küpfer *et al.* (1981) have shown, using a pseudoracemate consisting of (S)-(4-[^{3}H]-phenyl) mephenytoin and the [^{14}C]-labelled (R)-enantiomer, that the oxidation to the corresponding (S)-4-hydroxy metabolite results in retention of the label and therefore provides good evidence for migration of the isotope, i.e. an NIH shift. It is of interest to note that the reversal of the isotopic composition of the pseudoracemate did not alter the urinary disposition of either enantiomer (Küpfer *et al.*, 1981).

Walle *et al.* (1983 a) have used two pseudoracemates of propranolol involving deuteration in both the aromatic ring (2,4-d_2) and in the isopropyl group (d_6). Analysis of the material in urine following the single oral administration of both pseudoracemates to dogs yielded results in good agreement, slight differences being observed in routes involving aromatic oxidation due to partial loss of deuterium.

A reversal of pseudoracemate composition has also been utilized by Gal *et al.* (1976) during studies on the *in vitro* metabolism of racemic amphetamine using rabbit liver homogenates. Individual incubation of the labelled and unlabelled enantiomers indicated enantioselective metabolism of (R)-amphetamine to both 1-phenylpropan-2-ol and N-hydroxyamphetamine, whilst incubation of both pseudoracemic mixtures resulted in the reverse enantioselectivity. The results obtained indicate the inhibition of either (S)-amphetamine, or one of its metabolites, on the metabolism of the (R)-enantiomer (Gal *et al.*, 1976).

Ideally, in studies of this type, the labelled material should be shown to be metabolically and pharmacokinetically identical to the unlabelled material prior to administration of the pseudoracemate. McMahon and Sullivan (1976) demonstrated the metabolic equivalence of deuterium labelled and unlabelled ($+$) and ($-$)-propoxyphene by the separate administration of isotope mixtures of the individual enantiomers to dogs. The ratio of isotope labelled to unlabelled material in plasma was found not to change from that present in the original mixture over 32 hours post drug administration. Similar studies have also been carried out using d_6- and d_0-($+$)-chlorpheniramine by Miyazaki and Abuki (1976).

This technique for enantiospecific analysis has been utilized with great benefit by Walle and co-workers in their extensive studies of the stereochemistry of metabolism of propranolol in both dog and man (Walle, 1985; see Table 5 and references therein) and also by Trager and co-workers (see Table 5 for references) in their studies on the stereochemistry of both metabolism and drug interactions with the coumarin anticoagulants.

Methodology of this type has obvious advantages of both sensitivity and specificity, particularly if mass spectrometry is used for enantiomer differentiation and must, therefore, represent the ideal approach for an examination of the metabolic and pharmacokinetic properties of many chiral drugs. One limitation of this approach would be metabolic inversion of chirality, e.g. the 2-arylpropionic acid NSAIDs; in this case a combination of both isotopic

Table 5. Enantiospecific analysis utilizing pseudoracemic mixtures.

Compound	Composition of pseudoracemate	Analytical method	Application	Reference
Amphetamine	$(R)-d_0 : (S)-d_3$ $(R)-d_3 : (S)-d_0$	SIM-GC-MS (EI)	Metabolism of individual enantiomers and pseudoracemic drug using rabbit liver homogenates	Gal *et al.* (1976)
Chlorpheniramine	$(-)-d_0 : (+)-d_6$	GC-MS (CI)	Enantiomeric disposition in man	Miyazaki and Abuki (1976)
Cyclophosphamide	$(+)-d_4 : (-)-d_0$ $(+)-d_0 : (-)-d_4$	DI-MS (EI)	Urinary disposition of the drug and metabolites in the mouse	Cox *et al.* (1977)
1-(2,5-Dimethoxy-4-methyl phenyl)-2-aminopropane	$(R)-d_0 : (S)-d_6$ $(R)-d_6 : (S)-d_0$	GC-MS (CI) DI-MS (CI)	N-oxidation by rabbit liver microsomal preparations *In vitro* metabolism by rabbit liver microsomal preparations	Gal *et al.* (1975) Weinkam *et al.* (1976)
Disopyramide	$(+)-d_0 : (-)-d_n$ (extent of deuteration unclear)	SIM-DI-MS (CI)	Plasma pharmacokinetics in man	Giacomini *et al.* (1986)
Drobuline	$(+)-d_6 : (-)-d_0$ $(-)-d_6 : (+)-d_0$	SIM-GC-MS (EI)	*In vivo* and *in vitro* disposition in dogs	Murphy *et al.* (1978)
Ephedrine	$(+)-d_0 : (-)-d_5$	GC-MS (CI)	Urinary disposition of drug and metabolites in man	Baba *et al.* (1986)
Hexobarbital	$(R)-d_3 : (S)-d_0$	SIM-GC-MS (EI)	Metabolism and disposition following administration to rats and the effect of enzyme inducing agents on clearance	Van der Graaff *et al.* (1985, 1987)
Methadone	$(R)-d_5 : (S)-d_3$	SIM-GC-MS (CI)	Enantiomeric disposition in long-term maintenance patients (d_0-levels also monitored)	Nakamura *et al.* (1982)
α-Methyldopa	$(R)-{}^{12}C : (S)-{}^{13}C$	DI-MS (CI)	Uptake and metabolism in rat brain	Ames *et al.* (1977); Castagnoli *et al.* (1978)
Mephenytoin	$(R)-[{}^3H] : (S)-[{}^{14}C]$ $(S)-[{}^3H] : (R)-[{}^{14}C]$	HPLC followed by double isotope LSC	Metabolism and disposition following single dose and chronic drug administration	Küpfer *et al.* (1981, 1982)

(*continued*)

Table 5. (*Continued*).

Compound	Composition of pseudoracemate	Analytical method	Application	Reference
Nirvanol	(R)-[^{3}H] : (S)-[^{14}C]	TLC followed by double isotope LSC	Metabolism and pharmacogenetic investigation in man	Küpfer et al. (1984)
Noradrenaline	(−)-[^{3}H] : (+)-[^{14}C]	LSC	Uptake by rat brain homogenates	Iversen et al. (1971)
Oxprenolol	(R)-d_2 : (S)-d_0	HPLC followed by DI-MS (CI)	Stereoselectivity of aromatic oxidation of oxprenolol following administration to rats	Burke et al. (1980)
Phenprocoumon	(R)-^{12}C : (S)-^{13}C	SIM-GC-MS (EI)	Disposition in man, effect of sulfinpyrazone on enantiomer disposition	Toon et al. (1985) Heimark et al. (1987 b)
Propoxyphene	(+)-d_2 : (−)-d_0 (+)-d_0 : (−)-d_2 (+)-d_7 : (−)-d_0	GC-MS	Disposition in dogs	McMahon and Sullivan (1976)
Propranolol	(S)-d_0 : (R)-d_2	MS (CI)	Disposition in man	Wolen et al. (1978)
	(S)-d_0 : (R)-d_2	GC-MS (EI)	Disposition in dogs	Ehrsson (1976)
	(S)-d_2 : (R)-d_0	GC-MS (EI)	Bioavailability following oral administration to dogs	Walle and Walle (1979)
	(S)-d_0 : (R)-d_6	HPLC followed by DI-MS (CI)	*In vivo* and *in vitro* formation of 4-hydroxypropranolol in the rat	Powell et al. (1980)
	(S)-d_0 : (R)-d_6 (R)-d_6 : (S)-d_2	GC-MS (EI)	Plasma protein binding and pharmacokinetics in dogs	Bai et al. (1983)
	(R)-d_2 : (S)-d_0 (R)-d_6 : (S)-d_0	GC-MS	Stereochemical composition of metabolites following administration to dogs	Walle et al. (1983 a)
	(R)-d_6 : (S)-d_0	GC-MS	Protein binding to α_1-acid glycoprotein and human serum albumin	Walle et al. (1983 b)
	(R)-d_2 : (S)-d_0 (R)-d_6 : (S)-d_0 (S)-d_2 : (R)-d_0 (S)-d_6 : (R)-d_0	GC-MS	Disposition and metabolism in man	Walle et al. (1984)

Drug	Label	Method	Study	Reference
Tocainide	(R)-d_2 : (S)-d_0 (S)-d_2 : (R)-d_0	GC-MS (EI)	N-dealkylation in vivo following administration to rat, dog and man and in vitro using rat liver homogenates	Nelson and Bartels (1984 a)
			Regio- and stereoselectivity of aromatic oxidation in vivo and in vitro in the rat	Nelson and Bartels (1984 b)
	(R,S)-drug (400 mg) together with (S)-[^{3}H] enantiomer (5.9 mg)	HPLC followed by LSC	Disposition in man	Hoffmann et al. (1984)
Verapamil	(S)-d_0 : (R)-d_2	SIM-GC-MS (EI)	Bioavailability following oral administration to man	Vogelgesang et al. (1984)
	(S)-d_6 : (R)-d_0	SIM-GC-MS (EI)	Regio and stereoselectivity of O-demethylation and N-dealkylation in liver homogenates from rat and man	Nelson et al. (1988)
Warfarin	(S)-d_5 : (R)-d_0 (S)-d_0 : (R)-d_5 (S)-^{13}C : (R)-^{12}C	SIM-GC-MS (EI)	Enantiomer pharmacokinetics in healthy volunteers	Nelson and Olsen (1988) Hignite et al. (1980)
		HPLC followed by DI-MS (CI)	Enantiomer pharmacokinetics following administration of pseudoracemate together with phenylbutazone or seconal	Howald et al. (1980)
		SIM-GC-MS	Warfarin–phenylbutazone interaction. Warfarin/sulfinpyrazone interaction. Plasma-protein binding interaction between warfarin and sulfinpyrazone	O'Reilly et al. (1980) Toon et al. (1986)
			Warfarin/rifampicin interaction	Toon and Trager (1984) Heimark et al. (1987 a)
Xibenolol	(−)-d_0 : (+)-d_5 (+)-d_0 : (−)-d_5 (−)-d_0 : (+)-d_9 (or d_5) (+)-d_0 : (−)-d_9 (or d_5)	SIM-GC-MS (EI)	Pharmacokinetic and metabolic studies in man	Honma et al. (1985)

analysis together with an alternative method of chiral analysis would be required. Again under these circumstances the obvious advantages of the pseudoracemate approach are evident as the pharmacokinetics and metabolism of both drug enantiomers and of 'inverted' and non-inverted material may be examined simultaneously. Some initial observations demonstrating the metabolic and pharmacokinetic equivalence of deuterated and non-deuterated (R)-ibuprofen have recently been published (Baillie *et al.*, 1989).

6. *Applications of isotopically labelled substrates for mechanistic investigations*

An examination of the chirality of metabolism of both prochiral and chiral drug molecules may yield valuable information concerning the binding of the substrate to the active site of the enzyme involved. Investigations of the stereochemistry of metabolism at prochiral centres in drug molecules is facilitated by the use of stereospecifically labelled substrates; determination of either retention or loss of the isotope during metabolism may also give useful information concerning the mechanism of the reaction involved.

McMahon *et al.* (1969) used a deuterium label to examine the stereochemistry of oxidation of ethylbenzene to 1-phenylethanol by rat liver homogenates. It was found on incubation of (S)-[1-d]-ethylbenzene that the product retained 86 per cent of the isotope present in the starting material and that the product was >90 per cent (R)-[1-d]-1-phenylethanol. The data demonstrated that the oxidation takes place with retention of configuration at the benzylic carbon atom via an insertion reaction (McMahon *et al.*, 1969; Sullivan and Franklin, 1988).

Similarly, Battersby *et al.* (1976) investigated the stereochemistry of dopamine hydroxylation, by dopamine β-hydroxylase (E.C.1.14.17.1) using tritium-labelled (2R)- and (2S)-dopamine. Using both the individual enantiomers and a racemic mixture of the two, to which [1-^{14}C]-dopamine was added as internal standard, these authors established that the reaction was stereospecific and proceeds with retention of configuration to yield (R)-noradrenaline with loss of the pro-(R) hydrogen from dopamine (Battersby *et al.*, 1976). Similar observations have been reported using (S)-amphetamine and phenylethylamine as substrates (Taylor, 1974; Bachan *et al.*, 1974).

Battersby *et al.* (1979) have used a similar approach to examine the deamination of (1R)- and (1S)-[1-^{3}H]-aminoheptanes by rat liver mitochondrial monoamine oxidase (E.C.1.4.3.4.). This deamination proceeds by oxidation resulting in removal of one of the α-hydrogen atoms to yield an imine which undergoes hydrolysis to yield the corresponding aldehyde. Using their labelled substrates, Battersby *et al.* (1979) were able to show that the pro-(R) α-hydrogen was stereospecifically removed from the substrate. More recently Yu and Davis (1988) have investigated the stereochemistry of the deamination of benzylamine, by a number of amine oxidases, using (R) and (S)-[α-d]-benzylamine. The benzaldehyde(s) produced were analysed by both GC-MS and also by HPLC as the deuterated and non-deuterated aldehydes may be separated using a reverse phase (C-18) column. Using this method the amine oxidases could be divided into three groups based on the stereospecificity of the reaction:

1. those enzymes removing the pro-(R) hydrogen, e.g. mitochondrial MAO-B isolated from rat and bovine liver and hog kidney;
2. those enzymes removing the pro-(S) hydrogen, e.g. soluble amine oxidase from rat aorta and hog kidney;
3. non-stereoselective enzymes, e.g. bovine plasma amine oxidase.

It is of interest to note that the MAOs are bound to the outer mitochondrial membrane and possess a flavine prosthetic group and presumably have a similar configuration at the active site, whereas the soluble enzymes do not contain the flavine group (Yu and Davis, 1988).

Several recent studies have utilized stable isotope methodology with prochiral substrates to probe the chirality of the active site of cytochrome P450.

White *et al.* (1986) have used unlabelled, $[1,1-d_2]$-, (R)- and (S)-$[1-d]$-ethylbenzene to examine the oxidation to 1-phenylethanol by the isozyme cytochrome $P450_{LM2}$. The enantiomeric composition of the product was determined by GC resolution of the diastereoisomeric esters formed on reaction with (R)-0-propionylmandelyl chloride. On incubation of ethylbenzene or the dideutero derivative, the products of the reaction were essentially racemic, whilst incubation of the (R) and (S)-monodeutero labelled substrates resulted in products which were found to consist of 42 and 72 per cent of the (R)-enantiomer of the alcohol respectively. Analysis of the isotopic composition of the products indicated a large deuterium isotope effect and indicated that the abstraction of the pro-(R) or pro-(S) hydrogen resulted in an alcohol of the opposite configuration to that of the original substrate. The abstraction of the pro-(R) hydrogen resulted in about 25 per cent of the (S)-alcohol, whilst the pro-(S) hydrogen abstraction resulted in about 40 per cent of the (R)-alcohol (White *et al.*, 1986). These data indicate that, following the stereoselective removal of either of the benzylic hydrogen atoms, an intermediate planar tricoordinate carbon centre is formed, which has sufficient freedom of movement at the enzyme active site to present either face to the iron-oxygen complex with subsequent formation of the alcohol (Figure 45). The authors concluded that the protein environment at the substrate binding site controls the stereochemistry of the cytochrome P450-dependent oxidations and is not an intrinsic characteristic of the oxidation mechanism (White *et al.*, 1986).

Two related studies, using prochiral substrates and utilizing GC-MS for enantiodifferentiation of the products, have been reported. Sugiyama and Trager (1986) investigated the oxidation of cumene (2-phenylpropane) to 2-phenylpropanol using (R)- and (S)-$[1-^{13}C]$-2-phenylpropane; Ichinose and Kurihara, (1987) examined the 0-demethylation of methoxychlor

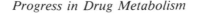

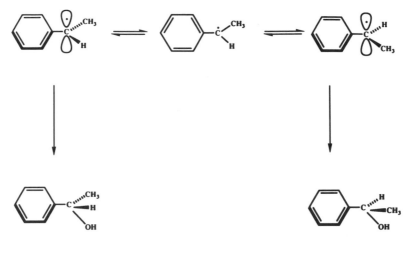

(S) - alcohol   (R) - alcohol

Figure 45. Inversion of the phenylethyl radical from enzymatic hydrogen abstraction from ethylbenzene resulting in formation of either (R)- or (S)-1-phenylethanol.

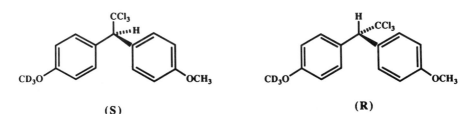

(S)   **(R)**

Figure 46. Structures of (R)- and (S)-[monomethyl-d₃] methoxychlor.

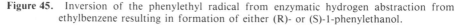

(2,2-bis(4-methoxyphenyl)-1,1,1,-trichloroethane) using (R)-, (S)- and racemic [monomethyl-d₃]methoxychlor (Figure 46).

With the use of control rat liver microsomal preparations, the oxidation of cumene at the pro-(R) methyl group occurred at about twice the rate of the pro-(S) group (Figure 47). With the use of microsomes induced with either phenobarbital or β-naphthoflavone, the product stereoselectivity changed with increasing oxidation of the pro-(S) methyl group. The results of this study were interpreted as indicating a small degree of incomplete equilibrium between two possible orientations of the compound at the enzyme active site, presenting the alternative methyl groups towards the active oxygen species (Sugiyama and Trager, 1986). Similar results were obtained by Ichinose and Kurihara (1987) for the demethylation of methoxychlor. In this case the interchange between the two large methoxyphenyl groups at the enzyme active site is relatively slow resulting in a large degree of incomplete equilibrium.

The above investigations indicate that product stereoselectivity of metab-

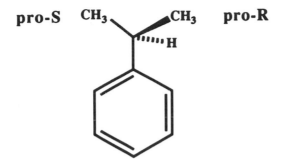

Figure 47. Structure of cumene

olism is a function of enzyme structure and chirality of the active site. The stereochemistry of the product is determined by the binding of the substrate and the conformational flexibility between possible orientations of the groups undergoing transformation at the active site. Such studies may yield useful data concerning the topology of the active site of the various isozymes of cytochrome P450 (Sugiyama and Trager, 1986).

7. Sample isolation and enantiomeric interactions

A number of potential analytical problems associated with the use of many of the techniques detailed above have been previously discussed: for example, differential detector responses of diastereoisomeric derivatives, the presence of trace organic contaminants in either the solvents or samples used for HPLC and the source dependence of enzymes used for the hydrolysis of diastereo-isomeric conjugates. This section is concerned with problems associated with sample manipulation and potential problems which may arise due to the so-called 'non-chiral differentiation' or dissymmetric effects.

It is frequently the case that samples of biological origin require an isolation and 'clean-up' procedure to be carried out prior to an analysis of drug or metabolite content. This is particularly true for studies involving the determination of enantiomeric composition for reasons stated previously. Such sample manipulations must be carried out to ensure that the enantiomeric composition of the analyte is unaffected. McErlane *et al.* (1987) found, in a study concerned with the determination of the enantiomeric composition of mexiletine in plasma, that both drug recovery and enantiomeric composition were influenced by the method of protein precipitation. The use of sodium hydroxide (2 M) both for precipitating protein and basifying samples prior to drug extraction, was found to result in a low recovery of the drug, but more importantly the enantiomeric ratio of the analyte(s) was altered, the recovery of the (R)-isomer being lower than that of the (S)-enantiomer. The problem was solved by the use of mixtures of zinc sulphate and barium hydroxide giving about 83 per cent recovery but maintaining the enantiomeric ratio (Figure 48).

The above situation indicates the problems associated with analysis of this type and also the need for careful observation of standard samples during analytical development. Of much greater difficulty are problems which arise due to enantiomer differentiation in non-racemic mixtures of isomers, a situation which occurs frequently in metabolic and pharmacokinetic studies. Preliminary sample 'clean up' procedures frequently employ an achiral chromatographic step which is generally regarded as non-enantiodifferentiating. Several examples have appeared in the literature recently in which enrichment of the isomer present in excess has occurred by achiral chromatography (Charles and Gil-Av; 1984; Cundy and Crooks, 1983; Tsai *et al.*, 1985).

The report of Cundy and Crooks (1983) is of particular interest. With the use of a sample of radiolabelled racemic nicotine (+)-bitartrate salt and a partisil-PXS cation exchange column, the racemic material eluted as one radiolabelled peak. Repeating the analysis coinjecting (−)-nicotine as a standard, the authors observed one UV peak, but the radiolabelled material eluted as two distinct peaks of similar area. Similarly on repeating the chromatography using (+)-nicotine as the standard, they noticed the same effect, but if racemic nicotine was used as a standard then both the 'cold' and radiolabelled material coeluted as one peak (Cundy and Crooks, 1983). The effect was investigated using unlabelled material of varying enantiomeric composition, alteration of the counter ion and using a reverse phase (C-18) column; in all cases resolution of the radiolabelled material was observed. Using this system it was possible to use preparative HPLC for the isolation of the individual isomers (Cundy and Crooks, 1983).

These so-called dissymmetric effects are not confined to chromatography; similar effects have been observed in polarimetry (Horeau, 1969) and also in NMR spectroscopy (Williams *et al.*, 1960; Dobashi *et al.*, 1986). This phenomenon is rationalized by self-association between the enantiomers, which may be due to hydrogen bonding and/or van der Waals interactions, to yield dimers or oligomers. The situation with regard to dimer formation may be illustrated thus:

$$E_R + E_S \rightleftharpoons E_R . E_S \text{ complex} \qquad (1)$$

$$E_R + E_R \rightleftharpoons E_R . E_R \text{ complex} \qquad (2)$$

$$E_S + E_S \rightleftharpoons E_S . E_S \text{ complex} \qquad (3)$$

The self-association of two enantiomers (E) of the opposite configuration forms a heterochiral dimer (equation 1) whilst association of two enantiomers of the same configuration results in formation of a homochiral dimer (equations 2 and 3). Evidence for dimer formation is supported by both NMR and IR data on amino acid derivatives (Dobashi *et al.*, 1986) and has been shown to be concentration-dependent (Williams *et al.*, 1969). In chromatography, such dimers may have differing affinities for the stationary and mobile phases of achiral systems or may occur only in an adsorbed layer, with the result that enantiomeric enrichment takes place (Cundy and Crooks, 1983; Charles and Gil-Av, 1984). However, in either case as one isomer is present in excess then the minor isomer is essentially placed in a chiral environment; it should perhaps therefore not be surprising that enantiodifferentiation takes place.

Such effects are of considerable significance in bioanalytical chemistry; for example if optical activity detectors are used in HPLC, is the optical purity

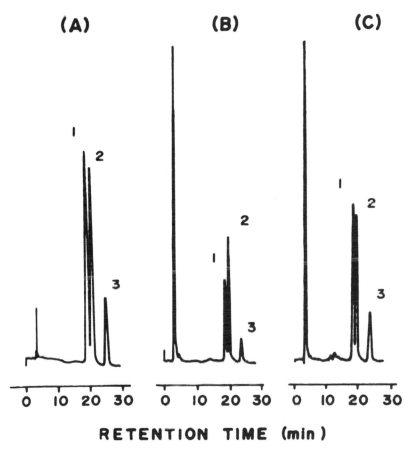

RETENTION TIME (min)

Figure 48. Effect of protein precipitation agent on recovery and enantiomeric composition of racemic mexiletine from plasma. Extraction of the racemate from (A) water, (B) plasma using sodium hydroxide for protein precipitation and (C) plasma using a zinc sulphate–barium hydroxide mixture. Chromatography was carried out using a Type I CSP; N-(3,5-dinitrobenzoyl)phenylglycine (ionic) as the 2-naphthamide derivatives of the analytes, peak (1) corresponding to (R)-mexiletine; (2) (S) mexiletine and (3) 1-(2,6-dimethylphenoxy)-2-ethanamine (internal standard) amide derivatives. Reproduced from McErlane *et al.* (1987) with permission of the authors and Elsevier Science Publishers BV.

directly related to enantiomeric purity? If solid phase extraction techniques are used, are both enantiomers extracted and liberated to the same extent? Caldwell and Testa (1987) and Caldwell *et al.* (1988 a) have addressed the above problems and others related to the various chromatographic techniques described above and proposed certain criteria as to the acceptability of evidence relating to the enantiomeric composition of drugs and metabolites. In the ideal case where samples of the individual isomers, of known enantiomeric purity, are available, then methods may be optimized with respect to isolation, derivatization and analysis. In the alternative situation where standards are not available, then Caldwell and Testa (1987) propose that data are acceptable only if the same analytical result is obtained utilizing two methodologies which rely on different principles for enantiodifferentiation, e.g. use of both a CSP and a CDA.

8. Conclusions

In, 1978 Beckett and Cowan wrote: 'A racemic mixture must be regarded as being comprised of two different compounds when metabolic studies are being considered'. Developments over the last decade have served to emphasize this statement and with the increasing realization that the biological properties and fate of the enantiomers of chiral drug molecules may be totally different, there will be increasing demands for the bioanalytical scientist to establish analytical methods capable of distinguishing between enantiomers.

Bioanalysis if one of the most difficult areas of analytical chemistry, being associated with small quantities of analyte(s) dispersed in highly complex media. To add to this situation, the problem of differentiation and quantitation of left- and right-'handed' molecules, compounds which until relatively recently have been extremely difficult to separate, requires an additional level of sophistication for analysis of this type. The problems associated with enantiomeric analysis are many and the effective use of the newer methods requires an appreciation of potential sources of error; also it may frequently be necessary to use a combination of techniques based on different physico-chemical principles.

It is clear from the above that our approach to enantiomeric analysis has changed dramatically over the last ten years and with the continual development of chiral chromatographic systems, elucidation of the mechanisms involved in the chiral recognition process and optimization of enantiomer resolution (Fell *et al.*, 1988), the situation will advance even more rapidly over the next ten years. Alternative techniques in the area of immunoassay methods and possible developments in biosensor technology (Hyland *et al.*, 1989) may also offer novel approaches for enantiomeric differentiation.

The development and application of the methodologies described above will contribute greatly to our knowledge and understanding of the critical role of stereochemistry in drug metabolism and the related areas of toxicology and clinical pharmacology, such that these disciplines no longer need to be considered as areas of 'flatland' science.

Acknowledgements

The author is grateful to Professor John Caldwell for helpful discussion, to those authors and publishers who gave their permission for the reproduction of figures and to Mrs Fay Green for expert preparation of the typescript.

Note added in proof

Since the completion of the manuscript there has been considerable interest in this area and the attention of interested readers is drawn to the edited volumes of Lough (1989) and Krstulovic (1989) and a comprehensive literature survey published by the Chromatographic Society (Wilson and Ruane, 1990).

References

Aaltonen, L., Kanto, J., Iisalo, E. and Pihlajamaki, K. (1984), *Europ. J. Clin. Pharmacol.*, **26**, 613.

Aberhart, D. J. and Cotting, J-A. (1988), in *Methods in Enzymology, Volume 166, Branched Chain Amino Acids* (R. A. Harris and J. R. Sokatch, eds), p. 14, Academic Press, New York.

Aboul-Enein, H. Y., Islam, M. R. and Bakr, S. A. (1988), *J. Liquid Chromatog.*, **11**, 1485.

Adams, J. D., Woolf, T. F., Trevor, A. J., Williams, L. R. and Castagnoli, N. (1982), *J. Pharm. Sci.*, **71**, 658.

Akrawi, S. H. and Wedlund, P. J, (1986), *J. Chromatog.*, **381**, 198.

Alak, A. and Armstrong, D. W. (1986), *Anal. Chem.*, **58**, 582.

Alembik, M. C. and Wainer, I. W. (1988), *J. Ass. Official Anal. Chemists*, **71**, 530.

Allenmark, S. (1986), *J. Liquid Chromatog.*, **9**, 425.

Allenmark, S. (1988), *Chromatographic Enantioseparation: Methods and Applications*, Ellis Horwood, Chichester.

Allenmark, S. and Thompson, R. A. (1987), *Tetrahedron Lett.*, **28**, 3751.

Allenmark, S., Bomgren, B. and Boren, H. (1983), *J. Chromatog.*, **264**, 63.

Alvarez-Coque, M. C. G., Hernandez, M. J. M., Camanas, R. M. V. and Fernandez, C. M. (1989), *Anal. Biochem.*, **178**, 1.

Ames, M. M., Melmon, K. L. and Castagnoli, N. (1977), *Biochem. Pharmacol.*, **26**, 1757.

Antonsson, A-M., Gyllenhaal, O., Kylberg-Hanssen, K., Johansson, L. and Vessman, J. (1984), *J. Chromatog.*, **308**, 181.

Ariens, E. J. (1984), *Europ. J. Clin. Pharmacol.*, **26**, 663.

Ariens, E. J., Soudijn, W. and Timmermans, P. B. M. W. M. (eds) (1983), *Stereochemistry and Biological Activity of Drugs*, Blackwell Scientific, Oxford.

Ariens, E. J., Van Rensen, J. J. S. and Welling, W. (eds) (1988), *Stereoselectivity of Pesticides, Biological and Chemical Problems*, Elsevier, Amsterdam.

Armstrong, D. W. (1984), *J. Liquid Chromatog.*, **7**, 353.

Armstrong, D. W. (1987), *Anal. Chem.*, **59**, 84A.

Armstrong, D. W., Ward, T. J., Armstrong, R. D. and Beesley, T. E. (1986), *Science*, **232**, 1132.

Armstrong, D. W., Han, S. M. and Han, Y. I. (1987 a), *Anal. Biochem.*, **167**, 261.
Armstrong, D. W., Yang, X., Han, S. M. and Menges, R. A. (1987 b), *Anal. Chem.*, **59**, 2594.
Avgerinos, A. and Hutt, A. J. (1987), *J. Chromatog.*, **415**, 75.
Baba, S., Kuroda, Y. and Horie, M. (1986), *Biomed. Env. Mass Spect.*, **13**, 141.
Bachan, L., Storm, C. B., Wheeler, J. W. and Kaufman, S. (1974), *J. Am. Chem. Soc.*, **96**, 6799.
Bai, S. A., Walle, U. K., Wilson, M. J. and Walle, T. (1983), *Drug Metab. Dispos.*, **11**, 394.
Baillie, T. A., Adams, W. J., Kaiser, D. G., Olanoff, L. S., Halstead, G. W., Harpootian, H. and Van Giessen, G. J. (1989), *J. Pharmacol. Exp. Ther.*, **249**, 517.
Ballard, K. D., Eller, T. D. and Knapp, D. R. (1983), *J. Chromatog.*, **275**, 161.
Banfield, C. and Rowland, M. (1983), *J. Pharm. Sci.*, **72**, 921.
Banfield, C. and Rowland, M. (1984), *J. Pharm. Sci.*, **73**, 1392.
Barnett, D. B. and Nahorski, S. R. (1983), *Trends Pharmacol. Sci.*, **4**, 407.
Barnett, D. B., Batta, M., Davies, B. and Nahorski, S. R. (1980), *Europ. J. Clin. Pharmacol.*, **17**, 349.
Bartos, F., Olsen, G. D., Leger, R. N. and Bartos, D. (1977), *Res. Commun. Chem. Path. Pharmacol.*, **16**, 131.
Battersby, A. R., Sheldrake, P. W., Staunton, J. and Williams, D. C. (1976), *J. Chem. Soc. Perkin Trans.*, **I**, 1056.
Battersby, A. R., Buckley, D. G., Staunton, J. and Williams, P. J. (1979), *J. Chem. Soc. Perkin Trans.*, **I**, 2550.
Beckett, A. H. and Cowan, D. A. (1978), in *Drug Metabolism in Man* (J. W. Gorrod and A. H. Beckett, eds), p. 237, Taylor & Francis, London.
Benschop, H. P. and De Jong, L. P. A. (1988), *Acc. Chem. Res.*, **21**, 368.
Benschop, H. P., Konings, C. A. G. and De Jong, L. P. A. (1981), *J. Am. Chem. Soc.*, **103**, 4260..
Benschop, H. P., Konings, C. A. G., Van Genderen, J. and De Jong, L. P. A. (1984), *Fund. Appl. Tox.*, **4**, S84.
Benschop, H. P., Bijleveld, E. C., Otto, M. F., Degenhardt, C. E. A. M., Van Helden, H. P. M. and De Jong, L. P. A. (1985), *Anal. Biochem.*, **151**, 242.
Benschop, H. P., Bijleveld, E. C., De Jong, L. P. A., Van der Wiel, H. J. and Van Helden, H. P. M. (1987), *Tox. Appl. Pharmacol.*, **90**, 490.
Berghem, L., Bergman, U., Schildt, B. and Sörbo, B. (1980), *Br. J. Anaesth.*, **52**, 597.
Berry, B. W. and Jamali, F. (1988), *Pharm. Res.*, **5**, 123.
Bertucci, C., Rosini, C., Pini, D. and Salvadori, P. (1987), *J. Pharm. Biomed. Anal.*, **5**, 171.
Bewick, D. W. (1986), *Pesticide Sci.*, **17**, 349.
Bilezikian, J. P., Gammon, D. E., Rochester, C. L. and Shand, D. G. (1979), *Clin. Pharmacol Ther.*, **26**, 173.
Bjercke, R. J., Cook, G., Rychlik, N., Gjika, H. B., Van Vunakis, H. and Langone, J. J. (1986), *J. Immunol. Methods*, **90**, 203.
Björkman, S. (1985), *J. Chromatog.*, **339**, 339.
Björkman, S. (1987), *J. Chromatog.*, **414**, 465.
Blaschke, G. (1986), *J. Liquid Chromatog.*, **9**, 341.
Blaschke, G. (1988), in *Chromatographic Chiral Separations*, (M. Zief and L. J. Crane, eds), p. 179, Marcel Dekker, New York.
Bobbitt, D. R. and Yeung, E. S. (1984), *Anal. Chem.*, **56**, 1577.
Bopp, R. J., Nash, J. F., Ridolfo, A. S. and Sheppard, E. R. (1979), *Drug Metab. Dispos.*, **7**, 356.
Brimfield, A. A., Hunter, K. W., Lenz, D. E., Benschop, H. P., Van Dijk, C. and De Jong, L. P. A. (1985), *Molec. Pharmacol.*, **28**, 32.

Brinkmann, U. A., Th and Kamminga, D. (1985), *J. Chromatog.*, **330**, 375.

Brooks, C. J. W. and Gilbert, M. T. (1974), *J. Chromatog.*, **99**, 541.

Buck, R. H. and Krummen, K. (1984), *J. Chromatog.*, **315**, 279.

Busker, E., Günther, K. and Martens, J. (1985), *J. Chromatog.*, **350**, 179.

Burke, R. R., Howald, W. N. and Nelson, W. L. (1980), *Res. Commun. Chem. Path. Pharmacol.*, **28**, 399.

Büyüktimkin, N., Büyüktimkin, S., Grunow, D. and Elz, S. (1988), *Chromatographia*, **25**, 925.

Caldwell, J. and Hutt, A. J. (1986), in *Progress in Drug Metabolism*, Vol. 9, (J. W. Bridges and L. F. Chasseaud, eds), p. 11, Taylor & Francis, London.

Caldwell, J., and Testa, B. (1987), *Drug Metab. Dispos.*, **15**, 587.

Caldwell, J., Darbyshire, J. F., Winter, S. M. and Hutt, A. J. (1988 a), in *Methodological Surveys in Biochemistry and Analysis, Volume 18, Bioanalysis of Drugs and Metabolites, Especially Anti-Inflammatory and Cardiovascular* (E. Reid, J. D. Robinson and I. D. Wilson, eds), p. 257, Plenum, New York.

Caldwell, J., Grubb, N., Sinclair, K. A., Hutt, A. J., Weil, A. and Fournel-Gigleux, S. (1988 b), in *Cellular and Molecular Aspects of Glucuronidation* (G. Siest, J. Magdalon and B. Burchell, eds), p. 185, Libbey Eurotext, London.

Caldwell, J., Hutt, A. J. and Fournel-Gigleux, S. (1988 c), *Biochem. Pharmacol.*, **37**, 105.

Caldwell, J., Winter, S. M. and Hutt, A. J. (1988 d), *Xenobiotica.*, **18** (Suppl. 1), 59.

Castagnoli, N., Melmon, K. L., Freed, C. R., Ames, M. M., Kalir, A. and Weinkam, R. (1978), in *Stable Isotopes, Applications in Pharmacology, Toxicology and Clinical Research* (T. A. Baillie, ed), p. 261, Macmillan, London.

Cayley, G. R. and Simpson, B. W. (1986), *J. Chromatog.*, **356**, 123.

Charles, R. and Gil-Av., E. (1984), *J. Chromatog.*, **298**, 516.

Choi, K. E. and Schilsky, R. L. (1988), *Anal. Biochem.*, **168**, 398.

Chu, Y-Q. and Wainer, I. W. (1988), *Pharm. Res.*, **5**, 680.

Cook, C. E. (1983), in *Topics in Pharmaceutical Sciences 1983* (D. D. Breimer and P. Speiser, eds), p. 87, Elsevier Science BV, Amsterdam.

Cook, C. E., Ballentine, N. H., Seltzman, T. B. and Tallent, C. R. (1979 a), *J. Pharmacol. Exp. Ther.*, **210**, 391.

Cook, C. E., Myers, M. A., Tallent, C. R., Seltzman, T. and Jeffcoat, A. R. (1979 b), *Fed. Proc.*, **38**, 742 (Abstract 2713).

Cook, C. E., Seltzman, T. P., Tallent, C. R. and Wooten, J. D. (1982), *J. Pharmacol. Exp. Theor.*, **220**, 568.

Cook, C. E., Seltzman, T. B., Tallent, C. R., Lorenzo, B. and Drayer, D. E. (1987), *J. Pharmacol. Exp. Ther.*, **241**, 779.

Cox, P. J., Farmer, P. B., Foster, A. B., Griggs, L. J., Jarman, M., Kinas, R., Pankiewicz, K. and Stec, W. J. (1977), *Biomed. Mass Spect.*, **4**, 371.

Crevat-Pisano, P., Hariton, C., Rolland, P. H. and Cano, J. P. (1986), *J. Pharmaceut. Biomed. Anal.*, **4**, 697.

Crowther, J. B., Covey, T. R., Dewey, E. A. and Henion, J. D. (1984), *Anal. Chem.*, **56**, 2921.

Cundy, K. C. and Crooks, P. A. (1983), *J. Chromatog.*, **281**, 17.

Cushny, A. R. (1926), *Biological Relations of Optically Isomeric Substances*, p. 1, Bailliere Tindall and Cox, London.

Dale, J. A. and Mosher, H. S. (1973), *J. Am. Chem. Soc.*, **95**, 512.

Dalgliesh, C. E. (1952), *J. Chem. Soc.*, **137**, 3940.

Däppen, R., Arm. H. and Meyer, V. R. (1986), *J. Chromatog.*, **373**, 1.

Davis, P. J., Yang, S-K. and Smith, R. V. (1985), *Xenobiotica.*, **15**, 1001.

Debowski, J., Jurczak, J. and Sybilska, D. (1983), *J. Chromatog.*, **282**, 83.

Degenhardt, C. E. A. M., Van den Berg, G. R., De Jong, L. P. A. and Benschop, H. P. (1986), *J. Am. Chem. Soc.*, **108**, 8290.

Delbressine, L. P. C., Van Bladeren, P. J., Smeets, F. L. M. and Seulter-Berlage, F. (1981), *Xenobiotica.*, **11**, 589.

Dieterle, W. and Faigle, J. W. (1983), *J. Chromatog.*, **259**, 311.

Dieterle, W., Faigle, J. W., Kriemler, H-P. and Winkler, T. (1984 a), *Xenobiotica.*, **14**, 311.

Dieterle, W., Faigle, J. W., Imhof, P., Sulo, M. and Wagner, J. (1984 b), *Xenobiotica.*, **14**, 303.

Dobashi, A., Saito, N., Motoyama, Y. and Hara, S. (1986), *J. Am. Chem. Soc.*, **108**, 307.

Dostal, L. A., Aitio, A., Harris, C., Bhatia, A. V., Hernandez, O. and Bend, J. R. (1986), *Drug Metab. Dispos.*, **14**, 303.

Drayer, D. E. (1986), *Clin. Pharmacol. Therap.*, **40**, 125.

Drummond, L., Caldwell, J. and Wilson, H. K. (1989), *Xenobiotica.*, **19**, 199.

Duke, C. C. and Holder, G. M. (1988), *J. Chromatog.*, **430**, 53.

Dumont, E., von Bahr, C., Perry, T. L. and Bertilsson, L. (1987), *Pharmacol. Tox.*, **61**, 335.

Edholm, L-E., Lindberg, C., Paulson, J. and Walhagen, A. (1988), *J. Chromatog.*, **424**, 61.

Ehlers, J., Konig, W. A., Lutz, S., Wenz, G. and Tom Dieck, H. (1988), *Angew. Chem. Int. Edn*, **27**, 1556.

Ehrsson, J. (1976), *J. Pharmacy Pharmacol.*, **28**, 662.

Einarsson, S., Folestad, S. and Josefsson, B. (1987), *J. Liquid Chromatog.*, **10**, 1589.

El-Mouelhi, M., Ruelius, H. W., Fenselau, C. and Dulik, D. M. (1987), *Drug Metab. Dispos.*, **15**, 767.

Enna, S. J. (1985), in *Neurotransmitter Receptor Binding*, 2nd edn (H. I. Yamamura, S. J. Enna and M. J. Kuhar, eds), p. 177, Raven, New York.

Ensing, K. and De Zeeuw, R. A. (1984), *Trends Anal. Chem.*, **3**, 102.

Euerby, M. R., Partridge, L. Z. and Rajani, P. (1988), *J. Chromatog.*, **447**, 392.

Faed, E. M. (1984), *Drug Metab. Rev.*, **15**, 1213.

Faraj, B. A., Israili, Z. H., Kight, N. E., Smissman, E. E. and Pazdernik, T. J. (1976), *J. Med. Chem.*, **19**, 20.

Fasth, A., Sollenberg, J. and Sörbo, B. (1975), *Acta Pharmaceut. Suecica*, **12**, 311.

Feitsma, K. G. and Drenth, B. F. H. (1988), *Pharmaceut Wkbl. Sci. Edn*, **10**, 1.

Feitsma, K. G., Bosman, J., Drenth, B. F. H. and De Zeeuw, R. A. (1985), *J. Chromatog.*, **333**, 59.

Fell, A. F., Noctor, T. A. G., Mama, J. E. and Clarke, B. J. (1988), *J. Chromatog.*, **434**, 377.

Ferkany, J. W. (1987), *Life Sci.*, **41**, 881.

Findlay, J. W. A. (1987), *Drug Metab. Rev.*, **18**, 83.

Findlay, J. W. A., Warren, J. T., Hill, J. A. and Welch, R. M. (1981), *J. Pharm. Sci.*, **70**, 624.

Fitzgerald, R. L., Blanke, R. V., Glennon, R. A., Yousif, M. Y., Rosecrans, J. A. and Poklis, A. (1989), *J. Chromatog.*, **490**, 59.

Foster, R. T. and Jamali, F. (1987), *J. Chromatog.*, **416**, 388.

Fournel, S. and Caldwell, J. (1986), *Biochem. Pharmacol.*, **35**, 4153.

Fournel-Gigleux, S., Hamar-Hansen, G., Motassim, N., Antoine, B., Mothe, O., Decolin, D., Caldwell, J. and Siest, G. (1988), *Drug Metab. Dispos.*, **16**, 627.

Francotte, E., Wolf, R. M., Lohmann, D. and Mueller, R. (1985), *J. Chromatog.*, **347**, 25.

Frank, H., Nicholson, G. J. and Bayer, E. (1978), *Angew. Chem. Int. Edn*, **17**, 363.

Fritz, S., Lindner, W., Roots, I., Frey, B. M. and Kupfer, A. (1987), *J. Pharmacol. Exp. Ther.*, **241**, 615.

Gal, J. (1977), *J. Pharm. Sci.*, **66**, 169.

Gal, J. (1985), *J. Chromatog.*, **331**, 349.

Gal, J. (1987), *Mag. Liquid Gas Chromatog.*, **5**, 106.

Gal, J., Gruenke, L. D. and Castagnoli, N. (1975), *J. Med. Chem.*, **18**, 683.

Gal, J., Wright, J. and Cho, A. K. (1976), *Res. Commun. Chem. Path. Pharmacol.*, **15**, 525.

Gazdag, M., Szepesi, G. and Huszar, L. (1986), *J. Chromatog.*, **351**, 128.

Gelber, L. R. and Neumeyer, J. L. (1983), *J. Chromatog.*, **257**, 317.

Gerding, T. K., Drenth, B. F. H., Van De Grampel, V. J. M., Niemeijer, N. R., De Zeeuw, R. A., Tepper, P. G. and Horn, A. S. (1989), *J. Chromatog.*, **487**, 125.

Giacomini, K. M., Nelson, W. L., Pershe, R. A., Valdivieso, L., Turner-Tamiyasu, K. and Blaschke, T. F. (1986), *J. Pharmacokin. Biopharmaceut.*, **14**, 335.

Gietl, Y., Spahn, H. and Mutschler, E. (1988), *J. Chromatog.*, **426**, 305.

Gil-Av, E., Feibush, B. and Charles-Siegler, R. (1966), *Tetrahedron Lett.*, **1009**

Goto, J., Goto, N., Hikichi, A , Nishimaki, T. and Nambara, T. (1980), *Anal. Chim. Acta*, **120**, 187.

Goto, J., Goto, N. and Nambara, T. (1982), *J. Chromatog.*, **239**, 559.

Goto, J., Ito, M., Katsuki, S., Saito, N. and Nambara, T. (1986), *J. Liquid Chromatog.*, **9**, 683.

Goula, R. J., Murphy, K. M. M. and Snyder, S. H. (1983), *Life Sci.*, **33**, 2665.

Grierson, J. R. and Adam, M. J. (1985), *J. Chromatog.*, **325**, 103.

Griffith, O. W., Campbell, E. B., Pirkle, W. H., Tsipouras, A. and Hyun, M. H. (1986), *J. Chromatog.*, **362**, 345.

Gross, S. J. and Soares, J. R. (1974), in *Immunoassays for Drugs Subject to Abuse* (S. J. Mule, I. Sunshine, M. Brande and R. E. Willetter, eds), p. 3, CRC Press, Boca Raton.

Gubitz, G. and Mihellyes, S. (1984), *J. Chromatog.*, **314**, 462.

Gunstone, F. D. (1975), *Guidebook to Stereochemistry*, p. 3, Longmans, London.

Gunther, K., Martens, J. and Schickedanz, M (1985), *Z. Anal. Chem.*, **322**, 513.

Gyllenhaal, O., König, W. A. and Vessman, J. (1985), *J. Chromatog.*, **350**, 328.

Hawkins, D. J., Kühn, H., Petty, E. H. and Brash, A. R. (1988), *Anal. Biochem.*, **173**, 456.

Heimark, L. D., Gibaldi, M., Trager, W. F., O'Reilly, R. A. and Goulart, D. A. (1987 a), *Clin. Pharmacol. Ther.*, **42**, 388.

Heimark, L. D., Toon, S., Gibaldi, M., Trager, W. F., O'Reilly, R. A. and Goulart, D. A. (1987 b), *Clin. Pharmacol. Ther.*, **42**, 312.

Helmchen, G. and Nill, G. (1979), *Angew. Chem. Int. Edn*, **18**, 65.

Helmchen, G., Nill, G., Flockenzi, D., Schukle, W. and Youssef, M. S. K. (1979), *Angew. Chem. Int. Edn*, **18**, 62.

Hermansson, J. (1983), *J. Chromatog.*, **269**, 71.

Hermansson, J. (1984), *J. Chromatog.*, **316**, 537.

Hermansson, J. and Eriksson, M. (1984), *J. Chromatog.*, **336**, 321.

Hermansson, J. and Eriksson, M. (1986), *J. Liquid Chromatog.*, **9**, 621.

Hermansson, J. and Schill, G. (1988), in *Chromatographic Chiral Separations* (M. Zief and L. J. Crane, eds), p. 245, Marcel Dekker, New York.

Hermansson, J., Iversen, T. and Lindquist, U. (1982), *Acta Pharmaceut. Suecica*, **19**, 199.

Hignite, C., Uetrecht, J., Tschanz, C. and Azarnoff, D. (1980), *Clin. Pharmacol. Ther.*, **28**, 99.

Hinze, W. L., Riehl, T. E., Armstrong, D. W., DeMond, W., Alak, A. and Ward, T. (1985), *Anal. Chem.*, **57**, 237.

Hoffmann, K-J., Renberg, L. and Bäärnhielm, C. (1984), *Europ. J. Drug Metab. Pharmacokin.*, **9**, 215.

Honma, S., Ito, T. and Kambegawa, A. (1985), *Chem. Pharmaceut. Bull.*, **33**, 760.

Horeau, A. (1969), *Tetrahedron Lett.*, **3121**.
Howald, W. N., Bush, E. D., Trager, W. F., O'Reilly, R. A. and Motley, C. H. (1980), *Biomed. Mass Spect.*, **7**, 35.
Huang-Chandler, M. H., Guttendorf, R. J., Blouin, R. A. and Wedlund, P. J. (1987), *J. Chromatog.*, **419**, 426.
Hutt, A. J. and Caldwell, J. (1983), *J. Pharmacy Pharmacol.*, **35**, 693.
Hutt, A. J. and Caldwell, J. (1984), *Clin. Pharmacokin.*, **9**, 371.
Hutt, A. J. and Caldwell, J. (1988 a), in *Metabolism of Xenobiotics* (J. W. Gorrod, H. Oelschläger and J. Caldwell, eds), p. 335, Taylor & Francis, London.
Hutt, A. J. and Caldwell, J. (1988 b), in *Methodological Surveys in Biochemistry and Analysis, Volume 18, Bioanalysis of Drugs and Metabolites, Especially Anti-Inflammatory and Cardiovascular* (E. Reid, J. D. Robinson and I. D. Wilson, eds), p. 115, Plenum, New York.
Hutt, A. J. and Caldwell, J. (1989), in *Xenobiotic Metabolism and Disposition* (R. Kato, R. W. Estabrook and M. N. Cayen, eds), p. 161, Taylor & Francis, London.
Hutt, A. J., Fournel, S. and Caldwell, J. (1986), *J. Chromatog.*, **378**, 409.
Hyland, R., McBride, J., Hanlon, G. W., Hutt, A. J. and Olliff, C. J. (1989), *Int. Symp. Electroanalysis in Biochemical, Environmental and Industrial Sciences*, Loughborough, UK, April 1989, Abstract.
Hyun, M. H., Baik, I-K. and Pirkle, W. H. (1988), *J. Liquid Chromatog.*, **11**, 1249.
Ichida, A. and Shibata, T. (1988), in *Chromatographic Chiral Separations* (M. Zief and L. J. Crane, eds), p. 219, Marcel Dekker, New York.
Ichida, A., Shibata, T., Okamoto, I., Yuki, Y., Namikoshi, H. and Toga, Y. (1984), *Chromatographia*, **19**, 280.
Ichinose, R. and Kurihara, N. (1987), *Biochem. Pharmacol.*, **36**, 3751.
Innis, R. B., Bylund, D. B. and Snyder, S. H. (1978), *Life Sci.*, **23**, 2031.
Itabashi, Y. and Takagi, T. (1986), *Lipids.*, **21**, 413.
Iversen, L. L., Jarrott, B. and Simmonds, M. A. (1971), *Br. J. Pharmacol.*, **43**, 845.
Jackman, G. P., McLean, A. J., Jennings, G. L. and Bobik, A. (1981), *Clin. Pharmacol. Ther.*, **30**, 291.
Jadaud, P., Thelohan, S., Schonbaum, G. R. and Wainer, I. W. (1989), *Chirality*, **1**, 38.
Jamali, F., Mehvar, R., Lemko, C. and Eradiri, O. (1988), *J. Pharmaceut. Sci.*, **77**, 963.
Jegorov, A., Triska, J., Trnka, T. and Cerny, M. (1988), *J. Chromatog.*, **434**, 417.
Johnson, D. M., Reuter, A., Collins, J. M. and Thompson, G. F. (1979), *J. Pharmaceut. Sci.*, **68**, 112.
Kaiser, D. G., Van Giessen, G. J., Reischer, R. J. and Wechter, W. J. (1976), *J. Pharmaceut. Sci.*, **65**, 269.
Kaminsky, L. S., Dunbar, D. A., Wang, P. P., Beaune, P., Larrey, D., Guengerich, F. P., Schnellmann, R. G. and Sipes, I. G. (1984), *Drug Metab. Dispos.*, **12**, 470.
Karush, F. (1956), *J. Am. Chem. Soc.*, **78**, 5519.
Kawashima, K., Levy, A. and Spector, S. (1976), *J. Pharmacol. Exp. Ther.*, **196**, 517.
Keller, J. W. and Dick, K. O. (1986), *J. Chromatog.*, **367**, 187.
Kemmerer, J. M., Rubio, F. A., McClain, R. M. and Koechlin, B. A. (1979), *J. Pharmaceut. Sci.*, **68**, 1274.
Knorr, H., Reichi, R., Traunecker, W., Knappen, F. and Brandt, K. (1984), *Arz.-Forsch.*, **34**, 1709.
König, W. A. (1987), *The Practice of Enantiomer Separation by Capillary Gas Chromatography*, p. 1, Huthig, Heidelberg.
König, W. A. (1988), in *Drug Stereochemistry. Analytical Methods and Pharmacology* (I. W. Wainer and D. E. Drayer, eds), p. 113, Marcel Dekker, New York.
König, W. A. and Ernst, K. (1983), *J. Chromatog.*, **280**, 135.

König, W. A., Steinbach, E. and Ernst, K. (1984), *J. Chromatog.*, **301**, 129.
König, W. A., Gyllenhaal, O. and Vessman, J. (1986), *J. Chromatog.*, **356**, 354.
König, W. A., Lutz, S., Mischnick-Lubbecke, P., Brassat, B. and Wenz, G. (1988 a), *J. Chromatog.*, **447**, 193.
König, W. A., Lutz, S. and Wenz, G. (1988 b), *Angew. Chem. Int. Edn*, **27**, 979.
König, W. A., Mischnick-Lubbecke, P., Brassat, B., Lutz, S. and Wenz, G. (1988 c), *Carbohydrate Res.*, **183**, 11.
Krstulovic, A. M. (1989) ed: *Chiral Separations by High Performance Liquid Chromatography: Applications to Pharmaceutical Compounds*, Ellis Horwood, Chichester.
Krstulovic, A. M., Gianviti, J. M., Burke, J. T. and Mompon, B. (1988), *J. Chromatog.*, **426**, 417.
Kuhn, H., Wiesner, R., Lankin, V. Z., Nekrasov, A., Alder, L. and Schewe, T. (1987), *Anal. Biochem.*, **160**, 24
Küpfer, A., Roberts, R. K., Schenker, S. and Branch, R. A. (1981), *J. Pharmacol. Exp. Ther.*, **218**, 183.
Küpfer, A., Desmond, P. V., Schenker, S. and Branch, R. A. (1982), *J. Pharmacol. Exp. Ther.*, **221**, 590.
Küpfer, A., Patwardhan, R., Ward, S., Schenker, S., Preisig, R. and Branch, R. A. (1984), *J. Pharmacol. Exp. Ther.*, **320**, 28.
Landsteiner, K. and Van der Scheer, J. (1928), *J. Exp. Med.*, **48**, 315.
Landsteiner, K. and Van der Scheer, J. (1929), *J. Exp. Med.*, **50**, 407.
Lee, E. D., Henion, J. D., Brunner, C. A., Wainer, I. W., Doyle, T. D. and Gal, J. (1986), *Anal. Chem.*, **58**, 1349.
Lee, E. J. D., Williams, K. M., Graham, G. G., Day, R. O. and Champion, G. D. (1984), *J. Pharm. Sci.*, **73**, 1542.
Lee, E. J. D., Aug, S. B. and Lee, T. L. (1987), *J. Chromatog.*, **420**, 203.
Lehr, K-H. and Damm, P. (1988), *J. Chromatog.*, **425**, 153.
Light, D. R., Waxman, D. J. and Walsh, C. (1982), *Biochemistry*, **21**, 2490.
Lin, J. H. and Hsieh, J. Y-K. (1988), *Drug Metab. Dispos.*, **16**, 540.
Lindeke, B., Weli, A. M. and Hermansson, J. (1987), *ISSX 2nd European Symposium on Foreign Compound Metabolism* (Frankfurt), Abs. C17.
Lindner, W., Leitner, C. and Uray, G. (1984), *J. Chromatog.*, **316**, 605.
Lindner, W., Rath, M., Stoschltzky, K. and Uray, G. (1989), *J. Chromatog.*, **487**, 375.
Lipkowitz, K. B., Demeter, D. A., Parish, C. A. and Darden, T. (1987), *Anal. Chem.*, **59**, 1731.
Lipkowitz, K. B., Demeter, D. A., Zegarra, R., Larter, R. and Darden, T. (1988), *J. Amer. Chem. Soc.*, **110**, 3446.
Liu, R. H. and Ku, W. W. (1983), *J. Chromatog.*, **271**, 309.
Lloyd, D. K., Goodall, D. M. and Scrivener, H. (1989), *Anal. Chem.*, **61**, 1238.
Lough, W. J. (1989) ed: *Chiral Liquid Chromatography*, Blackie, Glasgow.
Lyle, G. G. and Lyle, R. E. (1983), in *Asymmetric Synthesis Volume 1. Analytical Methods* (J. D. Morrison, ed), p. 13, Academic, New York.
Maeda, M. and Tsuji, A. (1981), *J. Pharmacobio-Dynamics.*, **4**, 167.
Maitre, J-M., Boss, G. and Testa, B (1984), *J. Chromatog.*, **299**, 397.
Maitre, J-M., Boss, G., Testa, B. and Hostettmann, K. (1986), *J. Chromatog.*, **356**, 341.
Mangold, J. B. and Abdel-Monem, M. M. (1983), *J. Med. Chem.*, **26**, 66.
Mannschreck, A., Koller, H., Stühler, G., Davies, M. A. and Traber, J. (1984), *Europ. J. Med. Chem.*, **19**, 381.
Martens, J., Gunther, K. and Schickadanz, M. (1986 a), *Arch. Pharmazie.*, **319**, 572.
Martens, J., Gunther, K. and Schickadanz, M. (1986 b), *Arch. Pharmazie.*, **319**, 461.
Masurel, D. and Wainer, I. W. (1989), *J. Chromatog.*, **490**, 133.

Matsukura, S., Sakamoto, N., Imura, H., Matsuyama, H., Tamada, T., Ishiguro, T. and Muranaka, H. (1975), *Biochem. Biophys. Res. Commun.*, **64**, 574.

McClanahan, J. S. and Maguire, J. H. (1986), *J. Chromatog.*, **381**, 438.

McDaniel, D. M. and Snider, B. G. (1987), *J. Chromatog.*, **404**, 123.

McErlane, K. M., Igwemezie, L. and Kerr, C. R. (1987), *J. Chromatog.*, **415**, 335.

McGilliard, K. L. and Olsen, G. D. (1980), *J. Pharmacol. Exp. Ther.*, **215**, 205.

McGilliard, K. L., Wilson, J. E., Olsen, G. D. and Bartos, F. (1979), *Proc. West. Pharmacol. Soc.*, **22**, 463.

McKay, S. W., Mallen, D. N. B., Shrubsall, P. R., Swann, B. P. and Williamson, W. R. N. (1979), *J. Chromatog.*, **170**, 482.

McMahon, R. E. and Sullivan, H. R. (1976), *Res. Commun. Chem. Path. Pharmacol.*, **14**, 631.

McMahon, R. E., Sullivan, H. R., Craig, J. C. and Pereira, W. E. (1969), *Arch. Biochem. Biophys.*, **132**, 575.

McMillan, D. C., Fu, P. P. and Cerniglia, C. E. (1987), *Appl. Env. Microbiol.*, **53**, 2560.

Meese, C. O., Thalheimer, P. and Eichelbaum, M. (1987), *J. Chromatog.*, **423**, 344.

Meese, C. O., Fischer, C. and Eichelbaum, M. (1988), *Biomed. Env. Mass Spect.*, **15**, 63.

Mehta, A. C. (1988), *J. Chromatog.*, **426**, 1.

Mehvar, R. and Jamali, F. (1988 a), *Pharm. Res.*, **5**, 53.

Mehvar, R. and Jamali, F. (1988 b), *J. Chromatog.*, **431**, 228.

Mehvar, R., Jamali, F. and Pasutto, F. M. (1988 a), *J. Chromatog.*, **425**, 135.

Mehvar, R., Jamali, F. and Pasutto, F. M. (1988 b), *Clin. Chem.*, **34**, 493.

Meinard, C., Bruneau, P. and Perronnet, J. (1985), *J. Chromatog.*, **349**, 109.

Midha, K. K., Hubbard, J. W., Cooper, J. K. and MacKouka, C. (1983), *J. Pharm. Sci.*, **72**, 736.

Miller, K. J., Gal, J. and Ames, M. M. (1984), *J. Chromatog.*, **307**, 335.

Miwa, T., Ichikawa, M., Tsuno, M., Haltori, T., Miyakawa, T., Kayano, M. and Miyake, Y. (1987), *Chem. Pharm. Bull.*, **35**, 682.

Miwa, B. J., Choma, N., Brown, S. Y., Keigher, N., Garland, W. A. and Fukuda, E. K. (1988), *J. Chromatog.*, **431**, 343.

Miyazaki, H. and Abuki, H. (1976), *Chem. Pharm. Bull.*, **24**, 2572.

Morrison, J. D. (ed) (1983), *Asymmetric Synthesis. Volume 1. Analytical Methods*, Academic, New York.

Mularz, E. A., Cline-Love, L. J. and Petersheim, M. (1988), *Anal. Chem.*, **60**, 2751.

Murphy, P. J., Williams, T. L., Smallwood, J. K., Bellamy, G. and Molloy, B. B. (1978), *Life Sci.*, **23**, 301.

Nagashima, H., Tanaka, Y. and Hayashi, R. (1985), *J. Chromatog.*, **345**, 373.

Nahorski, S. R., Batta, M. I. and Barnett, D. B. (1978), *Europ. J. Pharmacol.*, **52**, 393.

Nakamura, K., Hachey, D. L., Kreek, M. J., Irving, C. S. and Klein, P. D. (1982), *J. Pharm. Sci.*, **71**, 40.

Nambara, T., Tanaka, T. and Numazawa, M. (1979), *J. Pharmacobio-Dynamics*, **2**, 151.

Nelson, W. L. and Bartels, M. J. (1984 a), *Drug Metab. Dispos.*, **12**, 345.

Nelson, W. L. and Bartels, M. J. (1984 b), *Drug Metab. Dispos.*, **12**, 382.

Nelson, W. L. and Olsen, L. D. (1988), *Drug Metab. Dispos.*, **16**, 834.

Nelson, W. L., Olsen, L. D., Beitner, D. B. and Pallow, R. J. (1988), *Drug Metab. Dispos.*, **16**, 184.

Nicoll-Griffith, D. A. (1987), *J. Chromatog.*, **402**, 179.

Nicoll-Griffith, D. A., Inaba, T., Tang, B. K. and Kalow, W. (1988), *J. Chromatog.*, **428**, 103.

Nichols, D. E., Barfknecht, C. F., Rusterholz, D. B., Benington, F. and Morin, R. D. (1973), *J. Med. Chem.*, **16**, 480.

Nimura, N., Iwaki, K. and Kinoshita, T. (1987), *J. Chromatog.*, **402**, 387.
Niwaguchi, T., Kanada, Y., Kishi, T. and Inoue, T. (1982), *J. Forensic Sci.*, **27**, 592.
Okamoto, Y. and Hatada, K. (1988), in *Chromatographic Chiral Separations* (M. Zief and L. J. Crane, eds), p. 199, Marcel Dekker, New York.
Okamoto, Y., Kawashima, M. and Hatada, K. (1984 a), *J. Am. Chem. Soc.*, **106**, 5357.
Okamoto, Y., Honda, S., Hatada, K., Okamoto, I., Toga, Y. and Kobayashi, S. (1984 b), *Bull. Chem. Soc. Japan*, **57**, 1681.
Okamoto, Y., Aburatani, R., Miura, S. and Hatada, K. (1987), *J. Liquid Chromatog.*, **10**, 1613.
Okamoto, Y., Aburatani, R., Hatano, K. and Hatada, K. (1988), *J. Liquid Chromatog.*, **11**, 2147.
O'Reilly, R. A., Trager, W. F., Motley, C. H. and Howald, W. (1980), *J. Clin. Invest.*, **65**, 746.
Pedrazzini, S., Zanoboni-Muciaccia, W., Sacchi, C. and Forgione, A. (1987), *J. Chromatog.*, **415**, 214.
Pescher, P., Caude, M., Rosset, R. and Tambute, A. (1986), *J. Chromatog.*, **371**, 159.
Pettersson, C. (1984), *J. Chromatog.*, **316**, 553.
Pettersson, C. and Josefsson, M. (1986), *Chromatographia*, **21**, 321.
Pettersson, C. and Schill, G. (1981), *J. Chromatog.*, **204**, 179.
Pettersson, C. and Schill, G. (1986), *J. Liquid Chromatog.*, **9**, 269.
Pettersson, C. and Schill, G. (1988), in *Chromatographic Chiral Separations* (M. Zief and L. J. Crane, eds), p. 283, Marcel Dekker, New York.
Pettersson, C. and Stuurman, H. W. (1984), *J. Chromatog. Sci.*, **22**, 441.
Pflugmann, G., Spahn, H. and Mutschler, E. (1987 a), *J. Chromatog.*, **416**, 331.
Pflugmann, G., Spahn, H. and Mutschler, E. (1987 b), *J. Chromatog.*, **421**, 161.
Pirkle, W. H. and Finn, J. M. (1981), *J. Org. Chem.*, **46**, 2935.
Pirkle, W. H. and Finn, J. M. (1983), in *Asymmetric Synthesis, Volume 1, Analytical Methods* (J. D. Morrison, ed), p. 87, Academic, New York.
Pirkle, W. H. and Hyun, M. H. (1985), *J. Chromatog.*, **328**, 1.
Pirkle, W. H. and McCune, J. E. (1988), *J. Liquid Chromatog.*, **11**, 2165.
Pirkle, W. H. and Pochapsky, T. C. (1987), in *Advances in Chromatography*, Vol. 27 (J. C. Giddings, E. Grushka and P. R. Brown, eds), p. 73, Marcel Dekker, New York.
Pirkle, W. H. and Pochapsky, T. C. (1988), *Chromatographia*, **25**, 652.
Pirkle, W. H. and Pochapsky, T. C. (1989), *Chem. Rev.*, **89**, 347.
Pirkle, W. H. and Welch, C. J. (1984), *J. Org. Chem.*, **49**, 138.
Pirkle, W. H., Finn, J. M., Schreiner, J. L. and Hamper, B. C. (1981), *J. Am. Chem. Soc.*, **103**, 3964.
Pirkle, W. H., Hyun, M. H. and Bank, B. (1984), *J. Chromatog.*, **316**, 585.
Pirkle, W. H., Pochapsky, T. C., Mahler, G. S. and Field, R. E. (1985), *J. Chromatog.*, **348**, 89.
Pirkle, W. H., Pochapsky, T. C., Mahler, G. S., Correy, D. E., Reno, D. S. and Alessi, D. M. (1986), *J. Org. Chem.*, **51**, 4991.
Pohl, L. R. and Trager, W. F. (1973), *J. Med. Chem.*, **16**, 475.
Powell, M. L., Wagoner, R. R., Chen, C-H. and Nelson, W. L. (1980), *Res. Commun. Chem. Path. Pharmacol.*, **30**, 387.
Purdie, N. and Swallows, K. A. (1989), *Anal. Chem.*, **61**, 77A.
Ramsay, O. B. (1981), *Nobel Prize Topics in Chemistry, Stereochemistry*, p. 43, Heyden, London.
Rathbone, E. B., Butlers, R. W., Cookson, D. and Robinson, J. L. (1989), *J. Agric. Fd Chem.*, **37**, 58.
Reid, J. M., Stobaugh, J. F. and Sternson, L. A. (1989), *Anal. Chem.*, **61**, 441.
Reitsma, B. H. and Yeung, E. S. (1986), *J. Chromatog.*, **362**, 353.
Ridgewell, R. E. and Abdel-Monem, M. M. (1987), *Drug Metab. Dispos.*, **15**, 82.

Rominger, K. L. and Albert, H. J. (1985), *Arz. Forsch.*, **35**, 415.
Roston, D. A. and Wijayaratne, R. (1988), *Anal. Chem.*, **60**, 948.
Roussel, C., Steine, J-L., Beauvais, F. and Chemlal, A. (1989), *J. Chromatog.*, **462**, 95.
Roy, S. D. and Lim, H. K. (1988), *J. Chromatog.*, **431**, 210.
Rubin, A., Knadler, M. P., Ho, P. P. K., Bechtol, L. D. and Wolen, R. L. (1985), *J. Pharm. Sci.*, **74**, 82.
Ruelius, H. W., Tio, C. O., Knowles, J. A., McHugh, S. L., Schillings, R. T. and Sisenwine, S. F. (1979), *Drug Metab. Dispos.*, **7**, 40.
Ruud-Christensen, M. and Salvesen, B. (1984), *J. Chromatog.*, **303**, 433.
Sallustio, B. C., Abas, A., Hayball, P. J., Purdie, Y. J. and Meffin, P. J. (1986), *J. Chromatog.*, **374**, 329.
Salvadori, P., Rosini, C. and Bertucci, C. (1984), *J. Org. Chem.*, **49**, 5050.
Salvadori, P., Rosini, C., Pini, D., Bertucci, C. and Uccello-Barretta, G. (1989), *Chirality.*, **1**, 161.
Schill, G., Wainer, I. W. and Barkan, S. (1986 a), *J. Liquid Chromatog.*, **9**, 641.
Schill, G., Wainer, I. W. and Barkan, S. (1986 b), *J. Chromatog.*, **365**, 73.
Schmitthenner, H. F., Fedorchuk, M. and Walter, D. J. (1989), *J. Chromatog.*, **487**, 197.
Schurig, V. (1984), *Angew. Chem. Int. Edn*, **23**, 747.
Schurig, V. (1985), *Kontakte (Darmstadt)*, **1**, 54.
Schurig, V. (1986), *Kontakte (Darmstadt)*, **1**, 3.
Schurig, V. and Weber, R. (1984), *J. Chromatog.*, **289**, 321.
Schuster, D., Woodruff-Modi, M., Lalka, D. and Gengo, F. M. (1988), *J. Chromatog.*, **433**, 318.
Scott, B. S. and Dunn, D. L. (1985), *J. Chromatog.*, **319**, 419.
Sedman, A. J. and Gal, J. (1983), *J. Chromatog.*, **278**, 199.
Seideman, P., Ericsson, O., Groningsson, K. and von Bahr, C. (1981), *Acta Pharmacol. Tox.*, **49**, 200.
Shibata, T., Okamoto, I. and Ishii, K. (1986), *J. Liquid Chromatog.*, **9**, 313.
Shimizu, R., Kakimoto, T., Ishii, K., Fujimoto, Y., Nishi, H. and Tsumagare, N. (1986), *J. Chromatog.*, **357**, 119.
Silber, B. and Riegleman, S. (1980), *J. Pharmacol. Exp. Ther.*, **215**, 643.
Simmonds, R. G., Woodage, T. J., Duff, S. M. and Green, J. N. (1980), *Europ. J. Drug Metab. Pharmacokin.*, **5**, 169.
Simonyi, M. (1984), *Med. Res. Rev.*, **4**, 359.
Singh, N. N., Pasutto, F. M., Coutts, R. T. and Jamali, F. (1986), *J. Chromatog.*, **378**, 125.
Sioufi, A., Colussi, D., Marfil, F. and Dubois, J. P. (1987), *J. Chromatog.*, **414**, 131.
Sisenwine, S. F., Tio, C. O., Hadley, F. V., Liu, A. L., Kimmel, H. B. and Ruelius, H. W. (1982), *Drug Metab. Dispos.*, **10**, 605.
Slégel, P., Vereczkey-Donath, G., Ladanyi, L. and Toth-Lauritz, M. (1987), *J. Pharmaceut. Biomed. Anal.*, **5**, 665.
Smith, R. L. and Caldwell, J. (1988), *Trends Pharmacol. Sci.*, **9**, 75.
Soine, P. J. and Soine, W. H. (1987), *J. Chromatog.*, **422**, 309.
Soine, W. H., Soine, P. J., Overton, B. W. and Garrettson, L. K. (1986), *Drug Metab. Dispos.*, **14**, 619.
Souter, R. W. (1985), *Chromatographic Separations of Stereoisomers*, CRC Press, Boca Raton.
Spahn, H. (1987), *J. Chromatog.*, **423**, 334.
Spahn, H. (1988 a), *J. Chromatog.*, **427**, 131.
Spahn, H. (1988 b), *Arch. Pharm.*, **321**, 847.
Spahn, H. (1988 c), *J. Chromatog.*, **431**, 229.
Spahn, H. (1988 d), *J. Chromatog.*, **430**, 368.

Spahn, H., Weber, H., Mutschler, E. and Mohrke, W. (1984), *J. Chromatog.*, **310**, 167.
Spahn, H., Krauß, D. and Mutschler, E. (1988 a), *Pharm. Res.*, **5**, 107.
Spahn, H., Spahn, I., Pflugmann, G., Mutschler, E. and Benet, L. Z. (1988 b), *J. Chromatog.*, **433**, 331.
Spahn, H., Iwakawa, S., Lin, E. T. and Benet, L. Z. (1989 a), *Pharm. Res.*, **6**, 125.
Spahn, H., Wellstein, A., Pflugmann, G., Mutschler, E. and Palm, D. (1989 b), *Pharm. Res.*, **6**, 152.
Srinivas, N. R., Hubbard, J. W., Cooper, J. K. and Midha, K. K. (1988), *J. Chromatog.*, **433**, 105.
Stoltenborg, J. K., Puglisi, C. V., Rubio, F. and Vane, F. M. (1981), *J. Pharm. Sci.*, **70**, 1207.
Straka, R. J., Lalonde, R. L. and Wainer, I. W. (1988), *Pharm. Res.*, **5**, 187.
Sugiyama, K. and Trager, W. F. (1986), *Biochemistry*, **25**, 7336.
Sullivan, H. R. and Franklin, R. B. (1988), in *Metabolism of Xenobiotics* (J. W. Gorrod, H. Oelschlager and J. Caldwell, eds), p. 145, Taylor & Francis, London.
Szepesi, G. and Gazdag, M. (1988), *J. Pharm. Biomed. Anal.*, **6**, 623.
Takagi, T. and Itabashi, Y. (1986), *J. Chromatog.*, **366**, 451.
Takahashi, H., Kanno, S., Ogatu, H., Kashiwada, K., Ohira, M. and Someya, K. (1988), *J. Pharm. Sci.*, **77**, 993.
Takeuchi, T., Asai, H., Hashimoto, Y., Watanabe, K. and Ishii, D. (1985), *J. Chromatog.*, **331**, 99.
Tamegai, T., Tanaka, T., Kaneko, T., Ozaki, S., Ohmae, M. and Kawabe, K. (1979), *J. Liquid Chromatog.*, **2**, 551.
Tamura, S., Kuzuna, S., Kawai, K. and Kishimoto, S. (1981), *J. Pharmacy Pharmacol.*, **33**, 701.
Tan, Y. K. and Soldin, S. J. (1987), *J. Chromatog.*, **422**, 187.
Tang, B. K., Kalow, W. and Grey, A. A. (1978), *Res. Commun. Chem. Path. Pharmacol.*, **21**, 45.
Taylor, K. B. (1974), *J. Biol. Chem.*, **249**, 454.
Te Koppele, J. M., van der Mark, E. J., Boerrigter, J. C. O., Brussee, J., van der Gen, A., van der Greef, J. and Mulder, G. J. (1986 a), *J. Pharmacol. Exp. Ther.*, **239**, 898.
Te Koppele, J. M., Dogterom, P., Vermeulen, N. P. E., Meijer, D. K. F., van der Gen, A. and Mulder, G. J. (1986 b), *J. Pharmacol. Exp. Ther.*, **239**, 905.
Te Koppele, J. M., van der Mark, E. J. and Mulder, G. J. (1988 a), *J. Chromatog.*, **427**, 67.
Te Koppele, J. M., Coles, B., Ketterer, B. and Mulder, G. J. (1988 b), *Biochem. J.*, **252**, 137.
Testa, B. (1986), *Xenobiotica*, **16**, 265.
Testa, B. and Jenner, P. (1978), in *Drug Fate and Metabolism, Methods and Techniques*, Vol. 2 (E. R. Garrett and J. L. Hirtz, eds), p. 143, Marcel Dekker, New York.
Testa, B. and Mayer, J. M. (1988), in *Progress in Drug Research*, Vol. 32, (E. Jucker, ed), p. 249, Birkhäuser, Basel.
Thompson, J. A., Hull, J. E. and Norris, K. J. (1981), *Drug Metab. Dispos.*, **9**, 466.
Thompson, J. A., Holtzman, J. L., Tsuru, M., Lerman, C. J. and Holtzman, J. L. (1982), *J. Chromatog.*, **238**, 470.
Tokuma, Y., Fujiwara, T. and Noguchi, H. (1987), *J. Pharm. Sci.*, **76**, 310.
Toon, S. and Trager, W. F. (1984), *J. Pharm. Sci.*, **73**, 1671.
Toon, S., Heimark, L. D., Trager, W. F. and O'Reilly, R. A. (1985), *J. Pharm. Sci.*, **74**, 1037.
Toon, S., Low, L. K., Gibaldi, M., Trager, W. F., O'Reilly, R. A., Motley, C. H. and Goulart, D. A. (1986), *Clin. Pharmacol. Ther.*, **39**, 15.

Topiol, S., Sabio, M., Moroz, J. and Caldwell, W. B. (1988), *J. Amer. Chem. Soc.*, **110**, 8367.

Tosolini, G. P., Moro, E., Forgione, A., Ranghieri, M. and Mandelli, V. (1974), *J. Pharm. Sci.*, **63**, 1072.

Trager, W. F. and Jones, J. P. (1987), in *Progress in Drug Metabolism*, Vol. 10 (J. W. Bridges, L. F. Chasseaud and G. G. Gibson, eds), p. 55, Taylor & Francis, London.

Tsai, W-L., Hermann, K., Hug, E., Rohde, B. and Dreiding, A. S. (1985), *Helv. Chim. Acta*, **68**, 2238.

Turk, J., Stump, W. T., Wolf, B. A., Easom, R. A. and McDaniel, M. L. (1988), *Anal. Biochem.*, **174**, 580.

Van Bladeren, P., Breimer, D., Seghen, C., Vermeulen, N., Van der Guy, A. and Cannet, J. (1981), *Drug Metabol. Dispos.*, **9**, 207.

Van der Graaff, M., Hofman, P. H., Breimer, D. D., Vermeulen, N. P. E., Knabe, J. and Schamber, L. (1985), *Biomed. Mass Spect.*, **12**, 464.

Van der Graaff, M., Vermeulen, N. P. E., Hofman, P. H. and Breimer, D. D. (1987), *Biochem. Pharmacol.*, **36**, 1321.

Van Giessen, G. J. and Kaiser, D. G. (1975), *J. Pharm. Sci.*, **64**, 798.

Vermeulen, N. P. E. (1989), in *Xenobiotic Metabolism and Disposition* (R. Kato, R. W. Estabrook and M. N. Cayen, eds), p. 193, Taylor & Francis, London.

Vermeulen, N. P. E. and Testa, B. (1988), in *Stereochemistry of Pesticides. Biological and Chemical Problems* (E. J. Ariens, J. J. S. Van Rensen and W. Welling, eds), p. 375, Elsevier, Amsterdam.

Virtanen, R., Kanto, J. and Iisalo, E. (1980), *Acta Pharmacol. Toxicol.*, **47**, 208.

Vogelgesang, B., Echizen, H., Schmidt, E. and Eichelbaum, M. (1984), *Br. J. Clin. Pharmacol.*, **18**, 733.

Wainer, I. W. (1988), *A Practical Guide to the Selection and use of H.P.L.C. Chiral Stationary Phases*, p. 1, Baker, Phillipsburg.

Wainer, I. W. (1989), *LC-GC Int.*, **2**, 14.

Wainer, I. W. and Alembik, M. C. (1986 a), *J. Chromatog.*, **367**, 59.

Wainer, I. W. and Alembik, M. C. (1986 b), *J. Chromatog.*, **358**, 85.

Wainer, I. W. and Doyle, T. D. (1984), *J. Chromatog.*, **284**, 117.

Wainer, I. W. and Drayer, D. E. (eds) (1988), *Drug Stereochemistry, Analytical Methods and Pharmacology*, Marcel Dekker, New York.

Wainer, I. W. and Stiffin, R. M. (1988), *J. Chromatog.*, **424**, 158.

Wainer, I. W., Brunner, C. A. and Doyle, T. D. (1983), *J. Chromatog.*, **264**, 154.

Wainer, I. W., Doyle, T. D., Donn, K. H. and Powell, J. R. (1984), *J. Chromatog.*, **306**, 405.

Wainer, I. W., Alembik, M. C. and Johnson, C. R. (1986), *J. Chromatog.*, **361**, 374.

Wainer, I. W., Jadand, P., Schonbaum, G. R., Kadodkar, S. V. and Henry, M. P. (1988), *Chromatographia*, **25**, 903.

Walle, T. (1985), *Drug Metab. Dispos.*, **13**, 279.

Walle, T. and Walle, U. K. (1979), *Res. Commun. Chem. Path. Pharmacol.*, **23**, 453.

Walle, T., Wilson, M. J., Walle, U. K. and Bai, S. A. (1983 a), *Drug Metab. Dispos.*, **11**, 544.

Walle, T., Walle, U. K., Wilson, M. J., Fagan, T. C. and Gaffney, T. E. (1984), *Br. J. Clin. Pharmacol.*, **18**, 741.

Walle, T., Christ, D. D., Walle, U. K. and Wilson, M. J. (1985), *J. Chromatog.*, **341**, 213.

Walle, U. K. and Walle, T. (1989), *Chirality*, **1**, 121.

Walle, U. K., Walle, T., Bai, S. A. and Olanoff, L. S. (1983 b), *Clin. Pharmacol. Ther.*, **34**, 718.

Wang, L., Chorev, M., Feingers, J., Levitzki, A. and Inbar, M. (1986), *FEBS*, **199**, 173.

Ward, T. J. and Armstrong, D. W. (1988), in *Chromatographic Chiral Separations* (M. Zief and L. J. Crane, eds), p. 131, Marcel Dekker, New York.
Weaner, L. E. and Hoerr, D. C. (1987), *Anal. Biochem.*, **160**, 316.
Weber, H., Spahn, H., Mutschler, E. and Möhrke, W. (1984), *J. Chromatog.*, **307**, 145.
Wedlund, P. J., Sweetman, B. J., McAllister, C. B., Branch, R. A. and Wilkinson, G. R. (1984), *J. Chromatog.*, **307**, 121.
Weinkam, R. J., Gal, J., Callery, P. and Castagnoli, N. (1976), *Anal. Chem.*, **48**, 203.
Wernicke, R. (1985), *J. Chromatog. Sci.*, **23**, 39.
White, R. E., Miller, J. P., Favreau, L. V. and Bhattacharyya, A. (1986), *J. Am. Chem. Soc.*, **107**, 6024.
Williams, K. and Lee, E. (1985), *Drugs*, **30**, 333.
Williams, T., Pitcher, R. G., Bommer, P., Gutzwiller, J. and Uskokovic, M. (1969), *J. Am. Chem. Soc.*, **91**, 1871.
Wilson, I. D. (1986), in *Methodological Surveys in Biochemistry and Analysis, Volume 16, Bioactive Analytes Including CNS drugs, Peptides and Enantiomers* (E. Reid, B. Scales and I. D. Wilson, eds), p. 277, Plenum, New York.
Wilson, I. D. and Ruane, R. J. (1990) eds: *Chiral Separations—Chromatographic Society Surveys*, The Chromatographic Society, Nottingham.
Wilson, M. J. and Walle, T. (1984), *J. Chromatog.*, **310**, 424.
Wing, K. D. and Hammock, B. D. (1979), *Experientia.*, **35**, 1619.
Wolen, R. L., Obermeyer, B. D., Ziege, E. A., Black, H. R. and Gruber, C. M. (1978), in *Stable Isotopes, Applications in Pharmacology, Toxicology and Clinical Research* (T. A. Baillie, ed), p. 113, Macmillan, London.
Wu, D-F., Reidenberg, M. M. and Drayer, D. E. (1988), *J. Chromatog.*, **433**, 141.
Wuis, E. W., Beneken Kolmer, E. W. J., Van Beijsterveldt, L. E. C., Burgers, R. C. M., Vree, T. B. and Van der Kleyn, E. (1987), *J. Chromatog.*, **415**, 419
Wurzburger, R. J., Miller, R. L., Boxenbaum, H. G. and Spector, S. (1977), *J. Pharmacol. Exp. Ther.*, **204**, 435.
Yamaguchi, T. and Nakamura, Y. (1985), *Drug Metab. Dispos.*, **13**, 614.
Yang, S. K. (1988), *Biochem. Pharmacol.*, **37**, 61.
Yang, S. K. and Weems, H. B. (1984), *Anal. Chem.*, **56**, 2658.
Yang, S. K., Mushtaq, M. and Fu, P. P. (1986), *J. Chromatog.*, **371**, 195.
Yang, Z-Y., Barkan, S., Brunner, C., Weber, J. D., Doyle, T. D. and Wainer, I. W. (1985), *J. Chromatog.*, **324**, 444.
Yeung, E. S. (1988), in *Metabolism of Xenobiotics* (J. W. Gorrod, H. Oelschlager and J. Caldwell, eds), p. 161, Taylor & Francis, London.
Yeung, E. S., Steenhoek, L. E., Woodruff, S. D. and Kuo, J. C. (1980), *Anal. Chem.*, **52**, 1399.
Yost, G. S. and Finley, B. L. (1985), *Drug Metab. Dispos.*, **13**, 5.
Young, M. A., Aarons, I., Davidson, E. M. and Toon, S. (1986), *J. Pharmacy Pharmacol.*, **38**, 60P.
Yu, P. H. and Davis, B. A. (1988), *Int. J. Biochem.*, **20**, 1197.
Zief, M. (1988), in *Chromatographic Chiral Separations* (M. Zief and L. J. Crane, eds), p. 315, Marcel Dekker, New York.
Zief, M. and Crane, L. J. (eds) (1988), *Chromatographic Chiral Separations*, Marcel Dekker, New York.
Zukowski, J., Sybilska, D. and Bojarsk, J. (1986), *J. Chromatog.*, **364**, 225.

Index